Teaching Today's Health

Second Edition

Teaching Today's Health

David Anspaugh
Memphis State University

Gene Ezell
University of Tennessee-Chattanooga

Karen Nash Goodman
Parthenon Pavilion Psychiatric Hospital, Nashville

Merrill Publishing Company

A Bell & Howell Information Company

COLUMBUS · TORONTO · LONDON · MELBOURNE

Cover Photo: Merrill Publishing/Bruce Johnson

Published by Merrill Publishing Company
A Bell & Howell Information Company
Columbus, Ohio 43216

This book was set in Serifa.

Administrative Editor: Jeff Johnston
Production Coordinator: Jeffrey Putnam
Cover Designer: Cathy Watterson

Photo credits (All photos copyrighted by the individuals or companies listed.): Strix Pix, 7, 81, 165, 178,
308, 379, 511; Merrill Publishing/photographs by Kevin Fitzsimmons, 27, 272, 278; by Celia Drake, 37,
247; by Julie Estadt, 257; by Larry Hamill, 402; by
Jerry Harney, 453; Paul Conklin, 52; Northshore Publishing, 95; Alan Cliburn, 169; Tom McGuire, 174;
Harvey Phillips/Phillips Photo Illustrators, 212; Jerry
Bushey/Trinity Photos, 227; Vivienne della Grotta,
235; Dan Unkefer, 254; Billy E. Barnes, 312; Jeremy
Rowe, 349; Richard Khanlian, 354; Paul Schrock,
422; ACTION/Foster Grandparents Program, 431,
443; Irma McNelia 449.

Library of Congress Catalog Card Number: 86-62079
International Standard Book Number: 0-675-20542-5
Printed in the United States of America
   4 5 6 7 8 9 92 91 90 89 88

To our parents,
and to our families,
Jill, Cindy,
Aimee, Jay, and Megan

Contents

Preface

Many of the health decisions that people make are based on the values that they developed when they were children. Consequently, the goal of health education must be to teach children to appreciate the value of making decisions that will lead to good health habits. Health education is more than the mere giving of information. The second edition of *Teaching Today's Health* presents both content and instructional techniques to elementary school teachers by providing chapters that contain concise coverage of health topics, followed by chapters that contain methods for teaching the concepts contained in these topics. The specific content areas are: body systems; personal health; mental health; nutrition; safety and first aid; alcohol, tobacco, and drugs; sex and family life; aging; consumer health; environmental health; and death and dying. The methods chapter that follows each of these includes sequencing of topics, value clarification activities, dramatization, decision stories, discussion topics, experiments and demonstrations, puzzles and games, and bulletin board ideas.

Teaching Today's Health includes many unique features that will facilitate the teaching of health education. The content chapters contain "Health Highlights" that expand or introduce the coverage of special topics. The content chapters also contain discussion questions and summaries that encourage students to learn and expand on the material presented. The methods chapters contain an outline of the concepts to be taught and a cycle plan that keys each topic to its proper grade level. The activities in the methods chapters are classified by the technique that is used in them. All these activities have been used in elementary classrooms.

We believe that *Teaching Today's Health* provides broader and deeper coverage of health science content than any other text available. For this reason, it provides a solid foundation for teaching elementary health. More importantly, the text stresses the necessity of establishing lifelong knowledge and habits when teaching health in the elementary grades.

We would like to thank our reviewers for their helpful suggestions: Cheryl Kolander, Idaho State University; Charlene Agne-Taub, George Mason University; Gary Lewers, New Mexico State University; Scott Scobell, West Virginia State College;

and Iris Brown, Norfolk State University. We also thank these people who responded to an information survey:

Kathy Koser, Cal-State—Long Beach

Rosalind Hill, University of Wisconsin—Stevens Point

Michael Hoadley, University of South Dakota

Ryda Rose, University of Pennsylvania

Margaret Smith, Oregon State University

Lorraine Davis, University of Oregon

Mary Milliken, University of Georgia

Royden Grove, Indiana University of Pennsylvania

Michael Godfrey, Cal-State—Northridge

Ted Coleman, Cal-State—San Bernadino

John Kully, University of North Florida

Charles Worland, Cal-State—Hayward

Cynthia Wolford, Pennsylvania State University

Frank Schabet, Iowa State University

Ada Gustaveson, Edinboro State

Joyce Donatelli, Wilson College

David Lohrmann, Syracuse University

Susan Lipnickey, Miami University

Eric Vlahov, University of Tampa

Phyllis Levenson, University of Houston

Carol Ann Holcomb, Kansas State University

Richard St. Pierre, Pennsylvania State University

Sue Habkirk, University of Arizona.

We hope this book will better equip you to deal with the many health problems that your students will face during their school years and for the rest of their lives. We have tried to provide you with the information you will need to assist children in making sound decisions for good health, as well as with the strategies for conveying that information to your students.

D.J.A.
G.O.E.

1. The Need for Health Education

Health and Intellect are the two blessings of life—Menander, *Single Lines*

THE EVOLUTION OF HEALTH EDUCATION

During the latter part of the nineteenth century, epidemics were taking a drastic toll among the school population of the United States. Children who survived these epidemic diseases often had a diminished capacity to learn as a result of their illnesses. Sanitary conditions in the schools also played a part in the spread of disease.

Alarmed, school physicians instructed teachers to become more involved with the health of their students. At that time, health education was not yet part of the school curriculum. In fact, there was no such thing as health education as we know it. The first efforts in this direction were more crisis oriented than preventive. Teachers were instructed to make daily health inspections of their students and report any suspected cases of serious disease (Haag, 1972). In some schools, lunch programs were also instituted so that students would be less susceptible to illness.

By the turn of the century, these concerns led to the realization of the need for health education. But actual measures were slow in coming. In 1924, only four states had certification requirements for health education teachers in the secondary school (Haag, 1972).

Formal health education first took the form of instruction in anatomy and physiology. Health was taught purely as a science, and emphasis was placed on cognitive information. As health education evolved, health teachers became more concerned with the attitudinal and behavioral aspects of students' health as well. Today, the emphasis is on a preventive approach, as opposed to the crisis-oriented approach of yesteryear.

Health education has come a long way since the beginning of the century. In most states, it is considered a vital part of the curriculum. In fact, currently, there are teacher preparation programs for health education in at least 43 of the 50 states (Eta Sigma Gamma, 1977).

Health Highlight

What Health Education Is Today

Health education is an applied science basic to the general education of all children and youth. Its body of knowledge represents a synthesis of facts, principles, and concepts drawn from biological, behavioral, sociological, and health sciences, but interpreted in terms of human needs, human values, and human potential. Acquisition of information is a desired purpose but not the primary goal of instruction. Rather, growth in critical thinking ability and problem solving skills are both the process and the product of instruction. Information can be quickly outdated, but cognitive skills remain an always dependable means of discovering fresh data when they are needed. The ultimate goal of health education is the development of an adult whose lifestyle reflects actions that tend to promote his or her own health as well as that of family and the community.

Currently the most widely accepted definition of health education is that proposed by Green and others (1980) as "any designed combination of methods to facilitate voluntary adaptations of behavior conducive to health." That works quite well in most settings. In the case of school health education it is acceptable only up to a point. First, because as Kreuter (1984) admits, although changing behavior is the long-range goal of all health education, teachers and schools can only be held accountable for students' command of health knowledge and skills, not their behavior. Second, even if schools could be expected to change actual behaviors, it should not be assumed that all health-related behaviors of students need to be changed. Carlyon and Cook (1981) recognize this difference in their own definition which says that health education is "any activity with clear goals planned for the purpose of improving health-related knowledge, attitudes, or behavior." They continue, "The prevalent notion that the sole purpose of health education is to change behavior is erroneous. It may be used to prevent, initiate, or sustain behavior as well."

What Health Education Is Not

Sometimes objects or phenomena of any kind are defined as effectively by explaining what they are not, as by describing what they are. Health education is not simply a minor aspect of physical education nor is it hygiene with a new name. It is not a program in physical fitness, although physical fitness surely is one of its goals. It is not the inculcation of health habits. It is not watered down anatomy, physiology, biology or any combination of these sciences. It is not one or two short units specific to certain health concerns and temporarily hosted by another course as a means of satisfying state requirements or local concerns with the health crisis of the month or year. It most certainly is not an assembly lecture program, a rainy day activity, or incidental teaching in response to momentary health problems or concerns.

Source: Pollock, M. & Hamburg, M. (1984, April). *Health Education: The Basic of the Basics.* Paper presented at Delbert Oberteuffer Centennial Symposium, Atlanta, Ga.

WHAT IS HEALTH?

Health is uppermost in the minds of many Americans today, most visibly in the wellness movement, which stresses self-responsibility for one's health.

Within this century a great many medical and health advancements have been made. For example, a person in 1900 had a life expectancy of 47 years. By 1980, that figure had risen to 73 years; the U.S. death rate dropped from 17 to 9 per 1000. Think of the relatively recent advancements we now rely on mater-of-factly: the discovery of insulin in 1921, penicillin in 1928, the mass production of antibiotics during World War II, the development of open heart surgery in 1954, a vaccination for polio in 1955, human heart transplants in 1967, and the artificial heart in 1984. The optimism of a healthy society was reflected in a 1965 Gallup poll showing 77 percent of those surveyed believed a cure for cancer would be found by 1985. By 1976 a Presidential Commissioner stated that overcoming all disease was within reach.

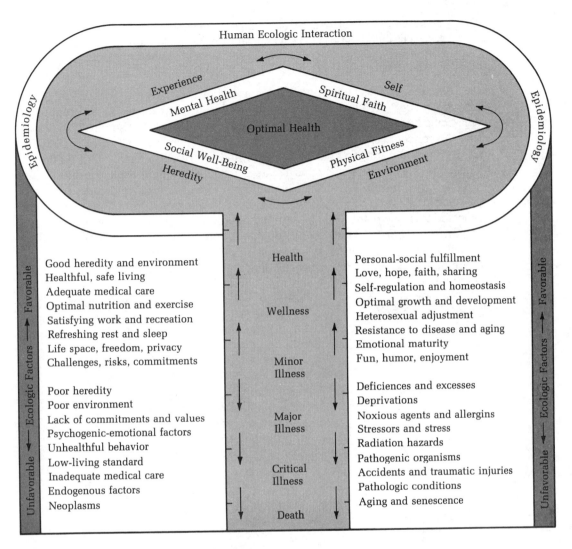

Figure 1.1
Hoyman's ecologic model of health and disease.

Source: Hoyman H. S., "Rethinking an ecologic-system model of man's health, disease, aging, death." *Journal of School Health*, vol. 45, no. 9, November, 1975, pp. 509–18. Copyright © 1975, American School Health Association, Kent, Ohio 44240.

Unfortunately, disease may always be present in society. Today we struggle with research on heart disease, cancer, herpes, and AIDS. Further, even if disease could be eliminated, would we be healthy? If we define health as continual optimum functioning, probably not.

Jonas Salk, who developed the vaccine for polio, believes we should view health not merely as freedom from disease, but as actively growing, developing, and evolving. He states

> By this I mean . . . the individual . . . may cope with the vicissitudes of life and function fully in the service of life in evolution.

. . . Just as certain diseases are contagious and are transmitted from person to person, let us think of health as being similarly transmissible. Also, just as some diseases arise endogenously, . . . [for example] birth defects . . . similarly the potential for health may be thought of as endogenous.

This concept goes far beyond the definition developed by the World Health Organization in 1947 (WHO, p. 3) of ". . . a state of complete physical, mental, and social well-being and not merely the absence of disease or infirmity." Hoyman (1975) stated that the concept of health had several dimensions, each having its own continuum. Each continuum ranges from desirable to undesirable, as illustrated in figure 1.1. The model portrays health, not as a state, but as a continually evolving process that is a result of behavior. The individual's ability to make decisions and interact socially, psychologically, and physically with society determines wellness. Dunn (1961) also reflected this viewpoint when he stated that optimal health or high level wellness is "an integrated method of functioning which is oriented toward maximizing the potential of which the individual is capable. It requires that the individual maintain a continuum of balance and purposeful direction within the environment where he or she is functioning." (p. 15).

The emphasis on personal volition is even stronger in Burt's Taxonomy of Life Styles (figure 1.2). His premise is that health behavior is determined by the courses

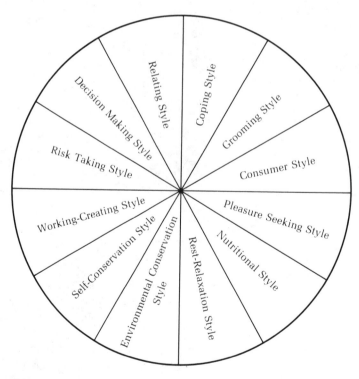

Figure 1.2
Burt's taxonomy of life styles.
Source: J. J. Burt, L. Meeks, & S. Pottebaum, *Toward a healthy life style through health education in the elementary school.* Belmont, Calif.: Wadsworth, 1980.

of action each of us chooses to follow. Burt contends that we must deal with each component of the taxonomy concurrently. He further contends that the 12 lifestyle factors shown in figure 1.2 form a framework for developing meaningful health education. The lifestyle approach involves three steps: (1) identifying the alternative lifestyle; (2) evaluating alternatives or reevaluating personal habits; and (3) intelligently selecting personal alternatives or change in lifestyle habits.

The 12 lifestyle factors can be defined as follows:

1. Coping style—This is the manner in which an individual learns to deal with lifestyles.
2. Relating style—An individual's relating style is the manner in which the person attempts to overcome feelings of aloneness and to gain recognition, appreciation, and a feeling of being needed.
3. Decision-making style—An individual can choose to make decisions, not make decisions, or allow someone else to make personal decisions.
4. Risk-taking style—Some individuals take many risks; others take few risks. Each person must weigh gratification against future rewards.
5. Work-creating style—This is the manner in which an individual chooses to be creative, productive, or destructive in work efforts.
6. Self-conservation style—An individual can increase or decrease the risk of a variety of health problems, ranging from dental caries to heart attacks depending upon lifestyle and attendant health habits.
7. Environment conservation style—Each individual should recognize a personal responsibility for protecting our natural environment and conserving our natural resources.
8. Rest-relaxation style—Options for rest and relaxation include transcendental meditation, biofeedback, and sleeping pills.
9. Nutritional style—What, when, where, and how much an individual eats reflects that person's nutritional style.
10. Pleasure-seeking style—This is the manner in which an individual determines not only what pleasures to seek but also determines when enough pleasure has been achieved or if more pleasure is needed.
11. Consumer style—This factor concerns how an individual evaluates the entire range of goods and services available, from clothing and food to medical care and health-related products.
12. Grooming style—An individual can choose to be well groomed and neat in appearance or slovenly.

Today, health is composed of many elements and "high-level health" requires a balance in and among all the factors which make up these elements. Eberst (1984) conceives of six dimensions of health (physical, emotional, mental, social, vocational and spiritual) and compares them to the six sides of Rubik's cube. He calls this framework the "health cube." Theoretically, total wellness (i.e. health) is achieved when the six sides are equal. Because human functioning is not static, the elements of the cube are constantly moving.

The cube model, like the others, stresses an important concept: no one can attain *perfect* health. Most people are at different levels for each element of health. As with Rubik's cube, there are millions of possible combinations of elements that can be

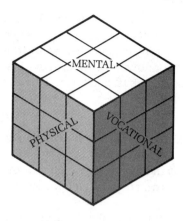
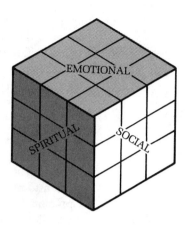

Figure 1.3
The "Cube" Model of Health.

Source: Eberst, R. M. "Defining health: A multidimensional model." *Journal of School Health*, vol. 54, no. 3, March 1984, pp. 99–104. Copyright © 1984, American School Health Association, Kent, Ohio 44240.

considered good health. Good health or high-level wellness is highly subjective and dependent on the values of the individual. An appropriate definition of health/wellness is *a way of life designed to achieve the highest degree for well-being.*

The younger children begin the lifelong process of becoming healthy, the greater the possibility they will be successful. Teachers must recognize that children bring to schools many values and behaviors. The elementary teacher must be aware of both the beneficial and negative aspects of a child's living practices. Teachers must also be aware of the powerful influence they exert on the lives of their students. Nowhere in the entire educational spectrum can a teacher make such an impression as at the elementary level. Consequently, the teacher should exemplify a lifestyle conducive to high-level wellness. If the teacher exhibits a style of living that is physically, socially, and psychologically pleasing, the chances are enhanced that students will attempt to incorporate those beneficial aspects in their own lives.

WHAT IS HEALTH EDUCATION?

Like the definition of health, the term *health education* has taken on new meanings over the years. While there are many ways of defining health education, the definition of the National Education Association (Wilson, 1971, p. 2) provides a framework for understanding what health education is. According to the NEA definition, health education is "the process of providing learning experiences which favorably influence understanding, attitudes, and conduct relating to individual and community health."

From the elementary teacher's perspective, health education is the process of developing and providing planned learning experiences in such a way as to provide information, change attitudes, and influence behavior. Put another way, health education is the process of helping elementary school children make intelligent decisions concerning health-related issues as these issues affect their own health, their

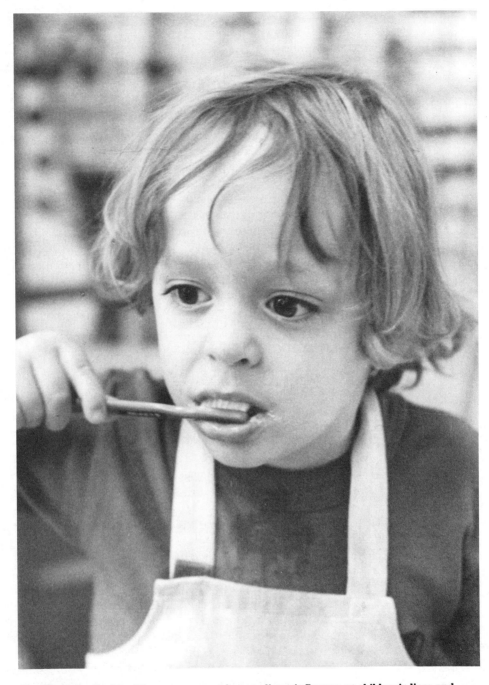

An effective school health program must have a direct influence on children's lives and behavior.

families' health, and their community's health. In theory, through this process the child learns individual responsibility for personal health, which will lead to health enhancement or high-level wellness. All this is accomplished by the teacher creating and facilitating learning experiences that develop the child's decision-making ability. With good decision-making skills, the child will better understand the personal, family, peer, and societal factors that influence quality of life.

Health education is a life-long process. A health-educated person

1. assumes responsibility for her health and health care; she participates in the decision-making process.
2. respects the benefits of medical technology, but is not in awe of medical equipment and tests.
3. seeks information regarding health matters.
4. tries new behaviors and modifies others.
5. is an active partner with the physician in the decision-making process.
6. is skeptical of health fads and trends.
7. asks questions, seeks evidence, and evaluates information.
8. strives for self reliance in personal health matters.
9. voluntarily adopts practices consistent with a healthy lifestyle.

ACCOMPLISHING HEALTH EDUCATION

With the school day already overcrowded, many elementary teachers wonder how they can find time to teach health education. But time *must* be found. Our nation's children are an invaluable resource. Health education can help ensure that this generation is fit physically, psychologically, and socially to assume the tasks of adulthood.

Still, the problem remains: When and how should health education be taught in the classroom? How can it be accomplished?

There are many approaches to teaching health, several of which will be discussed in chapter 4. However, the responsibility rests with each teacher to create and facilitate direct instruction in health and to correlate other health-related topics whenever the opportunity arises.

Time must be allotted for direct health instruction during the school day. There is no substitute for this. However, if the time that can be allotted is minimal, health instruction can be incorporated into other parts of the curriculum—reading, mathematics, science, geography, art, social studies, and physical education. Actually, there are some advantages to integrating a part of health instruction into other subject areas, including opportunities for a great deal of creativity in learning.

To accomplish health education, the topic selected must be appropriate to the developmental level of the child. Health must be taught every semester at every grade level from kindergarten through grade 6. Only in this way can it become a meaningful part of each child's learning experience.

To be meaningful, health education must influence a child's decision-making skills. To do this, health instruction must blend information-giving with attitudinal experiences. Brown (1974, p. 4) describes this balance as *confluent education,* which he defines as "the integration of cognitive learning with affective learning." In short, a child will be better able to make personal decisions concerning health behavior if the teacher has provided cognitive and affective opportunities for growth.

Presenting factual information alone—the cognitive aspect of health education—is not enough. Knowledge alone does not lead to changes in behavior. The failure of so many cognitive drug education programs in the past is evidence of this. The knowledge must become personalized—the affective aspect of health education. Strategies for accomplishing this will be presented throughout this text.

The American Medical Association (1982) has pointed out that, to be efficient, health instruction must be

1. Sequential: Health should be taught from kindergarten through twelfth grade, in a sequence that introduces concepts at appropriate learning levels. The curriculum at each grade should build on what has been learned in previous years, and should be the basis for curricula in future years.
2. Planned: Health instruction should have stated goals, objectives, activities, and evaluation criteria. It should be given scheduled time within the total curriculum, not taught sporadically or used as a substitute for other subjects.
3. Comprehensive: Instruction in only one or several health topics (e.g., drugs, nutrition, or sexuality) is not adequate for an understanding of health. A comprehensive health curriculum includes instruction in growth and development, mental/emotional health, personal and family lifestyles, nutrition, disease prevention and control, safety, drug use and abuse, and consumer and community health. More important than the individual subjects, however, is a study of how all subjects are interrelated and how all affect the quality of life.
4. Taught by qualified health teachers: An elementary school teacher requires training to teach health concepts and to relate these to the wellness of the students. Junior/senior high school teachers and school health coordinators should be professionally prepared health educators. State Departments of Education have information regarding certification requirements in each state.

In 1985, it was reported that the average fourth grader spends only 22 minutes a day in health instruction (O'Rourke, 1985). Perhaps it is encouraging to think that the elementary-school child is receiving at least 22 minutes per day. However, it is important to remember that, in the last twenty years, topics such as drug abuse, smoking, heart disease prevention, teenage pregnancy, adolescent suicide, stress control, incest, child abuse and CPR have been added to an already long list of topics such as nutrition, disease, mental health, sexuality, personal health, environmental health, first aid, and quackery (Purdy & Tritsch, 1985).

WHY HEALTH EDUCATION?

Perhaps the best argument for teaching health education is that health behaviors are the most important component of health status. Since health-related behaviors are both learned and amenable to change, what better time to start formal health education than in the early elementary school years, when the child is more flexible and more apt to accept positive health behaviors? In addition, many of the negative aspects of a lifetime of abuse could be avoided. This avoidance becomes increasingly important with increasing evidence that most health problems are due to smoking, poor nutrition, overweight, lack of exercise, stress, abuse of drugs and alcohol, and unsafe personal behavior (O'Rourke, 1985).

Unfortunately, health education still suffers from a lack of importance in the school curriculum and a lack of adequately trained teachers. If we wish to help prevent many of the conditions that are now the leading causes of death (cardiovascular disease, cancer, accidents, etc.), then we must emphasize prevention in our educational efforts. Children receive nearly 12,000 hours of education in grades K–12, yet less than 30 percent of a child's total schooling is in health (ERS, 1983). There is only 1 qualified health educator per 21,500 students, or 1 for every 50 schools (NCES, 1984).

Here is a list of some of the problems our society faces. The list, taken from the American School Health Association's *A Healthy Child: The Key to the Basics* (1983), underscores the need for better health education.

1. Between 1960 and 1977, the death rate among 15–19 year olds increased by 10 percent, largely because of increases in deaths from external causes such as suicide, homicide and motor vehicle accidents.

2. More school-age children now die of accidents than of diseases. In 1978 for example, accidents caused 51 percent of the deaths of children, 5–14; 26 percent of these deaths were by motor vehicle accidents, followed by death from drownings (7 percent) and fires (4 percent).

3. About 17 percent of the injuries to children occur at school, while more than half occur in or around the home. In the 1975–76 school year, for every 100 boys of school age, there were 51 injuries and 50 days lost from school, and for every 100 girls there were 29 injuries and 22 days lost. Most school injuries occurred during physical education class or interscholastic sports.

4. Respiratory conditions are leading causes of disability and restricted activity, including loss of school days, for school-age children and youth. In 1975–76, acute respiratory illness accounted for 61 percent of the school days missed. Asthma and chronic bronchitis were leading chronic conditions limiting children's activity.

5. Tooth decay also stands high among major health problems. Because of the multiple uses of flouride by children of all ages, dental caries has significantly declined in the United States over the last decade. Despite this fact, the average child aged 5–17 still experiences 4.8 decayed, missing or filled tooth surfaces. Nearly 12 million children have periodontal (gum) disease.

6. Nutritional problems, although they have changed in nature, continue to exist. Fewer children are undernourished. Today's nutrition problems are more likely to be related to over-consumption and imbalances in the types and amounts of foods consumed. Many children consume diets high in sugar, fat, and salt, and thus increase their risk of becoming obese and of acquiring diabetes, heart disease, hypertension, and other chronic degenerative diseases later in life.

7. Vision and hearing problems continue to exist among children and youth. In 1981, state maternal and child health agencies reported that over one quar-

ter of a million school-age children who received vision screening were found to require treatment.

8. Substance abuse is a problem of many school-age children. In a 1980 survey of high school seniors, nearly all of the students (93 percent) had tried alcohol; the great majority (72 percent) had used it in the previous month.

9. Alcohol-related accidents are the leading cause of death among adolescents. Most highway traffic fatalities (60 percent) among young people are related to alcohol.

10. Since 1966 the number of high school students intoxicated at least once a month has more than doubled from 10 percent to more than 20 percent.

11. When more than 3,000 high school students were surveyed to determine health needs with which they might want help, the top five were acne, sex education, depression, overweight, and getting along with parents.

12. Physical health problems of adolescents are: diabetes, kidney disease, heart disease, epilepsy, dental caries and gum disease, asthma, acne, vision problems, and scoliosis. However, if we were to look at the death rate among adolescents, we would have a different list. This list would include accidents, homicides, and suicides as the leading killers of teenagers.

13. The 1979 report of the Surgeon General, entitled *Healthy People,* indicates that one-fourth of all teenage girls have had at least one pregnancy before they reach the age of 19.

14. Of reported cases of a sexually transmitted disease, 75 percent were in the age group between 15 and 24.

15. Prior to 1962 the use of any kind of illicit drug was limited to 2 percent of the population. In 1977, 60 percent of 18 to 25 year olds had tried marijuana. Of the 12 to 17 year olds, 30 percent had tried it. About 19 percent of high school students smoke marijuana every day.

16. Of all children in single-parent families headed by a woman, more than 50 percent are living below the poverty level. Many of these children are at risk for emotional problems and may lack adequate health and other aspects of health care.

17. Surveys have shown that children in low-income families are more likely to be in poor health, lose more school days due to chronic health problems, have been hospitalized, and remain in the hospital longer than high-income children.

18. Child abuse and neglect is increasing. Statistics indicate that about one million children in America are abused and neglected. Between 100,000 and 200,000 are physically abused, 60,000 to 100,000 are sexually abused, and the remainder are neglected.

This list is not complete; many other health problems affect today's children. Let's look at some specific problem areas.

Degenerative Diseases

Cardiovascular diseases are the leading cause of death in the United States and Canada. The risk of these diseases is increased or decreased by lifestyle choices that individuals make. For example, the type of diet, the amount of physical activity engaged in, and the decision to smoke or not to smoke are all lifestyle choices that correlate highly with the incidence of cardiovascular diseases. There is a clear association between cardiovascular diseases and high cholesterol diets, being overweight, lack of physical activity, and smoking. Health education can make these facts known to students while lifestyles are still developing.

Lifestyle choices can also increase or decrease the chances of developing certain forms of cancer. For example, the link between smoking and lung cancer has been demonstrated by numerous studies. There is also some evidence that stress can increase the chances of contracting some forms of disease. Health education can assist individuals to find effective methods of dealing with stress, and thus perhaps lower the chances of developing disease. Further, health education can emphasize the importance of regular physical checkups, Pap tests, and cervix examinations, as well as regular self-examinations. In this way, early detection of disease can lead to cure or remission.

Personal Health Problems

Degenerative diseases are not the only health problems that can be reduced through proper health education. Personal health problems can also be lessened. Such problems range from mental disorders, stress, alcoholism, drug abuse, and obesity to personal safety and even dental caries.

Mental Health Problems.   According to Frederick (1977) more than 20 million people in the United States are estimated to be depressed or poorly adjusted to their environment. As many as 50 percent of the hospital beds in this country are filled by mental patients. The suicide rate is 12.5 per 100,000 population.

Stress.   Excessive or inappropriate stress can reduce the motivation, as well as the actual ability, to do tasks. In addition, both short-term and long-term impairments created by death, divorce, or other family situations are difficult to assess. Teachers learn quickly about how these problems impair learning and behavior.

Alcohol Abuse.   Alcohol abuse is the nation's number one drug problem. Twelve million Americans are alcoholics. Alcohol is involved in 50 percent of all fatal traffic accidents. Problem drinkers cost the nation billions of dollars each year in lost work time. Additionally, Hanson (1977) notes that pregnant women who drink as little as two ounces of alcohol a day may cause their offspring to suffer from fetal alcohol syndrome, which can manifest itself in growth deficiency, low brain weight, facial abnormalities, cardiac disorders, and mental retardation.

Drug Abuse.   Marijuana usage has increased rapidly among students in the United States. Younger and younger children are beginning to experiment with this drug. An Eta Sigma Gamma (1980) report notes that the active ingredient, THC (delta-9-tetrohydrocanabinol) is associated with lowering the body's natural defense system, altering cell metabolism, reducing the male hormone (testosterone) and the growth hormone, and diminishing motivation and constructive energy. THC has also been shown to impair the ability to drive or to perform other complex tasks. Marijuana, of course, is just one of the many drugs that cause health problems in our society. Even a simple listing of abused drugs would fill this page.

Obesity.   Many factors contribute to obesity. These include psychological, cultural, and genetic traits. Family eating patterns and physical activity play an important role in the development of childhood obesity. Obesity occurs in 10 to 20 percent of school-age children, and obese children tend to become obese or overweight adults. Anywhere from 20 to 40 percent of lower socioeconomic-level children are thought to be obese. One-fourth of higher socioeconomic level children are obese. Among these children, poor self-esteem, frequent fasting, and other related nutritional problems inhibit cognitive performance. (Charney, Goodman, McBride, Lyon, & Pratt, 1976; Garn & Clark, 1976).

Dental Caries. Another important health concern for the elementary school child is dental caries. By age 10 the average child has five carious teeth. Almost 100 million American adults have at least half their teeth decayed, filled, or missing. Perhaps 20 percent of adults are completely without teeth. Needless to say, a child with dental caries may be irritable and inattentive in the classroom.

Accidents and Poisonings. Accidents are the greatest threat to life and well-being in childhood. According to the National Safety Council (1978), they are the number one cause of death in children ages 5 to 14 years. Unsafe playing conditions, improper supervision, and unknowing neglect all contribute to childhood accidents. For example, four out of five bicycle accidents are believed to be associated with poor safety practices. Poisonings are almost an equal threat. Ingestion of medicines, particularly aspirin, is one of the most common forms of accidental poisoning, especially with children under five years of age.

Other Personal Health Problems. Additional health problems that require the attention of the elementary teacher include skin conditions, vision and hearing problems, communicable diseases, and child abuse. The list could go on and on. But by this point it should be clear how wide the range of health education must be. A brief look at yet another area of health education, community health problems, will make even clearer the scope of health education.

Community Health Problems

Health problems of the community include environmental concerns, sexually transmitted diseases and teenage pregnancies, and consumer health. Let's look at each of these areas.

Environmental Health. One of the major problems facing the United States today is environmental pollution—specifically air, water, chemical, radiation, and noise pollution. Each of these types of hazards lowers the quality of life.

Air pollution can be caused by carbon monoxide, sulfur oxides, hydrocarbons, smoke, and dust. Aesthetically, the resulting haze is ugly, but the effects of air pollution on individuals with bronchitis, emphysema, and heart problems can be life-threatening. Through health education, children must become aware of the importance of keeping our air breathable.

Water is a precious resource. Yet for years, sewage, industrial, and agricultural wastes were allowed to pour freely into our rivers and lakes. The oceans, too, were used as a dumping ground. By the 1960s, Lake Erie had become so badly polluted that it could no longer support many types of fish. Beaches in Hawaii and California had to be closed to swimmers because of water-borne bacteria from sewage outflows. Pesticide residue runoff from farms had made the water in many rivers unsafe to drink even after treatment.

The picture is somewhat better today because of tough environmental regulations. But there is pressure from some interest groups to ease these regulations. The result could be a return to serious water pollution throughout the nation. Environmental health education can help ensure that this does not happen.

Dangerous chemicals are also an environmental threat. Industrial waste products have caused cancer, birth defects, and a host of other health problems. Radiation is a similar threat. Children must be made aware of these dangers so that as adults they can make informed decisions about how best to protect our environment.

Yet another problem is noise pollution. Noise is more than a simple annoyance. It can lead to gastrointestinal disorders, high blood pressure, hearing loss, and other disorders. Noise can also affect the ability to concentrate, think, and learn.

Sexually Transmitted Diseases and Teenage Pregnancies. Unfortunately, pollution is not our only community health concern. Sexually transmitted diseases and unwanted teenage pregnancies are also major problems today. Sexual activity has led to high rates of sexually transmitted diseases. Each year, around 80,000 cases of syphillis and between 1.6 and 2 million cases of gonorrhea are reported in the United States (HEW, 1979). Of course, not all of the afflicted are teenagers, but the highest rate of sexually transmitted diseases is among individuals from 12 to 20 years of age.

Ignorance plays a large part in the transmission of such diseases. Many people do not even know that such diseases can be transmitted through sexual intercourse. Others are unaware that cures are available for most of these maladies. Still others are ignorant of the existence of some diseases, such as herpes, which is currently incurable.

Another problem is that of teenage pregnancies. More than a million teenagers become pregnant each year. Approximately one-third of these girls terminate their pregnancies through legal abortions. Many of these youngsters are nonetheless traumatized by the experience. For those who carry their babies to full term, there are other problems.

Maternal mortality among mothers under 15 is two and half times the rate than for mothers aged 20 to 24. Infant mortality is twice that of babies born to mothers aged 20 to 24. Mothers aged 25 and younger are also twice as likely to have low birth weight babies. Low birth weight is associated not only with infant mortality but also with birth injuries and neurological defects.

Social costs are also high. The majority of teenage mothers never finish high school. Marriage disruption is three times more likely for teenagers as for later child-bearers. Further, as of 1975 about half of the $9.4 billion in federal aid to families with dependent children went to families where the woman had given birth as a teenager. Nearly 1.6 million children five years old and younger live in families headed by mothers aged 14 to 25. Two-thirds of these families are living below the designated poverty level (Planned Parenthood, 1981).

Although teenage pregnancies and sexually transmitted diseases are being addressed in our schools, a mandate for sex education is needed in every state. This mandate must provide for sex education beginning in the elementary school. Until that time our children will remain uninformed and defenseless about their own sexuality.

Consumer Health

Young and old alike need to be informed about purchasing health services and products. Misconceptions about weight reduction, cancer cures, vitamins, hypertension, and arthritis are too numerous to mention. Every day another fad diet or some form of quackery preys on the misconceptions, gullibility, and superstition of the consuming public. Individuals must start learning how to be wise consumers from childhood on so that they can effectively evaluate the many forms of consumer information they receive. This process involves making appropriate decisions and must be started while in elementary school.

Not every area of concern in a comprehensive health education program has been touched upon here. But it is hoped that the pressing need for health education has been established. The scope of health education is a broad one. Personal, family, and community problems must be effectively addressed if we are to live personally and socially satisfying lives.

Elementary school children are at a point in development where they are acquiring habits that will remain with them throughout life. It is far easier to acquire desirable patterns of living early rather than to change ingrained habits later in life. The part played by health education holds great potential if early in life a sense of values coupled with knowledge and appropriate decision-making skills are developed.

THE COMPREHENSIVE SCHOOL HEALTH PROGRAM

A total school health program is needed if the elementary school is to function as an effective institution for promoting high-level wellness. A comprehensive school health program can be divided into three component parts: health services, healthful school environment, and health instruction. These three components are outlined in Table 1.1. Each component has a planning, administration, and evaluation aspect. Adequate planning for all three components ensures the comprehensiveness of each component. Effective leadership coordinates between the components and ensures proper staffing, budgeting, policy fulfillment, and evaluation.

School Health Services

The basic responsibility for the health of the child lies with the parents, but the school plays an important role, sometimes primary, sometimes secondary, in maintaining the health of each child.

All teachers should be concerned with student health, as any deviation from normal health is a possible deterent to the ability to learn effectively. Even minor disturbances such as a cold or stomachache can impair a student's ability to concentrate and therefore the ability to learn. The primary role of the teacher in this part of the health program is in observation, record-keeping, referral, and follow-up. You can also become involved in screening the students for various health functions, such as vision and hearing. Prepare the students for any screening examination they might be taking in the near future. This preparation will serve two purposes. First, student anxiety regarding the testing will be reduced if the fear of the unknown is removed.

Table 1.1
The School Health Program

School Health Services	Healthful School Environments	School Health Instruction

1. School readiness programs including preschool health screening and assessment of emotional and social readiness
2. Health appraisal by observation and periodic examination
3. Health counseling about physical and emotional problems for pupils and families, with referral and follow-up
4. Consultation with teachers relating to physical and emotional problems encountered, and recommendations regarding participation in physical education, special education programs and other school activities.
5. Emergency policies, facilities and first aid
6. Immunizations, tests and communicable disease procedures
7. Dental examinations, fluoride treatments and care
8. Cumulative records including health, accidents and social developments
	1. Friendly staff and pupil relationships
	2. Healthful school schedule
	3. School site of adequate size, location and safety
	4. School construction meeting standards for size, sanitation, safety features, lighting, furniture, acoustics, heating and ventilation
	5. Safety inspection, drills and patrols with pupil planning and participation
	6. Proper school maintenance
	7. Adequate and safe physical education and recreational facilities and staff
	8. School lunch and milk programs that meet standards
	9. Safe bus operation
		1. Planned health curriculum:
		  a. broad program goals
		  b. health instruction with teaching-learning objectives for all grade levels
		2. Adequate teacher preparation and in-service
		3. Resource materials and consultation for teachers
		4. Health education for parents and other adults
		5. Educational adaptations for handicapped children
		6. A comprehensive physical education program

Second, the screening exam then becomes a learning experience in health education for the students. The actual screening examination should be supervised by the school health nurse. The classroom teacher and school nurse should cooperate in all three areas of the comprehensive school health program, but particularly in the school health services area these two professionals can form a vital team in promoting the health of the child.

Areas where the classroom teacher can be particularly helpful to the school nurse are listed below. (Wilson, 1971)

Observation.   Observe the verbal and nonverbal behavior of each student for any deviation that might indicate a health problem. Has a normally outgoing child become withdrawn? Does a child strain to see what is written on the chalkboard? Does a child show undue irritability? Aggressiveness? Apathy? These are all signs of possible health problems, either physical, psychological, or social.

Teachers are in an excellent position to appraise the health of their students. The teacher sees the child for several hours each day in a variety of situations—in the classroom, the cafeteria, and on the playground. Teachers should be familiar with the expected growth and development patterns of students and are more likely to be objective in their appraisal than someone more closely identified with a student, such as a parent.

When a child poses a possible threat to the health of the other students, for example because of a contagious upper respiratory infection, appropriate steps to remove the child from the classroom should be taken. When children are allowed to attend school with contagious diseases, epidemics ensue.

Record Keeping. Keep an individual card file for each student. This file can be used as a referral source and can also be useful when discussing specific behaviors with parents or other members of the school health team. Objectivity should be the goal when making card file notes. Refrain from making value judgments about a child's behavior or condition. Also avoid attempts at diagnosing the student's condition; this is the responsibility of others on the health team. However, school health records for each student should be referred to since this information could be valuable in understanding the child's behavior. The health records can also familiarize you with any specific condition, such as diabetes or epilepsy, that might require emergency care in the classroom. Keep in mind that all information contained in a student's health records is confidential, and should not be shared as public knowledge in the teacher's lounge.

Referral. Upon noticing any detrimental change in a student's health or behavior, place the child under the school nurse's care, or in a situation where a school nurse is not immediately present, notify the appropriate member of the administrative staff. As a classroom teacher you should be able to help the school nurse, physician, or psychologist understand the everyday behavior of the child. For instance, while the physician might see the child in an isolated situation, you can provide input relative to the history of the student's behavior and explain whether the present behavior is usual or represents a drastic change.

You should also be familiar with health-related agencies in the community that can provide assistance for specific health problems. This knowledge could be valuable to parents in getting help if they are not able to afford the services of a private physician.

Follow-up. A dedicated teacher will continue to follow the student's case even after observation and referral have been completed. If the child is absent from school for any length of time, check with parents or the school physician concerning the child's health. When the student returns to the classroom, resume careful observation to aid in the child's recovery.

A good example of a teacher employing observation, record-keeping, referral, and follow-up is the instance where a teacher observed that a student had recurring injuries on various parts of his body. The teacher carefully noted the injuries in her personal card file on the student. After several weeks of observing, she referred the case to the assistant principal of the school. The teacher, nurse, and administrator met with the parents, who described the child as "accident prone." As part of the follow-up, the school nurse reviewed the teacher's anecdotal records on the student. In turn, the physician gave his findings to juvenile authorities, who tried and prosecuted the parents for child abuse. This dedicated teacher, operating within the school health program and in cooperation with the school nurse, played a significant part in promoting the health of her student in a difficult situation. She was careful not to make any diagnosis, nor did she accuse the parents of any wrongdoing. However, she did keep an accurate file on the student, referred the situation to the proper authority, and followed up the case to its conclusion.

Healthful School Environment

The school and classroom environment should be an outstanding example of health excellence for the students. When school officials demonstrate care in planning and maintaining the school, students learn a valuable health lesson. The teacher can play a critical part in conveying the appropriate message to the students concerning a healthful environment. If you demonstrate an interest in the environment, the students are more likely to do the same. If you are lackadaisical, however, the students will share this attitude.

Teachers should require a quality environment in which to work. This is important, not only for the teaching-learning process, but also for teacher and student morale. Whenever possible, volunteer as a consultant in planning and maintaining the school site and surroundings. Foster a cooperative relationship with the custodial staff, lunchroom staff, and administrators in charge of the various aspects of the environment. Work with the custodians by keeping your own classroom sanitary and by diplomatically suggesting positive improvements. The lunchroom and cafeteria are excellent locations for learning opportunities in nutrition and sanitation.

Teach students the importance of safe, sanitary, and aesthetically-pleasing surroundings in which to live and study. Teach the proper ways to maintain the school site—such as treating property with respect and demonstrating good manners in the cafeteria. Motivate students to enjoy and maintain their school environment.

Few teachers are fortunate enough to be able to work in ideal situations. However, you should do all that you can to enhance your teaching environment. The classroom should be physically adequate, pleasant, attractive, and comfortable for the students. When the classroom setting is bright, lively, and dynamic, morale is improved.

The psychological setting within the classroom is just as important as the physical. As the teacher, you are responsible for establishing the emotional tone within the classroom. The overall atmosphere should be one of acceptance, one in which you know the students well and are sensitive to their individual needs. The classroom should be nonthreatening. Stress is reduced when there is a relaxed approach to instruction, one in which there is less emphasis on competition that pits student against student. Students should feel free to express their true feelings without fear of ridicule or rebuke. They should also feel free to fail occasionally without punishment.

Be kind but just in promoting teacher-pupil relationships. Set reasonable goals for each student. Give praise for positive behavior. Challenge the students within their capabilities, and tolerate occasional frustration.

Allow the students to assist in planning health learning opportunities. If they are involved in planning, they will become more interested in the subject matter. When students are interested, discipline is less likely to become a problem. Discipline problems can be minimized by developing a warm, caring relationship with each pupil and by teaching self-discipline, maturity, and responsibility for one's own actions. If a student does misbehave, allow that student to analyze his or her own behavior, judge the behavior, and choose from among alternatives the means for changing that behavior. Avoid establishing a dangerous psychological set by using schoolwork as punishment; this procedure will encourage a negative attitude toward learning.

Additional suggestions for creating a pleasing psychological environment include the following:

1. Call each student by name.
2. Give positive reinforcement for appropriate academic and classroom behaviors.
3. Talk with each student every day.
4. Correct student behavior in a one-to-one conference.
5. Ask "feeling" questions as well as "knowing-the-answer" questions.
6. Make sure every student gets to perform as a helper in classroom maintenance activities.
7. Be pleasant, smile, and use direct eye contact when talking with students.

School Health Instruction

The third area of the school health program is actual health instruction, in which information is presented to students in a way that fosters desirable health knowledge, attitudes, and practices. Strategies, information, and methods concerning this aspect of a comprehensive school health program will be described later in the text.

Health educators should consider themselves as part of a team whose main mission is to provide optimal conditions to enhance the wellness of each student. Each member of the health team has a particular role to play. Like a chain, the health team is only as strong as its weakest link. Everyone involved with the health of students—including the students themselves—must take that personal responsibility seriously. Each member must work cooperatively with other members in order to reach the ultimate goal of total health.

SUMMARY

The quality of life that each individual ultimately is to have is determined in part by the health decisions the person makes. Our health is continually evolving and changing as a result of our behavior and decisions. Health is not a state, but a process through which we seek to feel at ease with our social, emotional, and physical environment. Health has many complicated, interrelated components that must be balanced if high-level wellness is to be achieved.

Health education is the process of developing and providing planned learning experiences that bring about effective decision-making. The process must provide a balance between cognitive and affective educational experiences. This balance, sometimes referred to as confluent education, is important for the presentation of knowledge. Factual information does not ensure behavioral change. Learning opportunities must be provided for discussion so that the information is personalized.

The need for health education is great. Many lifestyle-related illnesses, such as cardiovascular diseases, could be significantly reduced if a comprehensive health education program achieved its goals. The need for health education can further be seen in mental illness, alcoholism, drug abuse, sexually transmitted disease, and teenage pregnancy rates. Other problems, such as poor nutrition, dental health, and physical fitness, illustrate the need for early health education. Children must learn to make wise health decisions as they grow so that community health problems can be effectively addressed.

An effective school health program has three components. They are: (1) health services, (2) healthful school environment, and (3) health instruction.

DISCUSSION QUESTIONS

1. Why is health a difficult concept to define?
2. How is health constantly changing?
3. What is the meaning of the term *high-level wellness?*
4. How can health education be justified in the elementary school?
5. What is health education?
6. Discuss why decision-making is such a vital part of health education.
7. What implications does Burt's Taxonomy of Life Styles have for health educators?
8. Name and discuss the three areas of a comprehensive school health program.
9. What role does the teacher play in each of the areas of school health?
10. Discuss how a negative classroom environment might affect the child.
11. What are some positive reinforcers the teacher can develop in the classroom?

REFERENCES

_____. *A national directory of college and university school and public health educators* (5th ed.). Muncie, Ind.: Eta Sigma Gamma Professional Health Science Honorary National Office, 1977.

_____. *Accident facts* (1978 ed.). Chicago: National Safety Council, 1978.

_____. *A healthy child: The key to the basics.* ASHA: Kent, Ohio, 1983.

American School Health Association. *Selected school health support statements.* ASHA: Kent, Ohio, 1983.

Brown, G. I. *Human teaching for human learning: An introduction to confluent education.* New York: Viking Press, 1974.

Burt, J. J., Meeks, L., & Pottebaum, S. M. *Toward a healthy lifestyle through elementary health education.* Belmont, Calif.: Wadsworth, 1980.

Carlyon, W. H., and Cook, D. E. "Science instruction and health instruction." BSCS Journal, *4,* 1, 1981.

Charney, E.; Goodman H.; McBride, M.; Lyon, B.; & Pratt, R. "Childhood antecedents of adult obesity: Do chubby infants become obese adults?" *New England Journal of Medicine,* 1976, *295:*6.

_____. Constitution of the World Health Organization, in *Chronicle of the WHO.* Geneva: World Health Organization, 1947.

Dunn, H. L. *High level wellness.* Arlington, Va.: Beatty, 1961.

Eberst, Richard M. "Defining health: A multidimensional model." *Journal of School Health,* March 1984, *54:*3, pp. 99–104.

Educational Research Service. "Local school district budget items by type of community." *Spectrum: Journal of School Research and Information,* 1983, *1:*3, p. 16.

_____. *Focus on alcohol and drug issues.* Muncie, Indiana: Eta Sigma Gamma, 1980, *3:*1.

Frederick, C, J. *Suicide in the United States. Health Education,* 1977, *8*:6.

Garn, S., & Clark, D. Trends in fatness and the organs of obesity. *Pediatrics,* 1976, *57*:4.

Green, L. W., Krueter, M. W., Deeds, S. G., and Partridge, K. B. *Health education planning: A diagnostic approach,* Palo Alto, Mayfield, 1980.

Haag, J. H. *School health program* (3rd ed.). Philadelphia: Lea & Febiger, 1972.

Hanson, W. "Even moderate drinking may be hazardous to maturing fetus." *JAMA,* 1977, *237*:24.

Hoyman, H. S. "Rethinking an ecologic-system model of man's health, disease, aging, death." *Journal of School Health,* 1975, *45*:9.

Krueter, M. W. "Health promotion: The public health role in the community of free exchange," 4th annual colloquium in health promotion, Columbia University, New York: March 21, 1984, p. 5.

National Center for Educational Statistics. "The condition of education." NCES Pub. No. 84-401, Washington, D.C.: U.S. Government Printing Office, 1984.

O'Rourke, T. W. "Why school health education? The economical point of view." *Why School Health Education?* Delbert Oberleuffer Centennial Symposium, April 21, 1985, Atlanta, Ga. Cosponsored by Association for the Advancement of Health Education and the Office of Disease Prevention and Health Promotion, pp. 25–28.

Purdy, C. & Tritsch L. "Why health education? The practical point of view." Delbert Oberleuffer Centennial Symposium, April 21, 1985, Atlanta, Ga. Cosponsored by the Association for the Advancement of Health Education and the Office of Disease Prevention and Health Promotion, pp. 25–28.

_____. *Teenage pregnancy: The problem that hasn't gone away.* New York: Planned Parenthood of America, 1981.

U.S. Department of Health, Education, and Welfare. *Sexually transmitted disease fact sheet.* Atlanta: Public Health Science, Center for Disease Control, 1979.

_____. "Why health education in your school?" *American Medical Association.* AMA: Chicago, 1982.

Wilson, C. C. (Ed.). *School health services.* Washington, D.C.: National Education Association, 1971.

2. The Role of the Teacher in Health Instruction

TEACHER

I am that most fortunate of men for I am eternal. Others live merely in the world of today; I live in the world of tomorrow. . . . .For I am charged with that most sacred mission—to transmit all that our forebears lived for, loved for, and died for to the next generation. . . . .I make wisdom live. . . . .I do not simply teach the mind, I reach the heart, and when I reach the heart, I touch the soul. . . .—Rabbi Zev Schostak (from Phi Delta Kappan, October, 1984, p. 115)

THE CHALLENGE OF HEALTH EDUCATION

No subject places more emphasis on the teacher's own behavior and attitudes than health education. Because elementary school children are so impressionable, you can teach skills and influence behavior that foster high-level wellness. You will become your students' role model, and you will have the opportunity to portray a healthy image through your behavior. If your students see you eating good, nutritious food in the lunchroom, they will realize that nutrition is important to you. What you do is as important as what you say. Don't forget that children are very observant. It is critical that you endorse healthful practices in your lifestyle. You cannot expect your students to become excited about health just because you are. You must inspire them by making your health instruction lively, creative, and well planned. Cornacchia and Staton (1984) state "Health education demands that students become participants, not spectators." You must emphasize to students that they cannot become healthy passively. Involving them in active learning opportunities will personalize their health education. Your students will be better able to make their own responsible choices of healthful activities.

Barriers to Successful Health Teaching

Elementary education majors in most colleges receive very little instruction in health content. Because the elementary school teacher must teach many subjects, most college programs necessarily emphasize methods and materials instead of specific subject areas. Therefore, many elementary education majors receive direct health instruction only if they take a health course as an elective. To overcome this barrier, take as many health courses as you can. Keep in mind that methods courses only instruct you how to teach; specific subject area courses are necessary so that you know what to teach.

In choosing subject area courses, also keep in mind that health education is interdisciplinary; it can include psychology, sociology, physical science, biology, and even religion. The better prepared you are in each of these disciplines, the better you will be able to relate them to teaching health concepts.

Your preparation does not end when you receive your degree. Because health information is constantly changing, staying current is vital to successful health instruction. Almost daily, newspapers, magazines, and professional journals carry reports of new findings in health-related areas. You have an obligation to follow these developments. One way to do this is to attend educational seminars and workshops.

Yet there are many areas in health matters where authorities differ. You will often encounter conflicting reports about such matters as vitamins, drugs, or coping with death. Which approach should you adopt? Which information should you teach? How should you answer students' questions about controversial health topics, about a cure for AIDS, for example? As you become increasingly knowledgeable about health, you will rely more on your own professional judgment. Sometimes, though, you will have to have the courage to simply say, "I don't know."

Teaching controversial topics, such as sexuality or death and dying, is another barrier to successful health education. Pressure from parents, administrators, school board members, and community organizations may make it almost impossible to even mention some controversial topics in class. There are no easy answers to overcoming this barrier. Ignoring controversial topics, or pretending that such topics are not a valid part of health education, is not a solution. Cornacchia and Staton (1984) recommend the following strategy:

1. Maintain a scientific, unbiased approach.
2. Avoid getting involved in personality conflicts.
3. Follow course and unit outlines recommended or approved by local school officials.
4. Seek the help of community groups such as the PTA, local medical and professional organizations, and qualified resource people such as public health officials. This help may be in the form of vocal or financial support.
5. Use materials that have been prepared by such reputable organizations as the American Alliance for Health, Physical Education, Recreation and Dance; American School Health Association; American Medical Association; and National Educational Association.
6. Use a scientifically sound, up-to-date textbook.
7. Maintain adequate records of student activities, questions, interests, and problems. This can be enhanced by keeping anecdotal files for each student, and adding to the file periodically or when a specific incident occurs.

Other Problems to Implementing Instruction

In areas such as math or geography, the teacher can evaluate the success of instruction with a quantitative paper and pencil test. This is more difficult in health education because the concepts taught often involve students at an affective level, which is difficult to measure. The desired outcome—positive health behavior—might not be observable until years after the concepts have been taught.

Students' backgrounds, cultures, attitudes, and practices must also be considered; understanding their social environments will help you understand why they do what they do in class. Many elementary school students have poor health attitudes and practices. Students often have misconceptions about health-related topics. Children acquire some of these false ideas from family members or friends, or from television, which often glamorizes poor health practices. Combatting these influences will be a challenge, especially when the student feels that your ideas conflict with those of parents or peer group.

Finally, administrators sometimes place a low priority on health education by allowing other activities to substitute for health instruction, or by not placing health education in the curriculum at all.

Despite these problems and barriers, you can make a significant difference in the lives of your students. You must be aware of the controversies and difficulties that you will face, and focus your efforts on quality health education for the students.

Health Highlight: The Image and Reality of Health Educators

According to Dr. Digby Anderson, the public has three major criticisms of health education teachers:

1. One of the most frequent criticisms is: "What are these interfering people going to allow us to do? They take away the foods we want to eat, as well as other luxuries." In other words, many health educators try to be missionizing social engineers, bent on wholesale change, rather than reformers suggesting a modest change in lifestyles.
2. A second objection is about health educators' overstretched claims to competence. Some health educators overstep the boundaries of their qualifications by suggesting changes in areas in which they have no expertise.
3. Health education teachers frequently operate with an unrealistically low assessment of what ordinary people can do. They treat people as "idiots and their choices as ignorant."

Much of the above criticism is leveled at mass-media health education, and has little to do with much of the daily work of health education teachers in the schools. However, the criticism is being applied to all health educators.

Source: Anderson, Digby (1984). "Interfering, unrealistic know-alls?" *Health Education Journal, 44*,1: 43.

PROFESSIONAL PREPARATION

Although standards for professional training of health educators have been set by several professional health education groups, much of the health education in today's schools remains ineffective. This is the result of several factors, but poor teacher preparation is certainly one of them. A poorly prepared teacher can actually work against an effective school health program.

Ideally, a preschool or elementary school health teacher should be a specialist. There are several reasons for this. Health is different from other subjects; the content comes from a variety of sources and is not limited to one distinct discipline. Also, the behavioral outcomes desired of the student in a health class differ remarkably from other subjects. Because these outcomes are not easily measured, a health teacher should have specific training in making empirical observations that indicate whether the desired outcomes are being acquired.

Even when a teacher is dually prepared, say in Health and Physical Education, the health portion is typically slighted in favor of the physical education portion. The reduced number of courses in this dual major hinders effective teacher preparation. Fodor and Dalis (1981) suggest that a minimal level of training for teaching health at the elementary level include: (1) a basic course covering the health problems of elementary school-age children in the United States; (2) a course in the teaching of health at the elementary level, and (3) a course in the function, purpose, and organization of the school health program.

A course dealing with the personal health of the individual is also desirable. In this course, prospective teachers learn more about their own health behavior, enabling them to help students understand their own personal behavior. Further, a basic course in first aid and emergency is very helpful.

The National Task Force on the Preparation and Practice of Health Educators, Inc. (National Task Force, 1983) suggests every health educator should be academically prepared to reach minimum levels of competence for teaching health. This type of professional preparation will help the teacher apply health concepts into professional practice. According to the National Task Force, the prospective health teacher should be sufficiently prepared, through a course of study, to be able to carry out the following:

1. Communicate health and health education needs, concerns, and resources
2. Determine the appropriate focus for health education
3. Plan health education programs in response to identified needs
4. Implement planned health education programs
5. Evaluate health education programs
6. Coordinate selected health education activities
7. Act as a resource for health education.

As discussed earlier, a teacher's preparation does not end upon receipt of a diploma and teaching certificate. You can continue to educate yourself by taking graduate courses, either in specific content areas or in advanced teaching methods, joining local, state, regional, and national health education professional organizations, such as the American School Health Association and the Association for the Advancement of Health Education, and attending professional health conferences. Staying current also requires reading up-to-date textbooks, journals and other health-education publications. Finally, in-service workshops that deal with health-related topics are extremely valuable.

PERSONAL QUALITIES OF THE HEALTH TEACHER

To be a successful teacher of any subject demands more than just knowledge of the subject and appropriate professional preparation. The personal attributes of the teacher are also significant. In health education, teachers must be certain of what they hold valuable and true in their own lives. Having this foundation will help teachers be objective about controversial topics, allowing different points of view as necessary for a balanced discussion.

The teacher should be a positive role model. This does not mean that a teacher must be perfect. Accepting one's faults and limitations is also part of being a good role model. A health teacher should present the image of a physically, mentally, and socially healthy individual. The teacher should embody the image of a person who is attempting to maintain a high level of physical health through a solid exercise regimen, good general health habits, and proper nutrition. The teacher should demonstrate enthusiasm about life generally and teaching specifically. The teacher should be outgoing and exhibit an appropriate sense of humor. The teacher must be able to handle the stressors that face every professional.

Health Highlight: Teachers' Attitudes Toward the Public Schools

A Gallup/Phi Delta Kappa survey polled teacher attitudes toward the public schools and compared teacher attitudes about key topics with the views of the general public, including parents of children enrolled in the public schools. American teachers give high marks to American public schools, awarding local schools an A or a B. Teachers also rated favorably other teachers. However, teachers are less positive about the performance of administrators in the public schools and about local school boards.

A major source of teacher dissatisfaction involves what teachers perceive as poor compensation. Nine teachers in ten state that their salaries are too low, and almost nine in ten say that low pay is the reason teachers are leaving the profession. Further, teachers oppose the idea of merit pay by a two-to-one margin because of the difficulties in evaluation and the morale problems that might be created with a merit pay plan.

American teachers feel that the most important problem facing local public schools is a lack of parental support, while the public perceives lack of discipline in the schools as the most important problem.

Teachers were divided on the issues of public school testing programs and school prayer.

Source: Gallup, Alec (1984, October). "The Gallup Poll of Teachers' Attitudes Toward the Public Schools." *Phi Delta Kappan, 66,* 2: 97-107.

THE TEACHER AS PART OF THE HEALTH TEAM

As a teacher of health, you are part of a team whose mission is to do all it can to enhance the wellness of each student.

For greatest effectiveness, each team member must work with other members. Each member has specific responsibilities. Let's look at some of the major responsibilities of the health teacher as a member of the health team.

Working with Students

One of the teacher's responsibilities is counseling students in health-related matters. Counseling should be straightforward, and free of moral judgment, preaching, or scare tactics. In the role of counselor, you must develop good listening skills and communication skills. Sometimes it is difficult to get to the heart of the problem; these skills will help you offer sound advice.

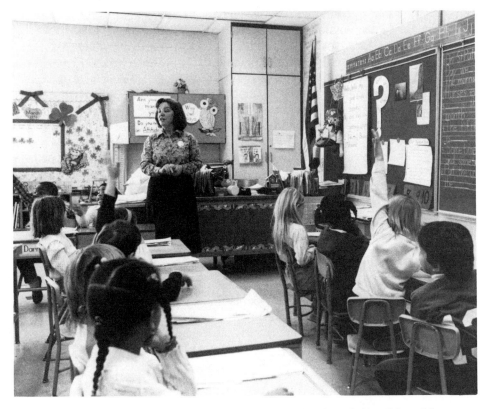

A teacher's personal attributes are as important as his or her knowledge of the subject.

No matter how concerned you are about a student's problem, you must recognize the limitations of your ability to help. If you cannot provide effective counseling, or if you realize that more help is necessary than you can give, refer the student to another teacher or an administrator. The student may also require additional guidance beyond the initial crisis counseling you can supply. Make sure you are familiar with available services in the school or community so you can refer the student to the most appropriate one. Most teachers are not professionally trained in counseling nor are they expected to replace those who are.

Working with Special Students

Because of advances in medical technology and pre-natal and post-natal care, many children with genetic defects, who would have died earlier, are now being born and living longer lives. These children, who were formerly segregated into separate schools or classrooms, are now mainstreamed into the public school classrooms. This integration of special students into the regular classrooms resulted from the passage in 1975 of Public Law 94–142, the landmark Education for All Handicapped Children Act. The law states that handicapped students have the same rights as all other students and that the education of the children must take place in the least restrictive environment.

The intent of P.L. 94–142 is to reject the idea of merely caring for or maintaining handicapped students. It emphasizes prevention and correction. Many special children still spend most, or even all, of their time in a special classroom because of their unique needs. But many others are taught in the regular classroom.

These special students bring with them complex physical, social, and psychological health problems. Their chances for optimal health and learning can be impaired if other students do not accept them socially. They can also have a difficult time coping with the emotional challenges of the regular classroom. In some instances, other students may ridicule them because of their differences.

As a teacher, you must be aware of these children's special health needs. Stress to all your students that each of them is unique and that they should strive to coexist with each other regardless of differences. Encourage positive behavior from the special students; emphasize what they can do rather than what they cannot do. Find a talent that each student has and encourage it to foster that student's feeling of self-worth. Look for every circumstance in which the special student can be included in social activities with other students. The special child should not be overprotected or pitied; this will serve only to alienate the child from the other students, hindering social and emotional adjustment. These positive actions will both help special students to adjust to the regular classroom, and encourage other students to accept them.

Working with Parents

Always notify a student's parents when an illness or serious deviation from normal health occurs. School policy should be followed when parents are notified. Some schools require teachers to contact parents through the administrative offices. A good policy is to ensure that a member of the school administration is present at any parent-teacher conference. The third party can clear up any confusion in communication and can serve as an arbitrator in case of misunderstanding. Explain to the parents the significance of the child's health condition, and encourage them to obtain needed care for the child. If a parent asks for guidance in seeking care, refer the person to the proper agency or individual. Be sure to take an active role in following up any case reported to parents.

Parents also need to be kept informed about curriculum changes and content, especially in controversial areas of health education. You can help educate parents how such modifications will benefit the students and the community.

Working with Other Teachers

A major responsibility of the health teacher is to keep the other teachers informed of health matters related to the community and students. This information will assist the other faculty members in understanding their students and also help them recognize the need for health education in the school.

The health educator can represent the faculty on health-related committees of teacher-parent and community organizations. You can help other faculty members be aware of the environmental conditions in the school that might be unhealthy to the students, staff, and faculty. You should also attempt to become involved in textbook selection committees. Look not only for sound, up-to-date content, but also beware of textbooks that propagate stereotypes.

Working with the School Administration

A primary duty of the health educator is to plan the health education curriculum and make recommendations to the administration regarding the health education program within the school. You can help interpret and implement any state requirement for the health curriculum. Also make suggestions concerning the health service program and health environment.

The teacher must also work closely with the school administration when notifying parents about a child's health, referring parents to appropriate health resources, and following up student cases. The teacher should keep the administration informed about a child's progress in school after returning from an illness.

Working with the School Nurse

Because of your daily observation of each child in your class, you can help the school nurse understand the health behavior of students. You can also assist the nurse in various aspects of the screening program—by preliminary screening in the classroom, by preparing students for screening tests to reduce their anxiety, and by referring students who are in particular need of screening. Teacher and nurse can cooperate in in-service workshops for the other faculty members. Finally, teachers who are properly trained can complement the school's emergency care program by offering their services when needed.

Working with Outside Agencies

One of your objectives should be to promote health education and awareness in the community. You can help volunteer organizations educate the community in health matters. Many of these agencies, such as the Heart Association and American Dental Association, have health curricula and need help to implement their programs in the schools. Through this cooperation, you can learn about other health professionals in your community and can acquaint yourself with the services offered to students by these agencies.

You should also become involved with the local public health department and cooperate with department staff members in providing services to the students and community. In addition, offer to serve on your community health council. If there is no health council, try to begin one. In such councils, interested health professionals meet regularly to discuss each other's programs. Such meetings are not only informational; they also can solve many problems related to duplication of services. When any two agencies have a similar program, the two organizations can cooperate in serving the community.

Finally, in this time of budget cuts and termination of health programs, you are strongly urged to become active in lobbying for health services and programs. Develop good relationships with individuals who make the decisions that affect health education in your community and state. Written correspondence helps, but face-to-face contact usually has more impact. Also, work with local teacher groups to educate legislators about health matters. Many voices can influence a legislator to introduce or to vote favorably for a bill. Health education professional organizations, such as the American School Health Association and the American Alliance for Health, Physical Education, Recreation, and Dance, also lobby on a national level.

SUMMARY

Teachers play an important role in their students' health. They have a tremendous opportunity to positively affect students by modeling their own health behavior, helping maintain students' health, and motivating students to make wise decisions concerning health behavior. Although teaching health can be challenging, it is also exciting and rewarding. Teachers should give a high priority to health education and use a scientific, objective approach in guiding students.

Unfortunately, many teachers do not receive much professional preparation for teaching health. But even if you are not training to be a health specialist, you should take specific courses dealing with health and receive appropriate training in observing health-related behaviors. You should also be a positive role model to further enhance students' health education.

The primary duty of the health teacher is designing and implementing learning opportunities that will enable students to make wise decisions concerning their own health. The teacher also works with other members of the school health team to promote and maintain student health through health services in the school. Teamwork with parents, the school nurse, the school physician, administrators, community organizations, and students is the key to a successful school health services program. In the team, the teacher observes each student for any deviation from normal health, reports to the proper authority within the school, and is available to refer the student and parent to the appropriate community resource or to counsel the student and/or parent concerning the child's health.

DISCUSSION QUESTIONS

1. Describe the challenges of the role of the elementary health teacher.
2. How does health education differ from other subject area instruction?
3. Discuss the evaluation of health education as a barrier to implementing good health instruction.
4. Briefly describe the recommended professional preparation of prospective health educators.
5. Why is it crucial for any teacher to be a positive role model in health behavior to the students?

6. Describe the role of the teacher in working with students to enhance their health.

7. Why are there more special students in the public schools today than before?

8. Why should an administrator be present at any parent-teacher conference?

9. List three ways a teacher can promote health education by working with outside agencies.

10. How can a teacher become more involved as a professional health educator?

REFERENCES

Anderson, D. "Interfering unrealistic know-alls?" *Health Education Journal, 1985, 44,* 1.

Cornacchia, H. J., & Staton, W. M. *Health in elementary schools.* (6th ed.). St. Louis: C. V. Mosby, 1984.

Fodor, J. T., & Dalis, G. T. *Health instruction: Theory and application,* (3rd ed.). Philadelphia: Lea & Febiger, 1981.

Gallup, Alec. "The Gallup Poll of Teachers' Attitudes Toward the Public Schools." *Phi Delta Kappan,* October 1984, *66,* 2.

National Task Force on the Preparation and Practice of Health Educators, Inc. A guide for the development of competency-based curricula for entry level health educators. New York: National Task Force on the Preparation and Practice of Health Educators, Inc., 1983.

3. The Nature of the Elementary School-Age Child

The youth gets together his materials to build a bridge to the moon, or, perchance, a palace or temple on the earth, and at length, the middle-aged man concludes to build a woodshed with them.—Henry David Thoreau

THE NEED FOR DEVELOPMENTAL UNDERSTANDING

To be effective, all teachers must have some awareness of the nature of their students at any given age level. Subject matter competency and teaching skill are not enough; teachers must also understand the developmental stages of childhood. This knowledge encourages teachers to look at the "whole" child, not simply viewing the child from an academic or instructional perspective. Better understanding of children's physical and emotional capabilities—and limitations—should help teachers apply instructional content in ways that are meaningful at a given grade level.

Almost all children enter school with a thirst for knowledge and abundant energy. You can foster these qualities by responding to your students with concern, love, and attention. Realistic expectations of students based on knowledge about the general nature of the school-age child will help accomplish this goal and promote positive educational experiences.

In this chapter the major aspects of child development are presented. These are physical growth and development, developmental difficulties, psychosocial needs, and learning theory.

PHYSICAL GROWTH AND DEVELOPMENT

Physical growth and developmental patterns are largely determined by genetic and environmental factors introduced prenatally and in early infancy. As a group, elementary school-age children exhibit "typical" trends during the maturation process. However, no one child is a textbook example who grows and develops exactly "on schedule." Nonetheless, the *sequence* of developmental stages remains consistent from individual to individual, even though the age or time span at which these changes occur varies greatly. By emphasizing this fact to both parents and children, you can do much to alleviate anxiety and concern about "normal" growth and development. Also point out that there are significant differences in developmental rates between boys and girls.

Height and Weight Changes

Growth is rapid during infancy. There is another period of rapid growth at the onset of adolescence. But between the ages of approximately 5 and 11 no dramatic growth increases are evident. The gradual and steady gains in height and weight for both boys and girls during this period go almost unnoticed. This is a time of relative developmental quiescence before the growth spurt that marks puberty and the resulting transition from childhood to adolescence. The growth spurt for girls usually occurs at about age 10, two years prior to that for boys. However, its duration is shorter than that for boys. Still, diversity in height and weight during the elementary school years varies more among individuals than among the sexes. The average heights and weights of children up to age 16 are shown in table 3.1. Note that the average increase in height during the elementary school years from the ages of 5 to 11 is approximately 2.5 inches per year! The average increase in weight per year varies from 4 to 6 pounds.

The body does not experience growth spurts uniformly; its parts grow at various rates. The slowest growing portion of the body is the trunk, while the hands and feet are among the fastest growing parts. The legs and arms develop more quickly than

Table 3.1
Average Height and Weight of Children to Age 16

Age in years	Boys				Girls			
	Inches	Centimeters	Pounds	Kilograms	Inches	Centimeters	Pounds	Kilograms
0	21.5	54	7.7	3.5	21.2	53	7.5	3.4
0.25			13.1	5.93			12.3	5.6
0.5			17.4	7.9			15.2	6.9
0.75			20.3	9.2			19.2	8.7
1	30.4	76	22.5	10.2	29.5	74	21.4	9.7
2	34.8	87	28.0	12.7	34.2	86	26.9	12.2
3	39.5	94	32.4	14.7	37.2	93	31.5	14.3
4	40.5	102	36.6	16.6	40.0	100	35.9	16.3
5	43.3	108	40.7	18.5	42.8	107	40.3	18.3
6	45.8	115	45.2	20.5	45.2	113	45.0	20.4
7	48.2	121	49.8	22.6	47.7	119	49.8	22.6
8	50.4	126	55.1	25.0	50.0	125	55.3	25.1
9	52.6	132	60.6	27.5	52.2	131	61.1	27.7
10	54.9	137	66.8	30.3	54.4	136	68.6	31.1
11	56.8	142	73.9	33.6	57.2	143	77.4	35.2
12	58.8	147	82.9	37.7	59.5	149	89.1	40.5
13	61.2	153	93.7	42.6	62.4	156	100.8	45.8
14	64.4	161	107.3	48.8	64.0	160	112.2	51.0
15	66.8	167	120.3	54.7	64.8	162	119.7	54.4
16	68.8	172	131.1	59.6	64.8	162	122.8	55.8

Source: J. M. Tanner, *Archives of diseases in childhood*, vol. 41, 1966, p. 613.

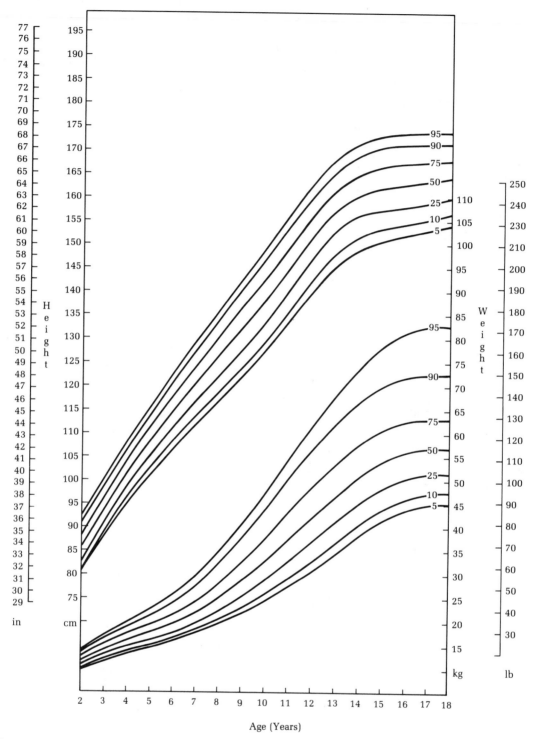

Figure 3.1
Physical growth of girls from ages 2 to 18.

Source: National Center for Health Statistics: NCHS Growth Charts, 1976. Monthly Vital Statistics Report. Vol. 25, No. 3, Supp. (HRA) 76–1120. Health Resources Administration, Rockville, Maryland, June, 1976. Data from the National Center for Health Statistics.

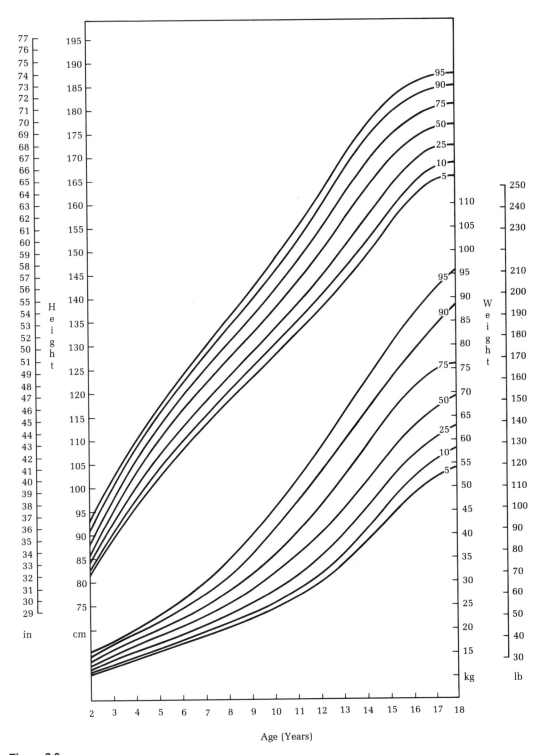

Figure 3.2
Physical growth of boys from ages 2 to 18.
Source: National Center for Health Statistics: NCHS Growth Charts, 1976. Monthly Vital Statistics Report. Vol. 25, No. 3, Supp. (HRA) 76–1120. Health Resources Administration, Rockville, Maryland, June, 1976. Data from the National Center for Health Statistics.

the trunk but more slowly than the extremities (Mercer, 1979, pp. 111–112). This may account for the fact that some older elementary school children appear more awkward or poorly coordinated than many of their peers. Figures 3.1 and 3.2 summarize the differences in physical growth patterns for girls and boys, respectively, according to percentile distribution for height and weight by age groupings.

Motor Coordination Patterns

The physiological changes that trigger growth of various body regions and gains in height and weight are almost always accompanied by advances in a child's motor skills and abilities. The occurrence of motor coordination landmarks in infancy and childhood (rolling over, grasping objects, walking, throwing a ball, hopping on one foot) is dependent upon skeletal development of the individual at a given stage of growth and appears to be directly correlated with height and weight measures. In other words, those elementary school children who are somewhat taller and experience earlier incremental gains in weight will likely appear to be somewhat better coordinated than their less physically mature peers.

Because the bones have not yet ossified, or hardened, at birth, a baby simply cannot exhibit sophisticated voluntary movements or control over muscular action and activity. For example, until the bones and muscles of an infant become well-developed in the neck region, the head will require support. This condition usually lasts until about two to three months after birth. Similarly, grasping and picking up objects cannot be accomplished until the bones of the hands and wrists harden. Since these bones are among the earliest to do so most infants can pick up objects with the palm of the hand by the time they are 7 to 10 months old (Ambron, 1975, p. 81). As physical maturation progresses, ossification and fusion of the bone ends also proceeds in a relatively predictable fashion. This leads to a greater degree of fine motor development throughout childhood among both boys and girls.

Like bones, the muscles of babies appear drastically different from those of children and adolescents, whose muscle mass increases because muscle fibers greatly lengthen and thicken during the first 15 years of life. Although people are born with all the muscle fibers they will ever have, these fibers must be developed in order to fully support and move the body. As a result, before about age 5, motor development revolves around use of the large muscle groups needed for gross motor movements such as standing, walking, and running. The muscle fibers of both elementary school girls and boys are of comparable length and thickness, thus accounting for the equal strength displayed by the two. However, following puberty and the growth spurt, the muscle tissue of males increases significantly in various body regions, particularly in the heart and lungs, producing greater absolute strength and endurance after adolescence because of greater oxygen transport capacity and a better physiological ability to neutralize the chemical by-products of muscular activity (Biehler, 1976, p. 459).

When considering muscular strength and endurance in relation to relative body size, however, the differences between males and females diminish (Matthews & Fox, 1976, pp. 462–466). Therefore motor coordination between the sexes in childhood is generally viewed as comparable or equivalent. While it is true that girls are slightly more advanced physically in terms of growth than are boys because they

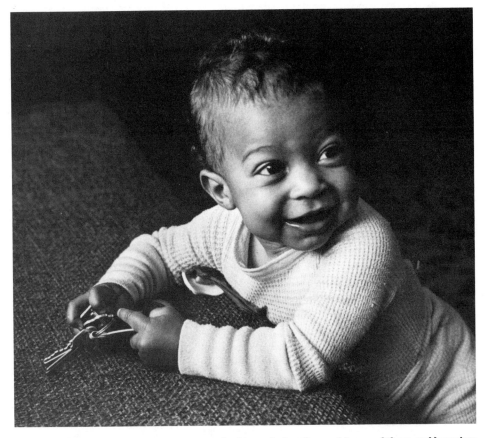

Preschool children are generally concerned with exploring the world around them and learning to perform tasks by themselves.

mature faster through an earlier adolescent growth spurt, the attainment and demonstration of motor skills and tasks seems more directly related to body size. Thus elementary school children as a whole, in their various grade groupings, will show many more similarities than differences in their motor skills and coordination.

Because fine motor skills—those requiring agility and defined special movement using smaller muscle groups—begin to develop around the time that children first enter school, children's need to exercise and participate in physical activity are heightened. Although muscular development and motor coordination appear to be a result of the maturation process itself and not due to "practice," the opportunity to exercise will improve development as well as enhance health and well-being.

Nervous System Development

Changes in height and weight along with sequential advances in motor coordination and development could not occur without the maturation of the nervous system. The brain and nervous system direct growth and functioning of all other bodily parts and

Table 3.2
Growth and Development Characteristics

GRADES K–3 AGES 5–8

PHYSICAL CHARACTERISTICS

Growth relatively slow.

Increase in large muscle coordination, beginning of development of small muscle control.

Bones growing.

Nose grows larger.

Permanent teeth appearing or replacing primary teeth; lower part of face more prominent.

Hungry at short intervals; may overeat and become fat.

Enjoys active play-climbing, jumping, running.

Susceptible to fatigue and limits self.

Visual acuity reaches normal.

Susceptible to respiratory & communicable diseases.

NEEDS

To develop large muscle control through motor skills.

To have play space and materials.

To use instructional tools & equipment geared to stage of development.

To establish basic health habits: toileting, eating, covering nose and mouth with cough, etc.

To have snack time and opportunity to develop social graces.

To have plenty of sleep and rest, and exercise interspersed with rest.

To have health examinations and follow-up.

To have visual and auditory checks.

To have dental attention.

Suggested Activities: Vigorous games emphasizing outdoor play with basic movement patterns and skills as well as singing games and rhythms.

EMOTIONAL CHARACTERISTICS

Self-centered, desires immediate attention to his/her problem—wants to be first.

Sensitive about being left out.

Sensitive about ridicule, criticism or loss of prestige.

Easily aroused emotionally.

Can take responsibility but needs adult supervision.

Parent image strong; also identifies with teacher.

Expresses likes and dislikes readily.

Questioning attitude about sex differences.

NEEDS

To receive encouragement, recognition, ample praise, patience, adult support.

To express inner feelings, anxieties and fears.

To feel secure, loved, wanted, accepted (at home & at school).

To be free from pressure to achieve beyond capabilities.

To have a consistent, cooperatively planned program of classroom control. Must have guidance.

To develop self-confidence.

To have some immediate desirable satisfactions.

To know limitations within which he can operate effectively.

To develop realistic expectations of self.

SOCIAL CHARACTERISTICS

Lack of interest in personal grooming.

Engages in imitative play.

Friendly, frank, sometimes aggressive, "bossy," assertive.

Generally tolerant of race, economic status, etc.

Gradually more socially oriented and adjusted.

Boys and girls play together as sex equals, but aware of sex differences.

NEEDS

To have satisfactory peer relationships; receive group approval.

To learn the importance of sharing, planning, working and playing together—both boys and girls.

To have help in developing socially acceptable behavior.

To learn to assume some responsibility; to have opportunities to initiate activities, to lead.

To work independently and in groups.

To accept sex role.

To develop an appreciation of social values, such as honesty, sportsmanship, etc.

INTELLECTUAL CHARACTERISTICS

Varied intellectual growth and ability of children.

Interested in things that move, bright colors, dramatizations, rhythmics, making collections.

Interested in the present, not the future.

Learns best through active participation in concrete, meaningful situations.

Can abide by safety rules.

Wants to know "why."

Attention span short.

NEEDS

To experience frequent success and learn to accept failure when it occurs.

To have concrete learning experiences and direct participation.

To be in a rich, stable challenging environment.

To have time to adjust to new experiences and new situations.

To learn to follow through to completion.

To develop a love for learning.

To learn without developing feelings of hostility.

To communicate effectively.

Source: A Pocketguide to Health & Health Problems in School Physical Activities, pp. 4–7. American School Health Association, © 1981. American School Health Association, Kent, OH. 44240.

Table 3.3
Growth and Development Characteristics

GRADES 4–6 AGES 8–11

PHYSICAL CHARACTERISTICS

Growth slow and steady.

Girls begin to forge ahead of boys in height and weight.

Extremities begin to lengthen toward end of this period.

Muscle coordination improving.

Continued small muscle development.

Bones growing, vulnerable to injury.

Permanent dentition continues.

Malocclusion may be a problem.

Appetite good, increasing interest in food.

Boundless energy.

Tires easily.

Visual acuity normal.

Menarche possible toward end of this period.

NEEDS

To develop and improve coordination of both large and small muscles.

To have plenty of activities and games which will develop body control, strength, endurance, and skills-stunts (throwing, catching, running, bicycles, skates).

To have careful supervision of games appropriate to strength and developmental needs; protective equipment.

To have competitive activity with children of comparable size.

To have sleep, rest, well-balanced meals.

To have health examinations and follow-up.

To have visual and auditory checks.

To have dental attention.

Suggested activities: More formal games with emphasis on body mechanics.

EMOTIONAL CHARACTERISTICS

Seeks approval of peer group.

Desire to succeed.

Enthusiastic, noisy, imaginative, desire to explore.

Negativistic (early part of period).

Begins to accept responsibility for clothing and behavior.

Increasingly anxious about family & possible tragedy.

Increasing self-consciousness.

Sex hostility.

Becomes "modest" but not too interested in details of sex.

NEEDS

To begin seriously to gain a realistic image of self and appreciate uniqueness of personality.

To be recognized for individual worth; to feel self-assurance and self-esteem.

To receive encouragement and affection; to be understood and appreciated.

To exercise self-control.

To talk about problems and receive reasonable explanations. To have questions answered.

SOCIAL CHARACTERISTICS

Learns to cooperate better in group planning and group play and abides by group decisions.

Interested in competitive activities and prestige. Competition keen.

Begins to show qualities of leadership.

Developing interest in appearance.

Strong sense of fair play.

Belongs to a gang or secret club; loyal to group.

Close friendships with members of own sex.

Separate play for boys and girls.

NEEDS

To be recognized and accepted by peer groups; receive social approval.

To have relationships with adults which give feelings of security and acceptance.

To assume responsibilities, have increased opportunities for independent actions and decisions.

To develop appreciation for others and their rights.

To learn to get along with others and accept those different from self.

INTELLECTUAL CHARACTERISTICS

Likes to talk and express ideas.

High potential of learning—in science, adventure, the world.

Eager to acquire skills.

Wide range of interests; curious, wants to experiment.

Goals are immediate.

Demands consistency.

Generally reliable about following instructions.

Attention span short.

NEEDS

To experiment, explore, solve problems, challenges, use initiative, select, plan, evaluate.

To receive individual help in skill areas without harmful or undue pressure.

To have opportunities for creative self-expression.

To have a rich environment of materials and the opportunity to explore it.

To participate in concrete, real-life situations.

To be able to accept one's self with strengths and weaknesses.

processes. Increases in height and weight, bone ossification and elongation, and muscular thickening would not proceed along expected, predictable lines if the nervous system itself failed to develop normally.

Although the brain at birth is, comparatively speaking, closer to its adult size than any other organ, it is developmentally more incomplete and inoperative than other systems. Maturation of the brain and nervous system is rapid during the first four years of life. The most highly developed section of the brain at birth is the midbrain, the area that controls involuntary reflexes such as attention, sleep, and elimination. However, the cerebrum, the center for cognition, motor control, and sensory awareness, becomes much more differentiated later. New cortical cells form after the first few months and enlarge to produce a heavier brain. As various portions of the cerebrum develop, more and more behaviors associated with thought, movement, and sensation are exhibited. Motor areas in the brain develop sequentially, accounting for the hierarchy of neuromuscular skills previously discussed. By age 4, development of the cerebrum is almost complete and serves to greatly influence fine motor development, intellectual activity, and perception throughout childhood.

At birth, the spinal cord is not completely covered by sheaths of myelin and therefore the transmission of nerve impulses is more primitive. This limits not only the child's motor functioning but also the ability to communicate and respond in various capacities. Myelinization occurs progressively in much the same way as cerebral development and is nearly completed by age 2 (Bee, 1978, p. 119). Because of the physiologically delicate nature of the brain and central nervous system through age 4 or 5, the child is more vulnerable to disease and environmental hazards at this time. Therefore, in infancy and during the first few years of elementary school, particular attention should be paid to any conditions that could have an adverse effect on neurological development and functioning.

Endocrine System Contributions

Human growth and development, while directed by the nervous system, is regulated by hormonal secretions from the endocrine system. The endocrine glands most directly concerned with physical changes in height, weight, skeletal-muscular maturation, secondary sex characteristics, and the like are the pituitary, thyroid, gonad, and adrenal glands.

Triggered by the hypothalamus, the pituitary gland secretes somatotropin, or growth hormone, which helps regulate growth of the skeleton and general body size. Children who exhibit extremes in height may have a problem with either an insufficient or overbundant amount of somatotropin being secreted. Maintenance of bone structure and skeletal growth is dependent upon secretions of thyroxin from the thyroid gland, which also helps to control the metabolic rate. Children exhibiting lethargy or extreme excitability may need to be checked for levels of thyroxin secreted.

The pituitary gland also releases hormones at the onset of adolescence that signal the reproductive organs or gonads to activate, thus initiating the development of male and female secondary sex characteristics in puberty. Although these hormonal influences among children are not generally in operation during the elementary school years, some girls at the fifth and sixth grade levels may begin showing signs of sexual maturation. Therefore it is essential for teachers to be well-informed about hormonal changes and their physical and emotional impact upon students.

Secretions of cortin and adrenalin from the adrenal glands are, respectively, important in affecting the speed of maturation and emotional adjustments made in times of stress. The adrenal glands, after decreasing in size immediately after birth, enlarge significantly up to age 5, whereupon stabilization is maintained until about age 11. From that time until a child reaches age 16, another rapid increase in size occurs, paralleling the growth spurt and influencing "teenage" emotions (Katachadourian, 1977, pp. 90–100). Further discussion of the physiological and psychological changes that occur during adolescence appears in chapter 19.

Cardiorespiratory Characteristics

Cardiorespiratory development parallels general physical growth patterns. There is rapid growth during infancy. Growth diminishes during childhood years, and then increases rapidly again during the growth spurt of adolescence. That is, a marked increase is observed in ages up to 5 and between ages 10 to 16. Heart rate and blood pressure may vary greatly from day to day for any given child because of the many factors that affect both. However, consistent, excessive deviations from the norm (i.e., 15 percent) may require special medical attention. Lung growth basically parallels cardiac growth and body growth in general. As older elementary school children begin to develop their chest muscles, breathing becomes more regular than that of younger students and is usually deeper and slower. Respiration rates also vary considerably among children and should not be a cause for alarm. As students progress through adolescence, cardiac output and lung size increase and show differences between males and females that are not evident at the elementary level. Tables 3.4 and 3.5 give age comparisons of cardiac and respiratory characteristics, respectively.

Table 3.4
Comparison of Heart Growth and Development from Birth to Adolescence, Averaged for Both Sexes.

	Birth	**1 yr**	**5 yr**	**7 yr**	**9 yr**	**10–16 yr**
Heart size compared to birth		2x	4x	5x	6x	7x–20x
Heart weight (g)	20–24	38–45	82–90	100	125	135–220
Heart rate (at rest)	150	110–115	100	95	90–95	82–85
Average systolic blood pressure (mm Hg)	52	96	99	105	110	115–120

Source: W. D. Sorochan and S. J. Bender, *Teaching elementary health science.* Reading, Mass.: Addison-Wesley, 1979, p. 41.

Table 3.5
Summary of Variations in Respiration With Age.

	Birth	**1 yr**	**5 yr**	**10 yr**	**20 yr**
Lung weight (increases as compared to birth)	1	3x			20x
Respiratory rates (min)	30–80	20–40	20–25	17–22	15–20
Tidal air (cc)	19	48	175	320	500

Source: W. D. Sorochan and S. J. Bender, *Teaching elementary health science.* Reading, Mass.: Addison-Wesley, 1979, p. 41.

DEVELOPMENTAL DIFFICULTIES

While the vast majority of children are born with good health and highly functional levels of well-being, some children are less fortunate and do not progress developmentally in a normal fashion. Developmental disabilities range from mild growth pattern lags in physical maturation or motor coordination that eventually diminish to severe physical, intellectual, emotional, or behavioral abnormalities that may be permanent. In between these two extremes are a wide array of disabilities that influence normal development, such as chronic illnesses, moderate physical handicaps, perceptual malfunctions, speech problems, learning disabilities, environmental deprivation, exposure to accidents, or communicable diseases.

It is not possible here to describe and discuss all the developmental difficulties that can occur prenatally, in infancy, or during childhood. However, because Public Law 94-142 requires the inclusion of children with various handicaps in the regular classroom whenever possible, you need to understand and be able to interact with children who have special needs. This portion of the chapter provides a broad overview of the more common developmental difficulties among infants and children.

Definition and Prevalence of Birth Defects

Any body function, structure, or metabolic process that exhibits an abnormality at birth is considered a birth defect. These disorders encompass both very noticeable structural conditions such as spina bifida, cleft lip and palate, hydrocephalus, or clubfoot as well as unseen defects in internal organs. In addition, blood, enzymatic, chemical, or genetic errors may be responsible for diverse bodily malfunctions that are evident at birth or shortly thereafter, but in some cases do not appear until adolescence or adulthood. Birth defects may be a result of inherited conditions, environmental insults to the fetus during pregnancy or the birth itself, or an interaction between the two.

According to The National Foundation-March of Dimes (1984), each year in the United States about 250,000 babies are born with a birth defect. This is 7 percent of all live births per year. Also, an estimated additional 500,000 babies die before birth as a result of a fetal abnormality. In addition, each year the death rate due to birth defects among children is 60,000.

Developmental difficulties arising at birth affect the daily lives of 15 million Americans: 4 million are diabetic; 3 million are mentally retarded; 1 million suffer with congenital bone, muscle, or joint disease; 750,000 have a congenital hearing impairment; 500,000 are born partially or totally blind; 350,000 exhibit heart or circulatory defects, and 100,000 have severe speech problems (National Foundation-March of Dimes, 1984).

Although medical advances have been made in treating, reducing, and preventing the occurrence of birth defects during the past few decades, a significant number of infants and school-age children continue to be faced with these problems. Thus knowledge of the etiology and nature of the more prevalent developmental disabilities is essential for educators at all levels.

Hereditary Factors

There are hundreds of structural and metabolic disorders that are passed on to children through their parents' chromosomes and the hundreds of genes each chromosome carries. The three major types of genetic disorders are chromosome defects, single-gene defects, and multifactorial defects.*

Chromosome Defects. Chromosomes are structures that determine inheritance and are located in the nucleus of cells. Most human cells have forty-six chromosomes in pairs. Sperm and egg cells have twenty-three chromosomes, which pair at fertilization. Chromosome defects occur when the cells have too many or too few chromosomes or when chromosomes have missing or extra parts or parts of a chromosome appear on another chromosome. Often chromosomal errors occur during formation of reproductive cells in the ovary or testis. As a result, the fertilized egg cell may contain chromosomes in abnormal number, structure, or arrangement. Once such an error occurs, it is repeated in the millions of cells that form the growing embryo, affecting various body structures and functions. Many chromosomal defects can be seen by microscope with the aid of special staining techniques. A karyotype, which is a photograph of chromosomes arranged in pairs according to length, permits the identification of specific chromosomal abnormalities.

Chromosome disorders affect both sexes and all ethnic groups in roughly equal proportions. Older women are more likely to have children with chromosome disorders than younger women. The risk is about 1 in 1,000 at age 34 or below, 6 in 1,000 at age 35 to 40, and 17.2 in 1,000 for women over 40 (National Clearinghouse, 1985).

The most common birth defect resulting from chromosomal error is Down syndrome, or mongolism. In Down syndrome there are three chromosomes—a trisomy—in pair number 21. Down children are mentally retarded and have facial and limb abnormalities. Often they have seriously malformed internal organs. The skin fold at the inner corners of the eyes gives the characteristic mongoloid appearance.

Ninety-five percent of Down syndrome cases are the result of random chromosomal error. However, about 5 percent of the cases occur in certain families at a higher rate than expected (Klug & Cummings, 1983). In familial (inherited) Down syndrome cases, normal-appearing parents transmit chromosomal abnormalities to their offspring who in turn exhibit the Down traits. For families in which inheritance of Down syndrome is suspected, chromosomal analysis may be necessary.

Down syndrome occurs in approximately 1 in 280 children born to women between the ages of 35 and 39. From age 40 to 44, the risk increases sharply, to one in every 80 children. If a woman is older than 44, her chances are 1 in 40 of bearing a child with Down syndrome. The risks are the same whether it is the woman's first pregnancy or not. (National Foundation 1984)

Single-Gene Defects. Normal development and functioning of every living being depends on genetic information transmitted by both parents at the moment of conception. Inborn characteristics from eye color to the parts of the nervous system are controlled by the action of one or more pairs of genes contained on chromosomes

---

*This discussion of hereditary factors is taken from *Health* by Hamrick, Anspaugh, and Ezell (Columbus: Merrill, 1986).

within the nucleus of all body cells. There are hundreds of genes, the basic units of heredity, on each chromosome. Among this vast number, a few are likely to be abnormal. It is likely that everyone carries some faulty genes that may or may not be expressed by certain physical traits.

Most traits require the interaction of many gene pairs, but for some only a single pair is involved. There are perhaps 3,000 known disorders caused by alterations in a single gene. The relative risk that a couple has of transmitting any one of the disorders depends on the frequency with which it appears in the family and on the kind of gene involved. For example, recessive diseases are named for the type of gene with which they are associated. An individual may be a carrier of a disease in this category—that is, she may possess the gene associated with the disease, but not the disease itself. The 1,117 diseases in this category tend to be severe and often fatal. They include cystic fibrosis (a disease affecting the function of mucus and sweat glands), phenylketonuria (liver enzyme deficiency), and sickle cell disease (a blood disorder primarily affecting blacks).

In the second category of single-gene diseases, affected individuals run a relatively high risk (at least 50 percent) of passing along the disease. Diseases in this category are called dominant diseases for the type of gene with which they are associated. They tend to affect both sexes equally, are structural rather than metabolic, and may show marked variability, with different individuals having different forms and symptoms of the same disease. Huntington's disease (progressive nervous system degeneration) and polydactyly (extra fingers or toes) are examples of dominant disorders.

Finally, there are diseases that are closely associated with an individual's sex. They are known as sex-linked disorders because they are controlled by genes located on the sex-determining chromosome. Sex-linked disorders are usually passed from mother to son. The mother may be a carrier, but her son will probably exhibit the trait. Among the 205 sex-linked disorders are color blindness (inability to distinguish certain colors), hemophilia (a defect in the blood-clotting mechanism), and muscular dystrophy (progressive wasting of the muscles).

Multifactorial Disorders. The majority of inherited disorders are caused by the interaction of many genes with other genes or with environmental factors. The pattern of transmission in this group is less well defined and the risk of recurrence is low—probably 3 to 5 percent if one child has been affected and 8 to 10 percent if two children have been affected.

The exact number of defects attributable to multifactorial inheritance is unknown. Defects that are thought to be multifactorial include

- cleft lip or palate
- clubfoot
- congenital dislocation of the hip
- spina bifida (open spine)
- hydrocephalus (with spina bifida)—water on the brain
- pyloric stenosis—narrowed or obstructed opening from stomach into small intestine

Detection and Diagnosis of Genetic Defects. The technology of prenatal diagnosis expands almost daily and can be extremely helpful to many couples at risk for transmitting a genetic disorder. At one time counselors were limited to a family pedigree to determine the risk of passing on defective genes. A pedigree is a diagram showing the ancestral history of a person for a particular trait. Now it is often possible to tell parents with certainty whether a fetus will become defective. Amniocentesis is the most widely used technique that makes this possible.

In amniocentesis, a sample of the fluid (amniotic fluid) in which the fetus floats is removed through a needle inserted through a woman's abdominal and uterine walls. It is usually performed after the fourteenth week of pregnancy. Chemical tests of this fluid can reveal most known chromosomal abnormalities, and more than seventy metabolic disorders. Up to 182 fetal conditions have been diagnosed prenatally using amniocentesis. It also is used in late pregnancy to determine the severity of Rh disease when the condition is suspected.

The usual procedure is to locate the placenta and position of the fetus with ultrasound equipment. This prevents injury when the needle is inserted into the amniotic sac. The entire procedure carries low risk for mother and baby, with one in 200 causing a pregnancy complication (National Clearinghouse, 1985).

About 97 percent of the high-risk women using amniocentesis find that the fetus is free of the suspected defect. If a defect is found, it may be possible to minimize damage through prompt action at or soon after birth. It is important to remember, however, that amniotic fluid found to be normal does not guarantee a healthy baby. Many birth defects cannot be detected through amniocentesis.

Ultrasound is used often as a prenatal diagnostic tool without amniocentesis. It provides a picture showing the location, size, and structure of the fetus in the uterus. It is particularly valuable in early diagnosis of multiple births and pregnancies that pose a threat to normal delivery.

Fetoscopy, insertion of a viewing instrument directly into the uterus to observe the fetus and take blood samples, is sometimes used for diagnosis of otherwise undetectable blood diseases and malformations. The method is still experimental and is available at only a few major medical centers.

Testing for carriers of genetic defects has been a major goal of genetic research. At present, carrier tests are available for a considerable number of potentially damaging genetic traits and more are being developed. For example, simple blood tests can identify carriers of thalassemia (Cooley anemia) and sickle cell disease. According to the National Foundation-March of Dimes, 10 percent of blacks in the United States are carriers of the sickle cell gene. Other tests have been developed for carriers of certain metabolic errors, such as Tay-Sachs disease. Practical and reliable carrier tests are still needed for several important genetic diseases such as cystic fibrosis, the most common genetic disease affecting the white population in the United States, and PKU (phenylketonuria), the inability to metabolize an amino acid, which results in brain damage.

Genetic counseling is available to couples who suspect that their future children may be at risk of inheriting a disorder. One or both parents may know of a history of birth defects in the family. They may belong to an ethnic or racial group at relatively high risk for a specific defect; have a history of radiation therapy, chemical, or hormonal exposure; have a history of numerous spontaneous abortions or stillbirths; or have had a previous child with a birth defect. The National Clearinghouse for Human Genetic Diseases indicates that most couples who are referred to genetic counseling centers meet one or more of these criteria:

- The mother is over thirty-five.
- A previous child was born with a chromosome abnormality.
- One of the parents has a chromosomal abnormality or rearrangement.
- A previous child was born with a metabolic defect.
- A previous child was born with a neural tube defect.

Metabolic Disturbances. Numerous genetic disorders result from an inborn error in fetal or neonatal metabolism. Like chromosomal abnormalities, many of these metabolic disturbances are poorly understood in terms of origin, effect, and treatment. Two of the most common metabolic disturbances are diabetes mellitus and muscular dystrophy.

Diabetes mellitus is not a contagious or infectious disease. It is the most familiar of the diseases caused by an endocrine gland disorder. The pancreas contains a group of cells called the islet of Langerhans, which produces the hormone insulin. This hormone enables the body to use sugar and starch after they have been converted into glucose by the digestive process. When there is a disturbance in the insulin mechanism, nourishment is seriously disturbed because glucose cannot be effectively used by the body. One factor leading to disturbance in the insulin mechanism is insufficient production of the hormone by the islet of Langerhans. Diabetes mellitus also may be the result of increased insulin requirement, or a decrease in the effectiveness of the insulin produced. Heredity is an important influence, as witnessed by the occurrence of the disease in members of the same family. Diabetes mellitus is more frequent in overweight people, occurs more often in women than men, and is more frequent in older people.

There are two types of diabetes mellitus: type 1, insulin-dependent and type 2, non-insulin-dependent. In general diabetes mellitus that appears in youth tends to be more serious than diabetes appearing later in life. There are screening tests to help detect diabetes. Any medical examination should include an analysis of the urine and blood for detection of the condition. Diabetes is treated through diet, insulin injection, or oral medications. The symptoms of diabetes are excessive thirst, frequent urination, unexplained loss of weight, weakness, listlessness, and fatigue. There may also be a decreased resistance to infection.

All types of muscular dystrophy appear to stem from the absence of one or more enzymes needed to metabolize food into glucose. No cure is available, but the use of antibiotics and physical therapy can help to prolong life and make movement somewhat easier. Nevertheless, death is inevitable and generally results from gradual weakening and failure of the heart or breathing process (Mordock, 1975, pp. 359–365).

Other Conditions

There are many other conditions which can affect children. Two of the most important are sickle-cell anemia and epilepsy.

Sickle-Cell Anemia. Sickle-cell anemia is an inherited blood disease which can cause pain, damage to vital organs, and, for some, early death. The effects of the disease vary greatly from person to person, but most people with the condition enjoy good health much of the time. Most cases of sickle-cell occur among blacks and Hispanics of Caribbean ancestry. Approximately one in 400 to 600 blacks and one in every 1000 to 1500 Hispanics inherits sickle-cell. The physical growth of children with the disease is often slower than normal.

Normally, the red blood cells are round and flexible. However, the red blood cells of a person with sickle-cell may change into a sickle shape within their blood vessels. The sickle cells tend to become trapped in the spleen and elsewhere and are destroyed. This results in a shortage of red blood cells which causes the person to be pale, short of breath, easily tired, and prone to infections. Viral infection and vitamin deficiency can worsen the condition.

When the cells become stuck in the blood vessels, they lose oxygen. This loss of oxygen causes severe pain in the abdomen and chest. If the condition is long lasting, damage to the brain, lungs, or kidneys, can even lead to death.

Sickle-cell anemia is not contagious, but it is inherited. Individuals may carry the disease (sickle-cell trait) but have no signs of the disease. When two persons who have the trait have a child, that child may inherit two sickle-cell genes and develop the disease. A test can identify people who either have the disease or carry the trait. Unfortunately, there is no medication or therapy which will correct the effects disease-causing gene. Progress in medical care has limited the damage from sickle-cell crises.

Epilepsy. The word *epilepsy* comes from the Greek word for seizures. Epilepsy is a disorder of the central nervous system characterized by sudden seizures, which usually last only a few minutes. Seizures are not always convulsive, and, even when they are, they are not as dangerous as they look. Epilepsy is not contagious, and, between seizures, epileptic children function normally. Seizures occur when there are excessive electrical discharges in some nerve cell of the brain. When this happens, the brain loses conscious control over certain body functions and consciousness may be lost or altered.

There are more than 20 different kinds of seizures. Only three will be described here: (Anspaugh, Gillilland, & Anspaugh, p. 80)

1. *General tonic clonic seizures (grand mal)* are the most disruptive in the classroom. The child becomes stiff and slumps to the floor unconscious. Rigid muscles give way to jerking, breathing is suspended, and saliva may escape from the lips. The seizure may last for several minutes, and the child will regain consciousness in a confused or drowsy state, but is otherwise unaffected.

For tonic clonic seizures:

(A) Keep calm. Ease the child to the floor and loosen his collar. You cannot stop the seizure. Let it run its course and do not try to revive the child.
(B) Remove hard, sharp, or hot objects which may injure the child, but do not interfere with his movements.
(C) Do not force anything between his teeth.
(D) Turn the child on one side for release of saliva. Place something soft and flat under his head.

(E) When the child regains consciousness, let him rest if he wishes.

(F) If the seizures last beyond a few minutes, or the child seems to pass from one seizure to another without gaining consciousness, call for medical assistance and notify his parents. This rarely happens but should be treated immediately.

2. *Generalized absence (petit mal) seizures,* most common in children, usually last only for 5 to 20 seconds. They may be accompanied by staring or twitching of the eyelids and are frequently mistaken for "daydreaming." The child is seldom aware he has had a seizure, although he may be aware that his "mind has gone blank" for a few seconds.

3. *Complex partial (psychomotor or temporal lobe) seizures* have the most complex behavior pattern. They may include constant chewing or lip smacking, purposeless walking or repetitive hand and arm movements, confusion, and dizziness. The seizure may last from a minute to several hours.

PSYCHOSOCIAL NEEDS

All children—boys and girls, toddlers and teens, those who have developmental difficulties and those who do not—need love and positive reinforcement coupled with prudent direction and discipline in order to promote feelings of self-worth and trust in others. A child entering school at age 5 or 6 will react and interact differently than a child who is 10 or 11 years old because of maturation level, the socialization process, and individual personality variables. Still, there appear to be universal needs, motivations, and tasks associated with predictable psychosocial development of children.

Preschool and kindergarten children are generally concerned with exploring the world around them and learning to perform tasks *for themselves.* They are beginning to assert their own autonomy and independence. According to Erik Erikson's (1950) eight stages of human development (table 3.6), at about age 4 or 5 children test role behavior while simultaneously focusing on activities that are pleasurable. Because of the creative and imaginative nature of the preschooler, fantasy and play become extremely important vehicles for this exploration. These activities also provide a safe arena in which to express ideas and feelings. Problems arise when a child's abundant energy and motivation spark ambitions that physically, intellectually, or emotionally exceed maturational ability to obtain them. A sense of failure and disappointment may occur when these initiatives are unsuccessful. Deep feelings of frustration, anxiety, and guilt may result if the child does not learn to come to grips with setbacks and accept them as part of individual limitations.

Teachers and parents should therefore provide young children with settings that present tasks which, with a little effort, can be accomplished. At school, this may take the form of asking students to help straighten their work areas, run errands, or rotate leadership roles like team captains. In other words, as a teacher you should help establish realistic and satisfying goals for students and allow them the opportunity to fulfill these goals. In this way, beginning students will learn to assert their initiative constructively and build upon prior successes when faced with a new or challenging situation. By meeting these challenges step by step, students will in turn

Table 3.6
Erikson's Eight Stages of Psychosocial Development

Age	Stage	Result of Success	Result of Failure
Early Infancy (birth to about 1 year) (corollary to Freudian oral stage)	Basic Trust vs. Mistrust	Trust results from affection and gratification of needs, mutual recognition.	Mistrust results from consistent abuse, neglect, deprivation of love, too early or harsh weaning, autistic isolation.
Later Infancy (1 to 3 years) (corollary to Freudian muscular anal stage)	Autonomy vs. Shame and Doubt	Child views self as person in his own right apart from parents but still dependent.	Child feels inadequate, doubts self, curtails learning basic skills like walking, talking, wants to "hide" inadequacies.
Early Childhood (about ages 4 to 5 years) (corollary to Freudian phallic locomotor stage)	Initiative vs. Guilt	Child has lively imagination, vigorously tests reality, imitates adults, anticipates roles.	Child lacks spontaneity, has infantile jealousy "castration complex," is suspicious, evasive, suffers from role inhibition.
Middle Childhood (about ages 6 to 11 years) (corollary to Freudian latency stage)	Industry vs. Inferiority	Child has sense of duty and accomplishment, develops scholastic and social competencies, undertakes real tasks, puts fantasy and play in better perspective, learns world of tools, task identification.	Child has poor work habits, avoids strong competition, feels doomed to mediocrity; is in lull before the storms of puberty, may conform as slavish behavior, has sense of futility.
Puberty and Adolescence (about ages 12 to 20 years)	Ego Identity vs. Role Confusion	Adolescent has temporal perspective, is self-certain, is a role experimenter, goes through apprenticeship, experiences sexual polarization and leader-follower, develops an ideological commitment.	Adolescent experiences time confusion, is self-conscious, has a role fixation, and experiences work paralysis, bisexual confusion, authority confusion, and value confusion.
Early Adulthood	Intimacy vs. Isolation	Person has capacity to commit self to others, "true genitability" is now possible, *Lieben und Arbeiten*—"to love and to work"; "mutuality of genital orgasm."	Person avoids intimacy, has "character problems," behaves promiscuously, and repudiates, isolates, destroys seemingly dangerous forces.
Middle Adulthood	Generativity vs. Stagnation	Person is productive and creative for self and others, has parental pride and pleasure, is mature, enriches his life, establishes and guides next generation.	Person is egocentric, nonproductive, experiences early invalidism, excessive self-love, personal impoverishment, and self-indulgence.
Late Adulthood	Integrity vs. Despair	Person appreciates continuity of past, present, and future, accepts life cycle and life style, has learned to cooperate with inevitabilities of life, "death loses its sting."	Person feels time is too short; finds no meaning in human existence, has lost faith in self and others, wants second chance at life cycle with more advantages, has no feeling of world order or spiritual sense, fears death.

Source: *Life and health*, 3rd ed., copyright © 1980 by Random House, Inc., Reprinted with permission.

develop a sense of control and mastery over the world around them and will feel less frustrated and guilty when success temporarily eludes them.

Keep in mind that kindergartners and first-graders are generally self-centered, which is quite natural developmentally. The world in which they have lived up to this point has been one in which their needs have been immediately and consistently met. Upon entering school, however, they are forced not only to compete against 20 or so other children for the teacher's attention, but they must also learn to socialize effectively during the school day. As a result, teachers who instruct younger elementary school students need to be aware of the seemingly monumental adjustments that the children must make. Young elementary school children may be faced with the conflict between meeting their own needs and being accepted by teacher and peers. Therefore it is crucial to exhibit sensitivity and understanding and provide as much attention and direct supervision as possible to each child.

As children mature they become more self-aware and much more concerned about peer group expectations and acceptance. During the middle to late elementary school years, the development of self-esteem, which begins in infancy, becomes paramount. Self-esteem is strongly linked to an individual's sense of accomplishment and feeling of being able to use abilities and talents in ways that are both personally rewarding and socially acceptable. This stage of psychosocial development, as outlined by Erikson (1950), usually begins around age 6 and lasts until puberty. At this stage, students exercise their feelings of industry through attempts to achieve academic and social accomplishments. Although Erikson sees this stage as an extension of the preceeding one, he notes that individuals now begin to place fantasy and play in a more realistic perspective and concentrate on further self-identification. Children at this age also begin to foster a deeper sense of obligation to family and friends and learn more concrete tasks that promote extended feelings of self-worth. On the other hand, children who do not realize their potential for industrious behavior and its rewards at this age may always be psychologically saddled with feelings of inferiority and futility. Of course, care should be exercised to prevent children at this developmental stage from focusing too strongly on work as the ultimate end. According to Erikson, if this happens individuals tend to view work as their primary duty and contribution to society or they may become rigidly conformed to a system that fosters excessive, unrealistic utilitarianism.

Thus, middle to late childhood, the years just before adolescence, are extremely crucial ones. During this time children first focus on others and display great interest in developing friendships. How successfully they do this may determine future adult social behavior. In addition, middle to late childhood is the time during which a child's value system begins to be internalized and impacts all other aspects of both the maturation and socialization processes.

Because self-role identity is forming, children at this age need role models who exemplify a strong sense of satisfaction with who they are as men and women and with their lives in general. Teachers must be particularly aware of their influence, either intended or unintended, on their students.

Positive reinforcement coupled with constructive criticism from you, the teacher, will do much to enhance self-esteem among students. Providing them with opportunities in a nonthreatening environment to clarify values, practice interpersonal communication skills, and achieve realistic social and academic competencies is of extreme importance for nurturing positive self-awareness and heightened self-worth.

LEARNING THEORY

No discussion concerning the nature of the elementary school-age child would be complete without at least a brief description of how children learn. It is, after all, learning that teachers are mainly concerned with and address day in and day out. A teacher who is knowledgeable about both child development and learning theory should be much better able to select instructional activities that capture the attention and fascination of children at a given level. In addition to helping teachers decide which activities to select, an awareness of the major principles of learning theory should enhance the teacher's ability to present these experiences in challenging and stimulating ways.

No one really knows exactly how learning takes place, and it is obvious that children learn in a variety of ways and from diverse experiences and opportunities. Learning itself is the lifelong process of accumulating, internalizing, and applying information to beliefs, attitudes, and practices. Learning allows people to achieve personal goals and interests and creates cognitive, affective, and behavioral changes that mature and broaden the individual.

Many theories about learning have been hypothesized, based on well-researched and documented facts and observations. The theories can generally be classified into two major categories: associative theories and cognitive or field theories. The associative theories of learning originated from Aristotle's perception that ideas become associated with one another on the basis of similarity or difference. More modern psychological thought presented the concept now known as behaviorism, which asserts that behavior is learned as a result of associating experiences with either pleasure or pain. On the other hand, cognitive or field theories are an outgrowth of the Gestalt movement begun in the early 1900s in Germany. These theories state that behavior is learned not in terms of separate experiences but rather in terms of an individual's perceptions, feelings, and interpretations of the experiences as they affect the individual overall (Mouley, 1973, pp. 25–26).

Associative Theories

The chief associative theories of learning are those of connectionism, developed by Edward L. Thorndike, and operant conditioning, an outgrowth of classical conditioning theory, developed by B. F. Skinner. Connectionism is the cornerstone of the associative theories and is based on Thorndike's work of more than 50 years in the field of educational psychology. On the basis of his detailed observation of animals, Thorndike concluded that learning takes place in a trial-and-error way in which random choices or selections are made to a given problem or situation until the "correct" response is discovered. When placed in the same situation or faced with a similar problem, experimental animals repeat the "correct" response until it becomes habit. According to Thorndike, this habit develops as a result of a connection, or bond, which forms as part of a neurophysiological reaction. Thorndike visualized a hierarchy of these stimulus-response behaviors that comprise what he called his Law of Effect. As repeated satisfying choices are made by the individual, the connection between the stimulus (situation) and response is increased or heightened so that in similar circumstances the "correct" response will be elicited and thus learned (Crow & Crow, 1963, pp. 229–231).

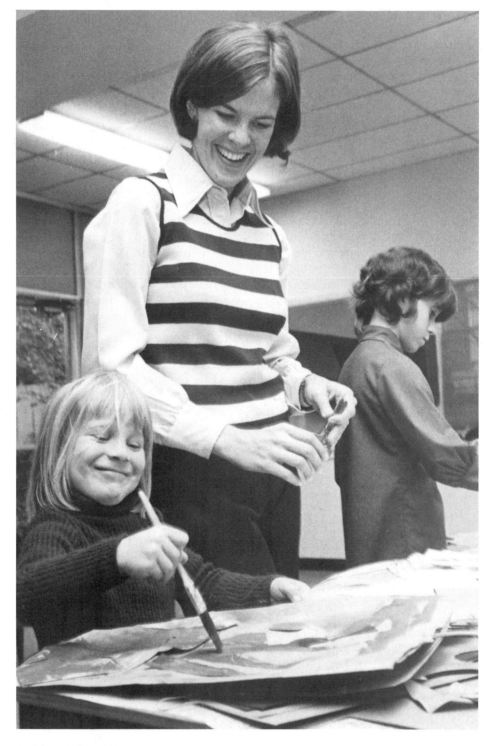

Positive reinforcement and constructive criticism from the teacher do much to enhance the student's self-esteem.

Based on Thorndike's work as well as Pavlov's famous experiments with dogs using classical conditioning (conditioned response), B. F. Skinner proposed that learning takes place when positive reinforcement of and immediate information about one's actions or behaviors are provided. That is, according to Skinner, a response (behavior) is learned, elicited, and repeated not because of a neurophysiological reaction, but because of positive reinforcement (praise, pleasure) that follows. In this way undesirable behavior may be changed or corrected if a meaningful reinforcement technique is used and feedback given. Skinner calls his theory operant conditioning and believes that only *positive* reinforcers promote learning (Edwards & Scannell, 1969, pp. 270–272).

The theories of Thorndike and Skinner have both been used by educators, either consciously or unconsciously, for years. Instructional methods that emphasize drills, repeated practice of a skill, rote memory lessons, and programmed instruction incorporate the ideas of associative learning with some degree of success for most students.

Cognitive or Field Theories

The cognitive or field theories of learning most frequently noted are those of Jean Piaget, John Dewey, Carl Rogers, and Abraham Maslow. The Swiss psychologist Jean Piaget believed that the individual gathers knowledge about the world in order to adapt to it through a progression of emphasis from motor activities, to perceptions, to conceptualization. He hypothesized that the first stage of learning focuses on one's awareness of and need to experience surroundings by mastering basic motor skills during infancy and early childhood. At the preschool level, children explore the world mainly through their perceptions and finally develop a logical, conceptual, cognitive framework for learning and behaving during middle to late childhood by viewing the total world (situation) with reason using all stages as a reference (Mueller, 1974, pp. 47–52).

The philosopher John Dewey suggested that problem-solving is directly dependent upon the social forces influencing the individual, so that learning must be viewed in terms of the child in relation to the social environment. Dewey believed that judgment and reason can only arise if children are placed in surroundings which allow *them* to make judgments. For example, children can only learn about democracy in a democratic classroom. Dewey was also concerned that the kind of problem-solving and learning that takes place in schools may not be readily applicable to real-life situations and surroundings (Lindgren, 1962, pp. 243–246).

The movement commonly known as humanism approaches learning from the standpoint that children must first be viewed as human beings and not students. The writings of psychologists Carl Rogers and Abraham Maslow, in particular, emphasize that personality formation and the ability to learn must have their roots in meeting both the biological and emotional needs of children. Both Rogers and Maslow are sometimes referred to as phenomenological psychologists because they believe that personal experience, not a standard human experience, is at the basis for problem-solving and decision-making and therefore is relative to individual feelings and perceptions. It is the total of one's experiences that produces patterns of learning and behaving, not isolated pieces of information or situations (Mouley, 1973, pp. 33–34).

Like the principles of learning hypothesized by the associative theories of Thorndike and Skinner, those proposed by cognitive theorists such as Piaget, Dewey, Rogers, and Maslow have been widely used by educators. Jean Piaget's work has been the foundation for many curricular implementations within schools all over the country because his ideas have proved to be effective. On the other hand, only in recent years have American educators accepted the suggestions of John Dewey. When he proposed major educational revisions at the turn of the century, he was considered both a revolutionary and a charlatan because, unlike the other theorists, he did not test his ideas. However, today Dewey's principles are widely acknowledged and accepted. In addition, the humanistic approach to learning postulated by Rogers and Maslow in the early 1960s seems to have gained a significant foothold within the American educational system, even though it has been criticized by some who favor a more traditional approach to learning.

SUMMARY

No teacher can be fully prepared to teach without knowing something about the characteristics of students at any given age. Although each child enters school with special and unique qualities, elementary school children are in many ways a homogeneous group. Up until about age 11, boys and girls differ little in physical characteristics such as height, weight, endurance, and strength, although there may be a wide range of individual differences among each sex. Growth and development at this time proceed at a gradual and steady pace. This changes at the onset of the adolescent growth spurt, which typically happens among girls first. Individual differences in growth and development may cause some children anxiety. By explaining the range of normal variation among individuals, which is due both to genetic and environmental factors, the teacher can help allay such fears.

Although most children are basically healthy and developing normally during the elementary school years, some have developmental difficulties or disabilities. With more such children in the regular classroom as a result of Public Law 94-142, the teacher must be prepared to assist these individuals achieve their full potential. Some disabilities are due to birth defects. Birth defects due to genetic aberrations can result in such conditions as Down syndrome and cystic fibrosis. Environmental influences can also result in birth defects, as can difficulties during childbirth. The specific causes of many birth defects, such as cerebral palsy, learning disabilities, and cleft palate, however, have not been identified and are assumed to be due to interactive influences.

Apart from the basic physical needs of food, clothing, shelter, and safety, to grow and thrive all children require love, attention, guidance, and support. These basic psychosocial needs must be met to mold and maintain self-identity and self-worth. To assist in providing psychosocial needs most effectively, the elementary school teacher should understand the psychosocial stages of human development.

The work of Erik Erikson is particularly relevant. Erikson notes that children enter school with an abundance of energy and curiosity. At this stage they are discoverers and explorers seeking to assert autonomy and independence. They are also, however, still quite self-centered and have not learned much social interaction. Further, children's ambitions at this stage sometimes exceed their abilities and failure may result in deep feelings of frustration and guilt. The teacher must structure the classroom environment and provide opportunities for success while at the same time helping children accept limitations due to ability or maturational level.

Older elementary school children appear less self-centered, are more interested in establishing friendships, and are concerned about social and academic accomplishments. At this stage, too, the teacher must help children set realistic goals and assist in building self-esteem. The teacher also serves as a powerful role model as the children's sex-role identities surface and values systems begin to be firmly established.

Understanding the principles of learning theory is important if the teacher is to be effective in providing knowledge. There are two main categories of learning theories: associative and cognitive or field. Associative theories, such as Thorndike's connectionism theory and Skinner's operant conditioning theory, view learning as a matter of association between a particular stimulus and response that is heightened through positive reinforcement and feedback. In contrast, the cognitive or field theories of Piaget, Dewey, Rogers, and Maslow arise from Gestalt theory and emphasize the need for providing meaningful experiences that are ultimately received and interpreted by the individual in context with the person's total perception of their relation to other experiences.

DISCUSSION QUESTIONS

1. Discuss several *general* reasons why you believe it is important for all teachers to have basic knowledge about child growth and development.
2. What are the major characteristics of elementary school-age children in regard to
   a. height and weight
   b. motor coordination
   c. nervous system and development
   d. endocrine system contributions
   e. cardiorespiratory characteristics
3. Define the term *birth defect*. Briefly outline the prevalence of birth defects among children in America.
4. Devise your own chart comparing the psychosocial needs of kindergarteners; first, second and third graders; and fourth, fifth, and sixth graders.
5. List the two chief associative theories of learning and their originators. Compare the main tenants of each of these.
6. Describe the chief cognitive or field theories of learning and their originators. How do the associative and cognitive theories or learning differ? Does this make one more credible in your opinion? Why?
7. Devise two hypothetical classroom situations in which your knowledge about learning theory could be helpful to both you and the student(s).

REFERENCES

Ambron, S. R. *Child development.* San Francisco: Holt, Rinehart, & Winston, 1975.

Anspaugh, D. J., Gilliland, M., & Anspaugh, S. J. "The student with epilepsy." *Today's Education,* September-October 1980, pp. 78–85.

Bee, H. *The developing child.* New York: Harper & Row, 1978.

Biehler, R. F. *Child development: An introduction.* Boston: Houghton Mifflin, 1976.

Crow, L. D., & Crow, A. *Educational psychology.* New York: American Book, 1963.

Dutton, G. *Mental handicaps.* London: Butterworth, 1975.

Edwards, A. J., & Scannell, D. P. *Education psychology: The teaching-learning process.* Scranton, Pa.: International Textbook, 1969.

Erikson, E. *Childhood and society.* New York: W. W. Norton, 1950.

Guthrie, H. E. *Introductory nutrition.* St. Louis: C. V. Mosby, 1975.

Katachadourian, H. *The biology of adolescence.* San Francisco: W. H. Freeman, 1977.

Kirkman, B., & Bicknell, J. *Mental handicap.* London: Churchill Livingstone, 1975.

Klug, W. S. & Cummings, M. R. *Concepts of genetics.* Columbus: Merrill, 1983, p. 254.

Lindgren, H. C. *Educational psychology in the classroom.* New York: John Wiley, 1962.

March of Dimes. *Birth defects, tragedy & hope* (pamphlet). White Plains, New York: 1984.

Matthews, D. K., & Rox, E. L. *The physiological basis of physical education and athletics.* Philadelphia: W. B. Saunders, 1976.

Mercer, J. *Small people: How children develop and what you can do about it.* Chicago: Nelson-Hall, 1979.

Mordock, J. B. *The other children: An introduction to exceptionality.* New York: Harper & Row, 1975.

Mouley, G. J. *Psychology for effective teaching.* New York: Holt, Rinehart & Winston, 1973.

Mueller, R. J. *Principles of classroom learning and perception: An introduction to educational psychology.* New York: Praeger, 1974.

National Clearinghouse for Family Planning. "Family planning and genetic counseling." *Health Education Bulletin,* no. 26. (August 1985), *24*:1.

National Foundation–March of Dimes. *Genetic Counseling.* White Plains, New York: 1984, *11.*

Winchester, A. M., & Martens, T. R. *Human genetics.* 4th ed. Columbus: Merrill, 1983.

4. Planning for Health Instruction

Walking into a classroom at any level without having first planned the day's objectives is like beginning an automobile trip with an empty gas tank.—Donald A. Read and Walter H. Greene, *Creative Teaching in Health*

CONTENT AREAS IN THE ELEMENTARY SCHOOL

Teaching health education, like teaching any subject, requires careful planning. You must know what to teach, when to teach it, and how to teach it so that the content is internalized, or personalized, by the students. First graders are vastly different from sixth graders. Health instruction at each grade level must be tailored to the maturational, intellectual, and interest levels of the students.

Virtually every state department of education has a health education syllabus that can be used as a guide for curriculum planning. Read it carefully. In it you will find a recommended list of topics to be presented at each grade level.

But effective planning takes more than just reading your state health education guide—far more. As Willgoose (1974, p. 439) puts it:

> Good planning for creative and innovative classwork requires long hours of reading about what others have accomplished; visiting other schools; participating in curriculum development; attending health workshops; evaluating new methodologies; working with school health services personnel; previewing films, slides, filmstrips, cassettes and video tapes; and preparing demonstration materials and displays. These are tasks that take considerable time primarily because health topics and health education methods are so multidisciplinary and multidimensional.

The general public often visualizes elementary health instruction merely in terms of rules for toothbrushing and bicycle safety. It is, of course, far more than that. Various health education authorities cite from 10 to 20 different content areas, depending on how areas are grouped or separated. Most health educators agree on the following content areas for elementary health instruction:

- Mental Health
- Body Systems and the Senses
- Nutrition
- Family Life
- Alcohol, Drugs, and Tobacco
- Safety and First Aid
- Personal Health
- Consumer Health
- Diseases: Chronic and Communicable
- Environmental Health
- Aging
- Death and Dying

Each of these content areas is composed of dozens of topics. For example, Personal Health encompasses dental care, personal care, exercise, rest, and physical fitness, to name just a few topics. Content areas and topics also change in emphasis to reflect current knowledge and health concerns. Further, community mores affect content areas. In some communities, for instance, sex education is considered a vital part of health education; in many other communities, it is felt that the subject should not be a part of the curriculum.

Grade Placment for Health Education Topics

Once you have charted basic content areas, you must determine how much emphasis to place on each area at each grade level. Emphasis should be based on the developmental level, health needs, and interest of the children. A planned cycle of presentation of content areas ensures that necessary topics will be included and will receive appropriate emphasis at each grade level. An example of a cycle plan based upon developmental needs is shown in table 4.1.

Table 4.1
Cycle Plan for Elementary Health Education Content Areas

Content Area	Grade Level						
	K	1	2	3	4	5	6
Mental Health	**	**	*	*	**	**	***
Body Systems and the Senses	**	**	**	**	*	*	*
Nutrition	*	*	**	*	**	*	**
Family Life	*	*	*	**	**	***	***
Alcohol, Drugs, and Tobacco	**	*	*	**	**	***	***
Safety and First Aid	**	**	***	**	**	**	*
Personal Health	**	**	*	**	*	**	***
Consumer Health	*		*	*	**	**	**
Diseases		*	*	**		**	***
Environmental Health		*	*	**	*		**
Aging		*	*	*	*		**
Death and Dying		*		*	*		**

Key: *** = major emphasis, ** = emphasis, * = touched upon or reviewed.

A cycle plan helps eliminate useless repetition and ensures that topics are covered to the depth necessary for a particular grade. It also prepares children for the subject matter awaiting them in junior and senior high school.

DEVELOPING SCOPE AND SEQUENCE

Content areas must not only be identified, they must also be ordered and organized. That is, the scope and sequence of the health education curriculum must be determined. Scope refers to the depth or difficulty of the material—the "what" to teach. Sequence refers to the order in which the material is to be covered—the "when" to teach it. Here again your state department of education health guide can be of great use. Such guides usually spell out the scope and sequence of health education for each grade level. They may also indicate what skills a child should possess after completing the course of study. Figures 4.1 and 4.2 show recommendations made by the Illinois Department of Education as to what health skills a child should have by the end of the third grade and the sixth grade.

Planned health instruction should attempt to ensure that each previous learning experience provides the basis for new learning. Topics should build upon one another, not be presented as discrete bits of information. Concepts within each lesson should relate to each other, lessons within a unit should relate to each other, and

---

By the end of the third grade, students should be able to do the following:

- Explain how trained medical personnel help protect an individual's health. (Consumer Health)
- Describe desirable health practices that will promote good dental health. (Dental Health)
- Explain how medicines, when used properly, are helpful for maintaining health. (Drug Use and Abuse, Alcohol)
- Discuss factors in one's surroundings that influence human health. (Human Ecology and Health)
- Explain the importance of personal health practices as they relate to the process of growing and developing. (Human Growth and Development)
- Explain how making friends and getting along with others make life more satisfying. (Mental Health and Illness)
- Understand the importance of a nutritional breakfast. (Nutrition)
- Describe how good posture affects appearance and body function. (Personal Health)
- Understand that children are susceptible to a variety of diseases and disorders. (Prevention and Control of Disease)
- Identify and describe community resources that affect health. (Public and Environmental Health)
- Understand that all injuries should be cared for immediately. (Safety Education and Disaster Survival)
- Understand that some substances that are commonly used can be harmful. (Smoking and Disease)

Figure 4.1
State of Illinois recommendations for health skills to be learned in grades K–3.

By the end of the sixth grade, students should be able to do the following:

- Understand that mass media may be misleading sources of health information. (Consumer Health)
- Realize that oral neglect affects appearance and social relationships. (Dental Health)
- Identify personal goals and practices established early in life that can help one to avoid the misuse of drugs. (Drug Use and Abuse, Alcohol)
- Describe new discoveries and inventions that create hazards in our environment. (Human Ecology and Health)
- Describe how differences in growth and development can affect feelings and social relationships. (Human Growth and Development)
- Explain how individuals react differently to stressful situations. (Mental Health and Illness)
- Understand that special foods or supplements are not usually required to meet normal nutritional needs. (Nutrition)
- Identify the benefits of rest and sleep to personal health. (Personal Health)
- Understand that the control of diseases and disorders depends upon individual action as well as advances in medical technology. (Prevention and Control of Disease)
- Identify public health regulations that promote individual and community health. (Public and Environmental Health)
- Understand that first-aid procedures help one to act quickly and correctly in emergencies. (Safety Education and Disaster Survival)
- Understand that individuals react differently to the chemicals found in tobacco. (Smoking and Disease)

Figure 4.2
State of Illinois recommendations for health skills to be learned in grades 4–6.

units within the course should relate to each other. In this way, students will see health education as a whole rather than seemingly unrelated fragments. This unity of relationships, as visualized by Fodor and Dalis (1981), is shown in figure 4.3.

Scope also refers to the arrangement of the curriculum from kindergarten through senior high school. As such, it serves as a reminder that everything done in the classroom should be built upon what has been accomplished previously so that initial learning becomes the basis for subsequent learning. This relationship is shown in figure 4.4 (Fodor & Dalis, 1981).

Relationship of concepts within a lesson	Concept 1 ←→ Concept 2 ←→ Concept 3
Relationship of lessons within a unit	Lesson 1 ←→ Lesson 2 ←→ Lesson 3
Relationship of units within a course	Unit 1 ←→ Unit 2 ←→ Unit 3

Figure 4.3
Sequential organization of the health curriculum.

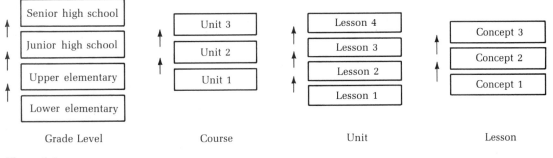

Figure 4.4
The scope of the health curriculum.

DETERMINING WHAT TO TEACH

Although your state health education guidelines are helpful in determining the scope and sequence of the health curriculum, they should not be your sole planning aid. In developing the curriculum, you must also consider such factors as the social mores of your community, student interest, student health needs, and available textbooks and courses of study.

Social Mores

The curriculum that you develop must be acceptable to the community in which you live. Ascertaining the social mores of the community calls for careful judgment. You have an advantage if you are well acquainted with the community, perhaps because of long-term residence. Even then, however, it may be difficult to assess feelings within the community about how best to teach certain health topics, such as substance abuse or sex education. Be sure to discuss controversial topics with administrators before implementing any course of instruction.

Another community influence on curriculum development comes from special interest groups, which may be national, state, or local. Their charge is to promote or protect their own philosophy or special interests. Most of these groups are sincere about bringing beneficial services to the children in a community, but such groups can also have a detrimental influence on curriculum development. For example, groups that form to stop sex education can be formidable opponents to the development of a comprehensive health education program.

Student Interest

Children are more interested in certain health topics than in others depending upon their age. For example, younger children are apt to be more interested in the parts and functions of their bodies than are slightly older children. Also, because primary age children are more self-centered, they are less concerned about social topics than are upper elementary children.

Questionnaires, checklists, and direct questioning can all aid you in determining student interest in your class. In fact, there is no substitute for interacting directly with your class to gauge interest in various topics. At the same time, familiarity with professional literature on the subject is equally important. As Byler, Lewis, and Totman (1969) demonstrated, there are basic health interests common to all students regardless of locality or socioeconomic class. Table 4.2 shows some of the questions these authors found in their study. Note how the children's questions at different grade levels reflect both inherent student interest at a particular age and the maturational and intellectual level of the students.

In planning the health curriculum, be sure that the scope and sequence of topics mirror student interest at each grade level. Keep in mind that younger children do not have the intellectual maturity to deal with abstract topics. Also recognize that younger children have shorter attention spans.

Student interest is directly tied to intellectual maturity. In the preschool years, children learn language and the ability to express themselves, but the concepts they are able to form are rather elementary, for example, big-little, good-bad, boy-girl, short-tall. All concepts, including these, are abstract generalizations. However, the ability to abstract is still quite limited in young children, and the concepts they form tend to be only those that relate to their immediate environment. Topics chosen for health instruction must reflect this fact.

Later in elementary school, children's abstract reasoning becomes better developed and students are capable of dealing with more than immediate life situations. Then, increasingly abstract health concepts such as pollution or aging, can be taught. Reasoning and insight into causal relationships also develop.

Table 4.2
Differing Interests of Elementary-Age Children

Grades K—2
How does my heart beat?
What makes blood?
What makes people cry and laugh?
How can you tell which is a cow and which is a bull?
What makes you stop growing?
What makes people smart?

Grades 3—4
How do ears work?
How does my brain work?
How can you walk, run, and bend?
How do people get fat?
Where does a baby come from?
Why do people die?

Grades 5–6
What are the best foods for a person to eat?
How does a girl get a baby?
How do I act happy or sad?
Why can't I get along with my brother or sister?
What do drugs do to the body?
How does air pollution affect people?

Source: Byler, Lewis, & Totman, 1969.

Health Needs

All children, regardless of community, have certain basic health needs. These include the need for love and nurturing, sound nutrition, intellectual stimulation, proper dental care, and safety. However, specific health needs vary from community to community, and the curriculum that you plan should take into account these special needs. For example, inner city children may need to receive emphasized instruction about the dangers of lead poisoning, as many inner city dwellings still contain lead-based paint. Similarly, the safety instruction provided will vary depending on whether the community is a rural or an urban one.

Textbooks and Courses of Study

Most elementary health textbooks contain detailed suggestions for developing curriculum. The teacher's editions of these texts provide outlines and units for teaching health and identify major concepts to be taught at a given grade level. Like your state health guidelines, however, textbooks cannot provide a course of study tailored to your specific community and your specific classroom. Because textbooks are developed for use nationally, they may lack sufficient depth of coverage on topics of particular relevance to your setting.

To supplement the textbook you use, you will probably wish to obtain pamphlets, filmstrips, and other learning aids from government or private health-related agencies such as the Department of Agriculture or the National Safety Council. A list of such resources is given in appendix A. Most health-related agencies will make classroom materials available free of charge or at a nominal cost. Be sure, however, to screen all materials before classroom use to determine their appropriateness, any possible bias, and up-to-dateness.

TEACHING FOR VALUES

A value is a highly prized belief about an idea or doctrine. Values give direction to life and determine behavior. As a society, we share many of the same values. However, each community, family, and individual has a more specific set of values. Values are closely linked with personal feelings and must be carefully considered when planning health instruction. Failure to do so can result both in the blocking of effective learning and opposition from parents and community organizations.

Values are learned through a variety of experiences and interactions with the environment. The family, peer group, school, church, and the media all influence personal value formation. In other words, value formation is a continual process. Yet many parents become concerned when formal teaching about values takes place in the schools. There is concern that values contrary to the parents' values will be inculcated. Any recommendation or point of emphasis by a teacher can be construed as the imposition of values. Conversely, to take no stand at all can imply an anything-goes attitude.

Therefore, in planning health instruction, you must make clear how values will be a part of your teaching. Your job is not to impose your own values; it is to help chil-

Health Highlight

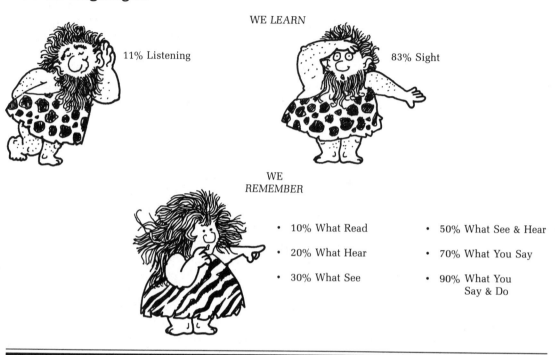

WE *LEARN*

11% Listening

83% Sight

WE
REMEMBER

- 10% What Read
- 20% What Hear
- 30% What See

- 50% What See & Hear
- 70% What You Say
- 90% What You
  Say & Do

dren develop their own values by making wise decisions about health-related matters. Keep in mind that children will form values with or without your assistance. You can aid them in making decisions that will lead to high-level wellness by providing factual knowledge about health and by allowing children to clarify their own feelings.

Remember that values and feelings are intertwined. If a balance between knowledge and and attitude toward health education is to be achieved, you must address student feelings in your teaching. In other words, the study of health must be personalized if it is to have an impact. By providing opportunities for children to identify feelings and personalize health information, you can help them understand how information, attitudes, and behavior affect the quality of life. In doing so, children become better equipped to deal with peer pressure, communicate more effectively, and develop sound decision-making skills.

Each person must weigh the importance or value of a decision against perceived rewards and costs involved in attaining goals. To brush one's teeth regularly, to smoke, to have regular physical examinations, and to experiment with drugs are all examples of decisions that affect health. Decisions must be made by the individual; consequently, you must make a planned effort to help children think through the possible consequences of health-related decisions.

CURRICULUM APPROACHES

As a beginning teacher, you will probably find many useful resources that will help you plan a course of health education for your class. As noted, these resources include the state health education guidelines, commerical health education textbook series, and materials from government and private health-related agencies. None of these, however, actually constitutes a developed health education curriculum.

To qualify as a health curriculum, a plan for teaching health must be worked out in great detail. Later in the chapter, an overview of this process will be presented. Rather than to develop an entirely new curriculum plan, you might adopt an existing one. Separate plans worthy of special mention are the School Health Education Study (SHES); the Health Activities Project (HAP); Health Skills for Life; Growing Healthy; You, Me & Others; and the Heart Treasure Chest.

School Health Education Study

SHES is mentioned because it holds historical significance and serves as a reference for several curriculum projects. Although somewhat dated, it still reflects an excellent conceptualization of health education.

SHES is a comprehensive K–12 health education curriculum that was developed in the 1960s. The project developers visualized health as having *physical, mental,* and *social* dimensions, as shown in figure 4.5. In this conceptual model, health is seen as "dynamic interaction and interdependence among the individual's physical well-being, his mental and emotional reactions, and the social complex in which he exists" (School Health Education Study, 1967).

This interaction and interdependence are reflected in the key concepts shown in the model; *growing and developing, interacting,* and *decision-making.* Growing and developing is defined as a dynamic life process by which the individual is in some ways like all individuals, in some ways like some individuals, and in some ways like no other individual. Interacting is an ongoing process in which the individual is affected by and in turn affects certain biological, social, psychological, economic, and physical forces in the environment. Decision making is a uniquely human process of consciously opting to take or not take an action or of choosing one alternative rather than another.

The scope of the SHES curriculum is embodied in the ten concept statements shown in figure 4.5 as C 1, C 2, and so on. These statements are as follows (School Health Education Study, 1967, pp. 21–23):

1. Growth and development influences and is influenced by the structure and functioning of the individual.
2. Growing and developing follows a predictable sequence, yet is unique for each individual.
3. Protection and promotion of health is an individual, community, and international responsibility.
4. The potential for hazards and accidents exists, whatever the environment.
5. There are reciprocal relationships involving man, disease, and environment.

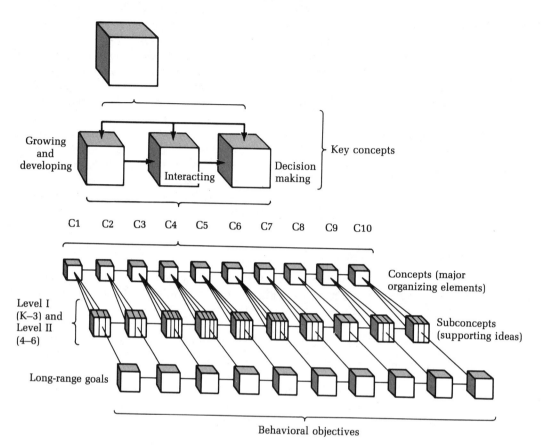

Figure 4.5
Conceptual model of the SHES curriculum.

6. The family serves to perpetuate man and to fulfill certain health needs.
7. Personal health practices are affected by a complexity of forces, often conflicting.
8. Utilization of health information, products, and services is guided by values and perceptions.
9. Use of substances that modify mood and behavior arises from a variety of motivations.
10. Food selection and eating patterns are determined by physical, social, mental, economic, and cultural factors.

Subconcepts of these ten conceptual areas serve as guides in the selection and ordering of subject matter as well as in the development of appropriate instructional or behavioral objectives. Each subconcept is viewed through physical, mental, and social dimensions. For each of the concepts, long-range goals are stated in terms of behavioral objectives. These goals represent desired student outcomes for the total sequential curriculum.

The SHES curriculum marked an important breakthrough in comprehensive K–12 health education. The emphasis is on the conceptualtization of concepts rather than facts, which tend to become dated or require constant revision.

Health Activities Project

HAP is currently under development at the University of California, Berkeley (Lawrence Hall of Science, 1987). At present it consists of 64 student-centered activities grouped into 13 modules for use in grades 4–8. Each module represents from six to eight weeks of classroom activity. Titles of the modules are as follows:

1. Breathing Fitness
2. Sight and Sound
3. Heart Fitness
4. Action/Reaction
5. Balance in Movement
6. Skin Temperature
7. Flexibility and Strength
8. Personal Health Decisions
9. Growth Trends
10. Consumer Health Decisions
11. Nutrition and Dental Health
12. Your Heart in Action
13. Environmental Health and Safety

HAP modules are packed in a kit, with each kit containing materials for 27 students (figure 4.6). Each module includes a teacher's guide that states the purpose of the activity, describes the activity itself, gives procedures for setting up, provides an introduction to the activity, and suggests evaluation follow-up procedures.

One advantage to the HAP materials is that they are reusable and can thus be shifted from class to class. Each module comes with the necessary apparatus, games, wall charts, and other materials used in the activity.

HAP is not an all-inclusive curriculum, but it is an excellent student-centered project that provides a wide range of low-cost activities. Additionally, the student-centered approach allows children to learn concepts that will better enable them to control their own health behavior.

Health Skills For Life

Health Skills For Life is a relatively new approach to health education. The emphasis is on skill acquisition rather than knowledge acquisition. Ten major health content areas consisting of 118 units are used in a comprehensive K–12 curriculum. The 10 content areas are

1. Health Services and Consumer Health, (6 units);
2. Fitness, (2 units);
3. Dental Health, (4 units);

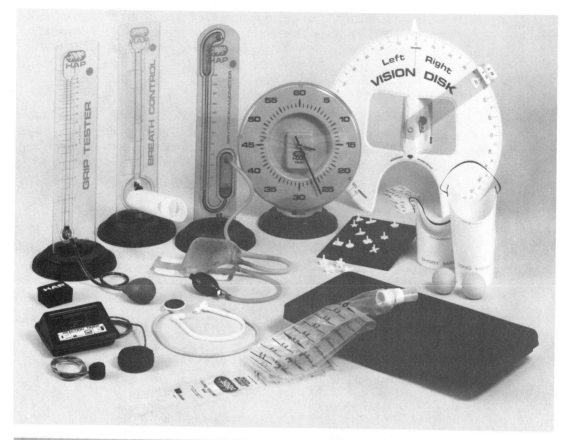

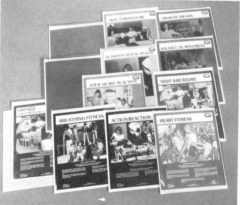

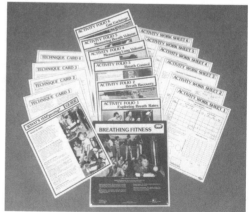

Figure 4.6
The HAP modules.

Source: Equipment and materials shown are from the Health Activities Project developed by the Lawrence Hall of Science and published by the HUBBARD Scientific Company of Northbrook, Illinois.

4. Environmental Health, (4 units);
5. Disease Prevention, (9 units);
6. Growth and Development, (12 units);
7. Nutrition, (12 units);
8. Substance Use and Abuse, (9 units);
9. Safety and First Aid, (27 units);
10. Mental Health, Family Life, and Human Sexuality, (33 units).

Each unit is independent of the other units in the curriculum. Any teaching aids needed for the program can be found locally. Units are bound in three-ring binders to facilitate revisions to the various units. Evaluation plans and tests for pretesting and posttesting, as well as skill tests, are included. An administrative guide is also included. A section of each unit includes the sequence for teaching, goals, performance indicators, estimated teaching time, content, student handouts, preparations needed, and integration with other subjects. The developers of the curriculum offer training to school districts which purchase the materials. The entire program was certified by the Oregon State Department of Education in 1982. The program is offered, either in parts or in its entirety, in more than 30 states. Figure 4.7 contains scope and sequence for the various units.

Growing Healthy

The Growing Healthy program has undergone several name changes over the years, but, like several other curriculum models, seeks to provide children with skills and information needed to live healthy and productive lives. The program has been used by 595 school districts in 41 states. What sets Growing Healthy apart from other programs is the variety of methods it employs. It is a multimedia, multidimensional, and multimethodological plan. The plan is designed to integrate with other subject areas and can be adopted to local needs and circumstances.

The curriculum seeks to provide a comprehensive sequence of courses for kindergarten through seventh grade in all aspects of health. Each grade level has a theme:

K: Happiness is Being Healthy
1: Super Me
2: Sight and Sounds
3: The Body—Its Framework and Movement
4: Our Digestion—Our Nutrition—Our Health
5: About Our Lungs and Our Health
6: Our Health and Our Hearts
7: Living Well with Our Nervous System

Instead of textbooks, the program uses films, slides, pamphlets, records, cassettes, books and resource people to supply information. Children receive hands-on learning experiences in small groups at learning centers located around the classroom. They investigate, share, teach, and learn from one another, and are encouraged to express their ideas and share feelings about their experiences.

Kindergarten	Grade 4
1. Seeking Adult Help 2. Toothbrushing and Dental Safety 3. Body Care 4. The Four Food Groups 5. Harmful Substances 6. School Fire Escape Routes 7. Traffic Signs and Signals 8. Use of Potentially Dangerous Objects 9. Communication and Making Friends	1. Being a Health Information Detective 2. Dental Flossing 3. Care of the Digestive and Excretory Systems 4. Selecting Foods for a Meal 5. Techniques to Deal with Peer Pressure 6. Predicting Consequences of Behavior 7. Developing Friendships with the Disabled and Elderly 8. Coping Skills for Family Changes

Grade 1	Grade 5
1. How Life Begins 2. Peer Influence on Safe Practices 3. Self Defense in Auto Accidents 4. Home Fire Escape Routes 5. First Aid for Scratches, Burns and Bee Stings 6. Different and Unique Individuals 7. A Child's Role in the Family	1. Reading Safety Information on Labels 2. Evaluating Community Environmental Health 3. Care of the Circulatory and Respiratory Systems 4. Reproductive Systems 5. Reading Food Labels 6. Comparing Fast, Fresh and Packaged Foods 7. Making Decisions about Drugs: Tobacco 8. Using a Safety Hazard Checklist 9. Water Safety and Rescue 10. Techniques for Controlling Fires 11. Bicycle Safety Precautions 12. Coping with Distress

Grade 2	Grade 6
1. Toothbrushing and Foods for Dental Health 2. Pollution and Your Health 3. Self Care 4. Selecting Carbohydrates, Fats and Proteins 5. Fire Escape Techniques 6. Proper Bike Riding Procedures 7. Communicating Feelings and Dealing with Hostility and Aggression	1. Personal Fitness Planning 2. Care of the Nervous System 3. Puberty 4. Drugs, Drug Effects and Drug Storage 5. First Aid for Shock Victims 6. First Aid for Bleeding Victims 7. First Aid for Breathing and Choking 8. First Aid for Poisonings 9. First Aid for Burns 10. Observing and Reporting Child Abuse 11. Communication Skills: Paraphrasing and Perception Checks 12. Wholistic Health Concepts and Planning Health Improvements

Grade 3
1. Introduction to Body Systems 2. Care of the Skin 3. Care of the Skeletal and Muscular System 4. Food Needed for Different Situations 5. Coping with Peer Pressure 6. Education for Natural Disasters 7. Expressing Love

Figure 4.7
Scope & Sequence of Unit Titles

Before school districts use the Growing Healthy program, teachers are trained at workshops on how to use the program. They then train others. The success of the program seems to depend on proper training of the teachers.

You, Me & Others

The March of Dimes Foundation developed You, Me, & Others to help elementary school students understand the basic concepts of genetics. The program consists of three different units. Unit One, *Variety,* is for kindergarten through second grade and emphasizes the normal variations in people and the things which make each person special. Unit Two, *Change,* is designed for grades three and four. It explores the nature of growth and development throughout the child's life. *The Chain of Life,* Unit Three, is for grades five and six. The unit follows the continuity of life from generation to generation and helps the student understand inherited characteristics. Each unit contains a teacher's guide, lesson plans, and reproductive masters. The series can be purchased from the March of Dimes at a very reasonable cost.

The Heart Treasure Chest

The Heart Treasure Chest was developed by the American Heart Association for children 3 to 5 years old. The chest consists of wall charts, stethoscope, recipe cards, activity and rest cards, and the "Healthy Heart Home Game." The recipe cards contain information to help students understand a healthy diet. The activity and rest cards identify behaviors which will help the child achieve cardiovascular fitness. The "Healthy Heart Home Game" is designed to provide information on exercise and diet in a board-game format. The program also provides informational newsletters called "Heart Rates" for parents. The Heart Treasure Chest has been tested in various school districts throughout the United States, and is available from the American Heart Association.

Other Teaching Materials

Agencies such as the American Cancer Society, American Heart Association, March of Dimes, American Red Cross, the American Dental Association, and the American Dairy Association provide free and inexpensive materials. Appendix A contains educational materials offered by some of the agencies. Contact your local affiliates for the latest materials available. Appendix A also lists sources of free and inexpensive health education materials.

DEVELOPING A HEALTH CURRICULUM

A health curriculum is a comprehensive K–12 plan designed to encompass pertinent health concerns and provide learning experiences throughout the school years. Such a plan should help promote responsible decisions and practices regarding personal, family, and community health.

A comprehensive school health education plan should be prepared for each local school district and then developed for the individual schools within the district. Although a district may elect to use a state-developed or other existing curriculum, in some cases the decision may be made to develop a new curriculum approach.

Designing and implementing a comprehensive program requires a great deal of expertise, time, and effort and must have input from community leaders, parents, teachers, students, and administrators. It cannot be developed in a summer or even a year. After the needs, interests, and comprehension abilities of the students have been determined, the following steps must be taken:

1. Development and writing of the first draft by grade level experts, who coordinate the lessons and units for scope and sequence
2. Evaluation and rewriting of the first draft
3. Field testing in representative schools of the second draft
4. Evaluation and rewriting of the second draft
5. Printing and distribution of the final draft for classroom use
6. Workshops and in-service training sessions to make the most effective use of the developed curriculum

Resource Unit

The goal of most curriculum projects is not to develop a substitute for commercially prepared textbooks. Instead, it is to develop a series of *resource units* based on the major concepts that should be taught at each grade level. A resource unit is a plan that can be used by teachers for presenting topics in an effective scope and sequence. It is strictly an aid for planning, not a teaching unit.

A resource unit contains general objectives, content suggestions, suggestions for learning experiences, evaluation procedures, and appropriate references for the teacher and the students. Because of its general nature, a resource unit is adaptable to a wide range of learning situations. Many resource units are divided by grade level, giving planning suggestions for kindergarten, grades 1–2, 3–4, and 5–6, or K–3 and 4–6. With the aid of a resource unit, the teacher can then develop actual teaching units.

Teaching Units

A *teaching unit* is an organized method for developing lesson plans for a particular group of students and thus can be tailored to each classroom. The resource unit serves as a guide, while the teaching unit is the plan for student learning. Unlike the resource unit, which is prepared by a curriculum committee, the teaching unit is developed by the classroom teacher. It is specific while the resource unit is general. The teacher selects the specific concepts to be studied, the objectives, content, learning experiences, evaluation methods, and references that will be used in class.

Given a well-developed resource unit that identifies major concepts, creating a teaching unit is fairly easy. In addition to the resource unit, the state health education guidelines, the teacher's edition of the classroom textbook, and various materials from health-related agencies can all be used to develop the teaching unit.

Title of Unit *Eating for Good Health*				
Grade Level *K-3* Conceptual Statement: *food selection and eating patterns are determined by social, economic and cultural factors*				
Objectives student will:	Content	Learning activities	Evaluation methods	References (a) Student (b) Teacher
Identify foods that belong to the four food groups.	*Food Groups A. milk 1. milk 2. cheese 3. ice cream 4. cottage cheese B. Meat 1. pork 2. beef 3. fish 4. eggs C. Fruit and Vegetables 1. citrus fruit 2. green vegetables 3. beets D. Bread and Cereal 1. whole grains 2. bread 3. rice*	*1. Discuss the four food groups, why they are important and what foods are in each group. 2. Have students play grocery store with empty cartons, cans etc. and place one food from each of the food groups in their sack. 3. By using wrappers from a fast food restaurant, the students pretend that they are at a fast food hamburger restaurant and they choose one food from each of the basic food groups to form a nutritious meal. Follow up with a field trip to a hamburger restaurant.*	*1. List four foods for each group. 2. From a group of pictures, ask the students to choose a food from each food group to form a nutritious menu for a day.*	*Student Films/Filmstrips "The Fruits and Vegetables" Encyclopaedia Britannica Educational Corporation, 1973 "Foods from Grains," Coronet Books Richmond, et.al., You and Your Health, II, Scott, Foresman, 1977. Chap. 3. Fodor, et.al., Being Healthy, Laidlaw Bros, 1980. Chap. 6. Teacher Richmond, et.al., You and Your Health, III, Scott, Fores, am. 1977. Chap. 3. Fodor, et. al., Being Healthy, I, Laidlaw Bros, 1980. Chap. 6.*

Figure 4.8
Typical unit format.

In preparing a teaching unit, a variety of formats can be used, depending on individual preference. Figure 4.8 illustrates a typical format. Regardless of format employed, the teaching unit should contain the following components:

1. Title of unit
2. Grade level
3. Conceptual statement
4. Objectives
5. Content
6. Learning activities
7. Evaluation
8. Resources for teacher and students

Title of Unit. The title of a teaching unit should describe what the unit is actually about. It should also serve as a motivational tool and suggest what direction the teaching will take. Examples of effective titles include "Good Food for Good Growth," "Keeping Me Clean," and "Safety Keeps You Smiling."

Grade Level. The grade level for which the unit is intended should be clearly identified. Some teachers even designate the room and school year in which the unit was used. Such a record can be valuable when units are revised for use with other classes.

Conceptual Statement. This section of the teaching unit defines the major concepts emphasized in the unit. The conceptual statement serves as a general information organizer and is rather abstract. That is, it does not contain facts about the unit but acts instead as a focal point for instruction. The conceptual statement is also a guide to the competencies that students should be able to demonstrate upon completion of the unit. Every conceptual statement should have a main theme, a consequence behavior, and future ramification, as in the following examples:

- It is essential to conserve our existing natural resources if we are to maintain a high quality lifestyle.

- Friendships provide an important avenue for dealing with our emotions and developing a positive self-image.

- Sports activities help develop many attributes and skills that are useful throughout life.

Objectives. An objective should describe what the student will be able to do after completing the unit. In practice, the terms *behavioral objective* and *instructional objective* are often used interchangeably. Objectives add direction to the conceptual statement by indicating what content should be taught and how it should be taught. The appropriate type of evaluation can also be determined in a properly stated objective.

Content. The content portion of a teaching unit should contain a summary of the facts needed to teach the unit. Content, which must be appropriate to the age of the students, is based on the conceptual statement and the objectives for the unit. The statement of content should also provide clear direction for the teacher, as in the following example from a Family Life teaching unit for grade 3:

I. Family members influence our feelings:
   A. Parents can make children feel sad by means of:
      1. Punishment
      2. Withholding privileges
   B. Children can hurt parents' feelings by:
      1. Breaking rules
      2. Not fulfilling expectations
   C. Family members can make each other happy by:
      1. Showing consideration
      2. Listening to one another
      3. Speaking kindly
      4. Showing concern for one another
II. Each family member has rights in the family unit:
   A. The right to respect from other family members
   B. The right to expect honesty from other family members
   C. The right to have obligations from family members fulfilled:
      1. Parents to grandparents
      2. Parents to children
      3. Children to parents
      4. Sibling to sibling
   D. The right of sharing with other family members
   E. The right to privacy

Learning Activities. Learning activities are experiences that help children internalize the content and form concepts. They provide the spark for discovery and examination of new ideas. Without effective learning activities, the best of concepts, objectives, and content have little impact. Because activities represent the point at which students come in contact with the actual curriculum, no unit can be effective if the learning activities are poorly planned or inappropriate.

Most resource units contain several suggestions for teaching the content. You should select those activities that you believe will work best in your own class. You must also feel comfortable using a particular methodology if the learning experience is to be successful. For example, teachers who have never used values clarification activities should become familiar with such activities in another setting before presenting such activities in their own classrooms.

In preparing learning activities, be sure to provide an adequate description of what should be done. The thoroughness of description tends to vary from one resource guide to the next. In developing a teaching unit, make sure that your description of learning activities is sufficient so that any other teacher reading the unit would know exactly what to do. Even if no one but you ever reads the description, you will find that sufficient detail will help set your thoughts about how to carry out the activity. For example, how would the following activity be handled from this description?

> Visit a farm or zoo where baby animals can be observed. Discuss how animals have their young.

A more detailed description is far more useful in conducting a successful learning activity. For example:

> Visit a farm or zoo where baby animals can be observed. Discuss how animals have their young. Note the ways in which baby animals resemble their parents and contrast the ways in which they are different. Discuss the ways in which different kinds of animals care for their young. Include mammals, birds, and reptiles. Ask the children to relate what they have observed to their own birth and family care. Compare and contrast similarities and differences.

Evaluation. There are two purposes to evaluation. The first is to determine if the student has developed the skill or assimilated the concepts of the unit. The second is to enable you to assess your own teaching effectiveness. Each objective must be evaluated. Resource units usually contain several suggestions for evaluating the main objectives of a unit. Select at least one method for evaluating each objective contained in the teaching unit.

References. The teaching unit should list two types of references. Student references are books, pamphlets, magazines, or chapters from texts that can be used by students to increase their understanding of the topic. Teacher references should help you develop greater understanding and insight into content and methodology for teaching the unit.

Lesson Plans

Once the teaching unit has been developed, you must plan how you will teach it by creating daily lesson plans that provide for logical progression of the unit from start

Unit title: _Mental Health - Getting to Know Me_   Date: _February 19, 1987_

                 Time: _10 a.m._

Conceptual statement: _There are healthy and_   Grade: _Three_

unhealthy ways to express emotions.   Teacher: _Goodman_

Objectives: _The student will identify several emotions and_
state acceptable ways to express them.

Teacher needs: _Pictures of people expressing emotions, crayons, paper._

Teaching points: _Write role-playing situations on index cards._

Content (progression)	Learning activities	Evaluation for activities

I. Emotions - the way we feel
    A. Anger   C. Sadness
    B. Love   D. Fear
             E. Excitement
 	
 II. Expressing emotions
 	
    A. Facial expression
      1) smile   3) tears
      2) frown   4) eyes
 	
    B. Talking
      1) soft voice   4) fast voice
      2) loud voice   5) slow voice
      3) excited voice
 	
    C. Body language
      1) using arms
      2) kicking
      3) clapping
	1. Discuss what feelings are and list on the board. Show pictures of people displaying different emotions. Several pictures that reflect a certain emotion.
	
	 2. Discuss ways we express emotions. Ask students to give ways that are acceptable / unacceptable means of expressing feelings. Have students role play these ways to express the various emotions.
		1. Give children a crayon and have them draw a face of the emotion requested.
		
		 2. Give the children a situation which speaks of expression of a particular emotion. Have them role play an acceptable way to express the emotion.

Teacher evaluation
1. Keep the lesson as taught?   yes _____   no _____   2. What I need to improve _____
3. Next time make sure _____   4. Strengths of lesson _____

Figure 4.9
Daily lesson plan.

to finish. Each lesson plan must be based upon concepts taught in previous lessons so that learning builds on the established base.

Figure 4.9 shows a typical daily lesson plan for grade 3. Notice that the format of this lesson plan parallels the format used for the teaching unit. A conceptual statement and objectives are stated for that day. The content outline provides a summary of the main topics to be covered. The learning activities are the heart of the lesson plan. They should be described in detail and listed in the order in which they are to be used.

The form shown in Figure 4.10 can be used as a supplement to your daily lesson plan. Writing down your learning activities strategy will help you focus more closely on the major concepts to be stressed. Use of such a form will also help you to develop lead-in questions or activities for the learning experience you wish to provide. Follow-up questions should also be listed on the form. These questions will reinforce the major concepts for your students.

As shown in the daily lesson plan example, each learning activity should be followed by an evaluation activity. Through this activity, you will be able to judge to some extent how well the students have learned the concept presented. Because the activity is a performance, it can also be used to determine how well your objectives have been achieved.

Following the daily lesson, you should also evaluate your own performance, as indicated at the bottom of the daily lesson plan example. How well have you presented the content? How effective were the activities? Did you fulfill your instructional objectives? From such an evaluation, you can improve your teaching skills and thus better meet the needs of your students.

DEVELOPING OBJECTIVES

The definitions of goals, behavioral objectives, and instructional objectives are not synonymous. A *goal* is a statement of instructional intent. Goals give direction and purpose to educational efforts. Goals are long-range and may take years to accomplish. They are useful in developing long-term objectives for curriculum and grade level expectations.

Behavioral objectives are for more than one lesson and are written for long-term or unit objectives. They do not tell the teacher what or how to teach, but do present a conceptual framework for selecting appropriate content, learning activities, and evaluation procedures. *Instructional objectives* indicate the learning or behavior to be demonstrated in a particular lesson. This objective is taught within the framework of each health class. The instructional objective is specific, short-ranged, and, if the time required to teach the objective is longer than one class period, it begins to resemble a behavioral objective.

The explicit task called for in the objective must be stated in measurable, action-oriented form (Kibler, Cegala, Barker, & Miles, 1974, p. 2) Instructional objectives are used as a basis for selecting content and learning activities and in planning evaluation. Objectives must be based on the developmental level of the children and on concepts appropriate to that developmental level. Properly constructed objectives will help you focus on what you want to accomplish. They also provide accountabil-

Name: _____ Bill Smith   6th Grade _____ Date: April 12 _____

Objectives: _____ The student will list six techniques _____
_____ used to influence tobacco use. _____
_____
_____

Introductory Questions. Comments, Activities
  1. What is a 'brand' name?
  2. What is a slogan? appeal?
  3. Do you think tobacco companies use appeals and slogans?
  4. What are some ways the tobacco companies appeal to us?
  5. Discuss appeals such as: love, fun, macho image,
     better taste, low tar and nicotine.
  6. Discuss slogans such as: You've come a long way, baby.

Learning Activity (Questions, Group Activities)
  Divide the students into groups and give each group
  a stack of magazines. Ask the group to find advertisements
  for tobacco products. What appeal or slogan is each
  advertisement using to get the consumers' attention?
  Discuss in groups and then with the entire class.

Major Concepts
  1. Tobacco industry uses appeals and slogans to sell
     products.
  2. Tobacco industry never mentions the diseases associated
     with tobacco use.
  3. Tobacco use is done because of the things advertisers
     attempt to connect with it.
  4. Advertising plays an important role in product use and selection.
  5. We should not be influenced by advertising claims.

Follow-up Questions

  1. Does use of a tobacco product really help you
     live a happier, healthy life?

  2. What does each cigarette package have on it?
     (A warning about dangers to health.)

Figure 4.10
Learning activity strategy format.

ity to administrators, parents, and students. All instructional effort should be based upon the objectives for the particular lesson or unit.

Classification of Instructional Objectives

With the foregoing criteria in mind, you should develop instructional objectives in three areas—the *cognitive,* the *affective,* and the *action domains.* As defined by Bloom (1956), the cognitive domain centers around knowledge. The affective domain emphasizes skills and attitudes. The action, or psychomotor, domain focuse', on skills and behavior.

Cognitive Domain. Bloom (1956, p. 8) describes the cognitive domain as "those objectives which deal with recall or recognition of knowledge and the development of intellectual abilities, skills." There are six progressive levels of development in the cognitive domain, ranging from simple to complex. These levels can be grouped into two divisions, low level and high level, as follows.

Low level:

1. Knowledge—Recognition and recall of information, terms, classes, procedures, theories, and structures. Some terms indicative of knowledge level objectives are define, recall, describe, identify, list, match, name, and recite.

2. Comprehension—Interpretation of what has been learned, change knowledge to another form, or predict outcomes and effects. Terms indicative of a comprehensive objective are explain, summarize, interpret, rewrite, estimate, convert, infer, translate, rearrange, and paraphrase.

High level:

3. Application—Use of knowledge in new situations.
   Terms used to construct this level of objective are change, compute, demonstrate, operate, show, use, and solve.

4. Analysis—Breaking whole units into regulated parts (deduction), understanding the organization and the relationship of its parts, noting similarities and differences. Terms used are outline, break down, subdivide, discriminate, diagram, order, categorize, and distinguish.

5. Synthesis—Combining elements into new wholes (induction), or integrating information, concepts. Terms used for constructing synthesis level objectives include combine, compile, compose, create, design, rearrange, plan, and produce.

6. Evaluation—Judging materials and methods, using standards of criteria to make a quantitative or qualitative judgment. Terms used to construct this level objective are justify, appraise, criticize, compare, support, conclude, and contrast.

Most instructional objectives in the cognitive domain fall in the low-level classification. However, you must also strive to develop higher level objectives if students are to progress beyond simple recall. High-level objectives help to promote decision-making and the personalizing of health information. By closely examining the nature of the four high-level areas of the cognitive domain, you will be better able to plan activities that will promote higher levels of cognitive development.

Affective Domain. The affective domain emphasizes the emotional processes of feelings, attitudes, values, and judgments. Development in this domain is also from the simple to the complex, with low-level and high-level divisions. The five stages of affective development, as described by Krathwohl, Bloom, and Masia (1964), are as follows:

Low level:

1. Receiving—Passive attention to stimuli (sensory inputs)
2. Responding—Reacting to stimuli (complying, volunteering, and so on)

   High level:

3. Valuing—Taking action consistent with a belief or value
4. Organizing—Commitment to a set of values (formulating values)
5. Characterizing—Total behavior conforming to internalized values and the integration of beliefs and attitudes into a philosophy of life

Preparing objectives in the affective domain is vital if students are to personalize your instruction. As Harbeck (1970) points out, there is a great need for instructional objectives that assess student attitudes and feelings:

> The affective domain is central to every part of the learning and evaluation process. Awareness initiates learning. Willingness to respond is the basis for psychomotor responses, and value systems provide the motivation for continued learning and for most of the individual's overt behavior. (p. 150)

One way to prepare affective objectives is to call for the weighing of the advantages and disadvantages, or possible rewards and penalties, of a health-related act. As with cognitive objectives, it is easier to prepare low-level affective objectives than higher level ones. Still, you should do all you can to assist students in developing affectively from lower to higher levels.

Measuring the results of affective objectives is difficult. You must rely largely on observation. Checklists and attitude scales are also of some help. However, children may respond to such devices with "approved" or teacher-advocated answers without actually incorporating the actual value or behavior.

Action Domain. The action domain deals with what the student actually does. Instructional objectives for health in this domain are concerned with the health practices and behavior the students are to exhibit immediately or in the future.

Three action behaviors described by the School Health Education Study (1967) are useful in preparing instructional objectives in this domain. They are observable health behaviors, nonobservable health behaviors, and delayed behaviors.

Observable health behaviors are those that can be seen and evaluated to some extent in the school environment. Examples include observing how a student relates to others, activities on the playground or in the classroom, personal appearance and grooming, and food selection in the school cafeteria.

Nonobservable health behaviors cannot be systematically observed in the school setting. Information about such behaviors can be derived by questioning the student

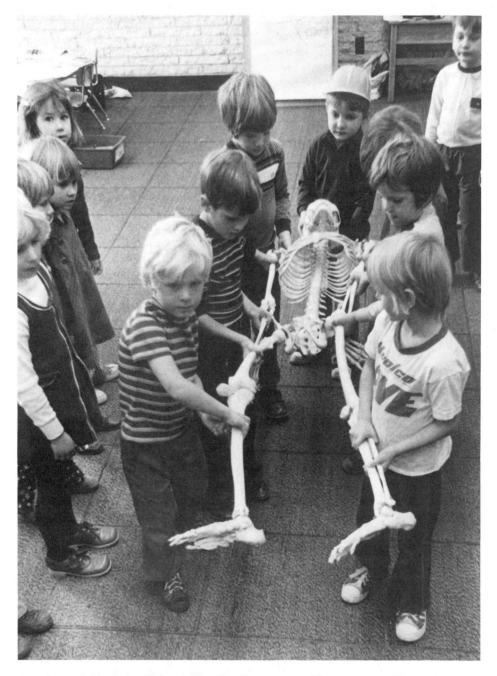

Learning activities help children internalize the content and form concepts. The teacher must select the activities that are best suited to each class.

and others aware of the student's health practices. Areas for questioning include nutritional practices, safety practices, social conduct, sleep habits, and exercise patterns. Substance abuse and family relationships are also important areas in this domain, but care must be exercised so not to invade the privacy of students or parents.

Delayed behaviors are health behaviors that will not or cannot be practiced in daily life until the student reaches adulthood, is confronted with the problem, or is in a position to assume greater responsibility for personal behavior. Examples of such behavior include maintaining a desirable weight, getting regular medical and dental checkups, and using community health services. In this area of the action domain, you can lay the groundwork for such positive behavior.

Obviously there is a great deal of overlap among the three domains. For example, the highest level in the affective domain is similar to behaviors in the action domain. Measurement of the higher levels of all three domains is difficult. What then should be your goal in evaluating the effectiveness of your instructional objectives? To consider important only that which can be measured results in the trivialization of instruction. Further, it is unrealistic to expect the student to receive information, process it (valuing), and incorporate it (action) in every instance. What *can* be accomplished through well-planned objectives is exposure to all three domains so that students make decisions that will enhance the overall quality of their own wellness throughout life. Children should be assisted to internalize information so that at some point it helps them to make decisions that lead to positive health behavior.

Writing Instructional Objectives

At first, writing instructional objectives may seem difficult. However, by following step-by-step procedures, you should become proficient with practice. Writing low-level objectives is easiest. In time, you should also be able to write effective higher-level objectives.

An instructional objective should contain five components. Following are definitions and examples of these components.

1. *Who*—The student or the one who is to exhibit the behavior. Usual terms used are *student, pupil,* or *learner.*
2. *Behavioral task*—The verbal statement of the outcome desired, usually stated in the future tense. The verb in this statement must be action-oriented rather than abstract. Use such verbs as as *write, construct, label, name, count, categorize,* and *organize.* Where possible, avoid vague terms such as *know, think, master, learn, grasp,* and *believe.* Such terms are difficult to evaluate and are open to broad interpretation.
3. *Product of the behavior*—The object of the action or what the student will actually do. For example: the student will define the terms; label the diagram; demonstrate bandaging.
4. *Conditions*—The specific conditions under which the student will be expected to do the activity. For example: on a test; orally; working in pairs.
5. *Standard of performance*—The minimum level of achievement, either quantitative or qualitative, that will be accepted as meeting the objective. For example: 80 percent correct; four out of five times; within six months; judged acceptable by a panel.

The following example illustrates how these five criteria are used in a properly constructed objective:

The student/will demonstrate/mouth-to-mouth respiration/
(Who)   (behavioral task)   (product of behavior)
using Resuscitation Annie/for three minutes without making any errors.
(conditions)   (standard of performance)

Limitations of Instructional Objectives

To be effective as instructional devices, objectives must be stated as precisely as possible. Properly developed, instructional objectives provide clarity of communication and help establish expectations for the learner. However, as Zais (1976) points out, instructional objectives also have limitations and drawbacks.

First, he notes, instructional objectives are practical only for specifying the lowest levels of learning. Higher level aspects of the three domains are difficult or even impossible to measure. Blind reliance on instructional objectives can lead to only the trivial (quantifiable) aspects of instruction being measured and considered important.

Second, instructional objectives tend to limit or restrict definitions of learning. For example, an objective may define the measurement of physical strength as the ability to do 20 pushups or to lift a 50-pound weight. However, there are many other indicators of strength. By its very precision and criterion for measurable performance, an instructional objective can obscure other valid indicators of a skill or ability.

Third, judgments made about abstract qualities, such as personal concern or appreciation, are based on subjective, indirect measures or observations. Zais argues convincingly that instructional objectives cannot be developed to measure such qualities adequately.

Although these limitations do not detract from the general usefulness of instructional objectives, they should always be kept in mind so that instructional objectives are not misused. Objectives should be seen as starting points, not terminal points. They should not be used to stipulate behavior in advance. An alternate behavior exhibited by the student at the end of instruction may be an equally valid indicator that learning has taken place.

SUMMARY

They key to effective curriculum construction is good planning. Good planning requires hours of investigating the literature and reviewing health education materials.

To be effective, the content areas in health education must be organized to ensure comprehensive coverage of grades K–12. Health topics should be based on the needs, interests, and comprehension level of the student. Community mores are also an important consideration when planning health education. A comprehensive health education program should take scope and sequence into consideration. To facilitate this, a cycle plan should be developed that focuses on the concept necessary for the children to understand at that point in their lives.

Effective health education requires a balance between the factual portion and the attitude or valuing portion of a curriculum. Time must be allotted for children to examine their feelings and to personalize the information under consideration. In this way, decision-making skills can be developed. The presentation of facts alone does not ensure learning, but the teaching of concepts helps to bring about long-term use of basic information.

Many useful commercial health education programs have been developed. SHES, HAP, and SHCP all represent innovations in health education. Most states have resource guides that teachers may use to develop teaching units. Each teaching unit should follow a prescribed format and be designed for a particular grade and group. From this unit, lesson plans for the daily activities are developed.

Instructional objectives are precise statements of intended learning outcomes. When stated properly, they facilitate communication and help focus the content, learning activities, and evaluation procedures. There are three types of objectives: cognitive, affective, and action. An instructional objective should contain five different components: who, the behavioral task, the product of the behavior, conditions under which the student performs, and the standard of performance.

DISCUSSION QUESTIONS

1. What are the advantages of sound planning?
2. Define scope and sequence and discuss their implications for health educators.
3. What criteria should curriculum developers consider?
4. What types of materials can agencies provide for teaching health?
5. What are values and how are they learned?
6. What are the advantages and disadvantages of using such programs as HAP or SHCP?
7. What are the differences between a resource unit and a teaching unit?
8. What purposes do well-developed objectives serve?
9. Why is it important that objectives be stated as precisely as possible?
10. What is the difference between a high-level and a low-level objective?

REFERENCES

Bloom, B. S. *Taxonomy of educational objectives, handbook 1: Cognitive domain.* New York: David McKay, 1956.

Byler, R., Lewis, G., & Totman, R. *Teach us what we want to know.* Hartford, Conn.: Connecticut State Board of Education, 1969.

Bureau of Health Education. *The school health curriculum project.* Washington, D.C.: U.S. Government Printing Office, 1977.

Fodor, J. T., & Dalis, G. T. *Health instruction: Theory and application* (3rd. ed.) Philadelphia: Lea & Febiger, 1981.

Harbeck, M. B. Instructional objectives in the affective domain. *Educational Technology,* January 1970. 10:49–52.

Kibler, R. J., Cegala, D. J., Barker, L. L., & Miles, D. T. *Objectives for instruction and evaluation.* Boston: Allyn & Bacon, 1974.

Krathwohl, D. R., Bloom, P. R., & Masia, B. B. *Taxonomy of educational objectives, handbook II: Affective domain.* New York: David McKay, 1964.

Lawrence Hall of Science. *Health activities project.* Northbrook, Ill.: Hubbard, 1987.

Read, D. A., & Greene, W. H. *Creative teaching in health.* New York: Macmillan, 1971.

School Health Education Study. *Health education: A conceptual approach to curriculum design.* St. Paul, Minn.: 3M Education Press, 1967.

Willgoose, C. E. *Health education in the elementary school.* Philadelphia: W. B. Saunders, 1974.

Zais, R. S. *Curriculum principles and foundations.* New York: Thomas Y. Crowell, 1976.

5. Techniques for Implementing Health Instruction

Effective teaching represents the culmination of a series of preparatory activities. Long hours of careful preparation often go into one class period. In setting the stage for effective instruction, the teacher must be a skillful predictor of events. Knowledge of students and a thorough knowledge of the subject field are necessary prerequisites to instructional excellence. Yet, of themselves, they are inadequate. The professional competence of a teacher rests on his ability to anticipate student needs and behaviors in advance of the actual experience. Instructional preparation, then, involves applied imagination in planning for the experience.—Kenneth H. Hoover, The Professional Teacher's Handbook

THE RELATIONSHIP OF METHODS TO LEARNING

Learning activities are things that make content and objectives come alive. This enlivening involves selecting methods and techniques that make learning exciting and motivating. Carrying this out is the direct responsibility of the teacher who, having established a working knowledge of the many methods available in health education, is limited only by his or her own creativity.

A method is any activity or experience that the teacher uses to interpret, illustrate, or facilitate learning. For the most effective learning to take place, you should seek methods that are student-centered and provide for group involvement. Additionally, you should use more than one method or activity for each major concept so that your instruction more fully encompasses the variety of student abilities and aptitudes.

The teacher must remember that selecting a variety of methods does not ensure learning. Several other factors influence effective learning and must be considered. For example, a good relationship with the students, conducive to learning, must be fostered. Treating students fairly is the first step in facilitating learning and creating a proper classroom atmosphere. Many techniques to help promote creative learning are available. With proper preparation, the methodologies listed in table 5.1 can be useful.

Table 5.1
Instructional Methods for Health Education

Audio	Audiovisual	Visual
Tape recordings	Motion pictures	Games
Records	Television	Bulletin boards
Debates	Filmstrips-recording	Filmstrips
Radio	Slide tape	Transparencies
Buzz groups	Talking tapes	Newspapers
Stories and storytelling	Plays	Demonstrations/
Brainstorming	Puppet shows	experiments
Values clarification	Show and tell	Magazines
Discussions		Charts/maps
Flannel, felt, and		Field trips
magnetic boards		
Computers		
Posters		

Factors Affecting Methodology

In selecting methods to provide learning experiences, keep the following criteria in mind:

1. *Select methods that contribute to total learning.* Some activities lend themselves to acquiring knowledge, while others are better suited to attitude assessment and decision-making. Ideally, the methods selected should help the student develop the ability to reason and assess the information being presented. Any method selected should involve the students as direct participants in the activity.

2. *The more complex the concept, the more activities needed to develop the concept.* As a general rule, for each concept, two methods or activities should be employed. If the material being studied is difficult, more than two methods or activities should be used. Another reason for using more than one method is that students learn in a variety of ways and through different means. Thus a variety of methods will help ensure that all students grasp the concept under examination.

3. *The methods selected should begin with the simple and move to the more complex.* Once you have prepared the class for the activity through a proper introduction, the students should become part of the learning activity. With simple activities, students should be able to learn by means of group involvement, self-assessment, and class-teacher interaction. As the students become better able to deal with more difficult topics, more complex methods can be used that require self-discovery or analysis of materials and conclusions.

4. *Audiovisual aids should be included whenever possible.* These can include models, classroom exhibits, films, filmstrips, and so forth. Audiovisual aids add another dimension to teaching concepts and are excellent for reinforcing learning.

Methods can be classified into many different categories. Some authorities distinguish between methods, media, and instructional materials, while others group all three into one category. Classification is unimportant as long as you can identify the strengths and weaknesses of each available technique. Your objective should be to select those methods that are most appropriate and effective with your class. The rest of this chapter is devoted to an examination of some of the many methods that can be used in health education.

VALUES CLARIFICATION TECHNIQUES

To personalize health concepts, students must relate to health instruction from the affective domain. An excellent method for achieving this end is through the use of values clarification activities. By examining and clarifying values, children can be assisted in fostering positive health behavior.

As mentioned earlier in the text, the use of values clarification techniques is not without some controversy. Values cannot and should not be avoided when teaching health education, but the teacher must be adequately prepared to do the job right.

Begin by recognizing that values are relative, personal, and often situational. You should not attempt to teach your own personal values or the "correct" values; instead, your goal should be to assist students in assessing and developing their own values so that these values lead to positive health behavior. It is essential that any value judgment made by the students be made through their own cognitive process. For a value judgment or health practice to evolve, according to Hochbaum, Rosenstock, and Kegeles (1960), the following criteria must apply:

1. Students must perceive the issue as being important.
2. Students must believe that they are susceptible to the problem.
3. Students must believe that the problem is serious.
4. The intensity of the threat and resultant anxiety must not be so great as to paralyze the ability to act.
5. There must be an action to take that the individual believes will be effective.

When engaging in any values clarification activity, sufficient time must be allotted for students to assess their own feelings about the issue under examination. Students must also feel free to assess their values without fear of being ridiculed or forced to pay lip service to the opinions of others, including the teacher's.

Keep these points in mind:

1. Values clarification activities do not lead to one "correct" solution to a problem; they are open ended. The purpose of these activities is to open the doors to additional assessment.
2. As a teacher, you are a participant in the activities and a role model for the students.
3. Every student has the right to decline from speaking, without having to give a reason for declining. Respect individual feelings and keep the activity non-threatening.

Many instructional devices are available for incorporating values clarification activities into the health curriculum. The ones that you choose should be appropriate for the developmental level of the students. As already discussed, young children are not capable of dealing with highly abstract issues. Further, they do not have the ex-

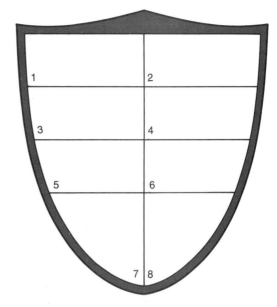

1. Name or draw something that you do well.
2. Name or draw something that you are trying to get better at.
3. Write down a feeling that would be very hard for you to change.
4. Write the thing you are most proud of having done.
5. Tell about a happy thing that happened to you.
6. Tell about a sad thing that happened to you.
7. Tell what you want to do with your life.
8. Write three words that best tell about who you are.

Figure 5.1
Shield activity for identifying and assessing values.

periential background to deal knowingly with topics far removed from their everyday world. Therefore it is not realistic to attempt to grapple with such values-related issues as euthanasia or world hunger at the primary level.

Simple Values-Related Techniques

One of the simplest and most appropriate activities for younger students involves what is known as shield activities. The major objective of these activities is to assist children in identifying values they have. A typical shield is illustrated in figure 5.1. Each child is given a prepared form as shown in the figure. The activity consists of filling in each segment of the shield with a values-related response, either in words or with drawings. For younger children, you should read the instructions aloud.

In presenting such an activity, it is essential that you thoroughly introduce, carry out, and summarize the experience. If this is not done, the activity becomes nothing more than a game. Through careful introduction, a psychological set is established so that the activity will be meaningful and the students will understand why they are doing it. By careful summation, you can help students assess their feelings and clarify existing values.

Asking children to complete open-ended statements is another simple values-related activity. This kind of activity is appropriate for children at a slightly higher developmental level. Examples of typical open-ended statements include the following:

I think that smoking is _____ .

If my friend did something wrong, I would _____ .

Decision Stories

Decision stories are open-ended vignettes that describe a values-related dilemma and ask students to suggest a course of action. The stories should reflect real-life circumstances and should be appropriate to the age level of the children. No easy answer should suggest itself in the story, but viable courses of action must be possible for the activity to be meaningful. If only unacceptable or repugnant alternatives seem possible, children will be unable to incorporate positive decision-making skills into their own behavior repertoires. A decision story that children can identify with and relate to can provide an excellent springboard for values discussion. A good decision story not only encourages students to sort out opinions, values, and feelings but also requires students to think about, test, and try them out. The real test of the importance of values comes with application.

In preparing decision stories, follow these guidelines:

1. The story should be between 50 and 150 words in length. It should include enough detail to establish realism and character, but it should not be so long as to obscure the central issue.
2. Establish a focus on the main issue with relevant supportive facts and events.
3. Do not slant the story so that only one solution or course of action is implied.
4. Provide a descriptive title.
5. End with a focus question that asks each student to suggest a course of action. This question is also the basis for discussion of the issue (Hamrick, Anspaugh, & Smith, 1980, p. 455)

Following are examples of decision stories.

Pressure

Jim and Paul are fifth graders in the same classroom. In the past few weeks they have become friends. One day while walking home from school, Jim and Paul meet some of Paul's other friends by the park. Paul's friends are all smoking. They offer Paul a cigarette. He takes it and lights up. Paul's friends also offer Jim a cigarette, but he says no. The boys start to make fun of him and call him a chicken. Even Paul is laughing at his friend.

Focus Question: What should Jim do?

Hot Spot

Mary's fourth grade class is taking an important arithmetic test. Mary has studied hard for the test. In the seat next to her is her friend Julia. Julia is worried that she will not pass the test. The teacher leaves the room for a minute. While she is gone, Julia asks Mary for some of the test answers. The other students see and hear this. The teacher will be back in the room soon.

Focus Question: What should Mary do?

Students are an excellent source for developing such decision stories. After exposure to a few models that you have written or located in values clarification materials, students are usually eager to write vignettes of their own. This should be encouraged, as student-developed stories are highly relevant and motivating to the students themselves.

Presenting Decision Stories in Class.   Begin by setting the stage for the story to motivate the class for the activity and to focus the inquiry. Discuss the title of the story and ask the children what it suggests to them. Stimulate the students' curiosity and get them involved from the start. For decision stories to be effective, students must be participants and not merely passive listeners.

After a few minutes of this warm-up phase, present the story itself. Most of the stories can be read aloud. However, you may also wish to give copies of the stories to the students so that they can consider the details of the presentation.

Then have the students offer individual responses to the focus question: What course of action does each student think most appropriate? Encourage thought and reflection on the matter, but do not force any student to respond unwillingly. A good way to get the students thinking is to have them each write their response on paper. The writing process facilitates thinking through the situation that has been presented. It also requires that each student make a commitment based on the information presented. Make it clear, however, that the written responses need not be shared with the class at this point.

Pooling Ideas.   Next, generate a list of all possible solutions to the decision story dilemma by asking students to share their responses with the class. This should be done on a volunteer basis. The teacher should not provide feedback to the students such as "That's good" or "I'm not sure that is such a good idea." Attempt to remain noncommital. Respond with such phrases as, "Thank you for sharing that idea with us," or by simply paraphrasing their responses. Then you can collect them and compile a list of solutions on the chalkboard without revealing which student offered any particular solution. You should also add possible solutions to the list that the students have overlooked.

Consider all the ideas put forth. Do not be judgmental and do not reject any solution out of hand. Remember that your role is to help students clarify their own values, not to impose values upon them.

Now, divide the class into small groups and have each group discuss the possible solutions to the dilemma. Allow time for each group to reach a consensus on the preferred solution. Encourage the students to offer reasons behind the solution they opt for.

Discussion and Reappraisal.   After each small group has come to some sort of agreement, have the groups present the results of their discussions. In all probability, different groups will opt for different solutions. Ask individual students why one solution seems better than another. Again, refrain from being judgmental. In accepting each opinion, you should display neutrality. Instead of commenting, "So you think that Mary should just pretend that she didn't hear Julia," you might say, "How could Mary have responded to Julia?"

Finally, have each student reconsider the decision story in light of the class discussion (Smith, Hamrick, & Anspaugh, 1981, p. 637). Some children will want to change their minds at this point. Others may modify their approach to the problem. Again have each student write down his or her solution to the problem along with reasons why the solution seems best. Have the students reflect on the ramifications of their decisions. Without necessarily requiring verbal responses, ask questions such as the following:

- Have you ever been in a situation like the one in the story?
- Did you come to the same solution then? Or would you come to the same solution?
- Did you or would you carry out your planned decision?
- What happened or what do you think would happen if you tried out this decision?
- How did this decision affect your own values? How were you affected by the decision? How were others affected?
- Would you always make a similar decision?

Using this structured approach to decision stories will help students develop decision-making skills. It will also assist them in applying rational thought to everyday problems involving values.

OTHER VERBAL AND DISCUSSION-ORIENTED METHODS

Values-clarification activities rely to a large part on discussion, as do many other classroom methods. Discussion is a useful technique, but it must be structured. Always keep in mind that your objective in employing any particular discussion method so that you do not lose the focus. Following are several other discussion-oriented methods that have been found to be effective in health instruction.

Brainstorming

Like values-clarification activities, brainstorming can be used to improve decision-making skills by having students generate many possible ideas concerning an issue. Freedom of expression and creativity are also encouraged. Possible topics for brainstorming sessions include:

- How can you get students to follow safety rules?
- How can students be encouraged to eat nutritious snacks instead of junk food?
- How can we make our physical environment healthier and more pleasant?

In conducting a brainstorming session, it is very important to follow these four rules:

1. The problem to be brainstormed must be well defined.
2. Any and all ideas must be accepted.
3. Criticism of any idea put forth is not allowed.
4. All ideas should be evaluated objectively when the session is over.

Brainstorming can be used effectively in the lower as well as upper elementary grades. The biggest drawback is that in a large class not every child may get a chance to express his or her thoughts. Nonetheless, the activity can be quite productive. By encouraging and accepting all opinions, new or novel possible solutions to a problem may be found. Even impractical suggestions can lead to new ways of thinking about an issue.

Follow-up is important. In the follow-up session, ask children to elaborate on their ideas. Present additional information that will be useful in making suggestions more practical or realistic. In doing so, emphasize to the class how the freewheeling brainstorming session led to many approaches to the problem.

Buzz Groups

Akin to brainstorming, buzz groups are an effective method for examining a specific problem. Generally this technique is productive if students are mature enough to use the format. It allows for student participation in an atmosphere conducive to discussion. The buzz group method should not be overused, however, since too much small group work can lessen student enthusiasm.

To use this approach, divide the class into groups of from three to five students. Have each group focus on a specific problem that you have introduced and discussed so that the children will have a knowledge base for their discussion. Each group should choose a chairperson and a recording secretary. The chairperson must keep the discussion on the topic, while the secretary records important points.

Allow 3–15 minutes for buzz group discussion. Suitable topics for this method include the following:

- How should an accident victim be handled?
- How can children get along better with brothers and sisters?
- What can be done to educate children to the dangers of smoking?
- What can be done about vandalism?

After the discussion time is over, ask the recording secretary for each group to present the results of that group's discussion. The more controversial the topic, the more likely it will be that many diverse opinions will be aired. In the summary discussion, encourage objective consideration of all approaches put forth.

Case Studies

Case studies are actual events that you can use in class for discussion. The decision story format lends itself well to the case study method. Just substitute the actual event for the hypothetical one. Good sources for case study materials are health journals, newspapers, news magazines, and television programs.

Debate

Debate focuses on the merits and problems associated with a proposed solution to a problem. Through the use of this technique, you can ensure that both sides of an issue are presented. Although debate can be used in the lower elementary grades, the method is more effective when used with older children, who are more articulate and better able to organize their thoughts for oral presentation. Students must also be able to work individually as well as cooperatively and in groups.

Topics suitable for debate include the use of nuclear power or its alternatives, the supposed merits of organic foods versus regular produce, and the use of laboratory animals in medical experiments. Environmental issues are also good debate topics.

Thorough preparation for a debate is essential. Students who volunteer to be part of a debate team should be given ample time to become knowledgeable about the issue they will discuss. You should engage the whole class in this preparation so that students not on the debate teams are prepared to deal with the pros and cons of the arguments objectively.

In selecting students for debate teams, be sure that both sides are well balanced in ability. Your role is that of moderator. You should keep both debate teams on the topic and also guard against emotions becoming too extreme during and after the debate.

Committee Work

This technique allows small groups of children to research a topic of interest. Each group member has an opportunity to do indepth research on the topic. For elementary school children, the work must be closely supervised and structured. It is very important that each member of the group contribute to the project if it is to be successful.

Projects that lend themselves well to committee work include the following:

- Investigating different types of pollution
- Collecting newspaper and magazine articles on a recent medical discovery or health approach
- Researching different kinds of foods used in different cultures as sources of essential nutrients

Results of the committee work are presented orally. Encourage committee members to use exhibits and audiovisual aids to reinforce their presentations.

This method can also be used on an individual basis. In such an instance, each student makes a presentation of research done.

Lecture, Group, and Panel Discussion

Discussion, in one form or another, is probably the most common technique used in education. Lecture discussion is usually thought of as a lecture delivered by the teacher. However, this method should not be limited to one-way communication. Lecture discussion can be from teacher to student, student to teacher, or student to student. The technique should be a means for achieving two-way communication.

For group discussion to be effective, the teacher must develop an atmosphere of freedom in the classroom and the discussion must be kept on course. Without a feeling of freedom, students will not state their true feelings. If the discussion is not kept on course, digression from the main topic will occur. Curtis and Papenfuss (1980, p. 139) offer the following suggestions for conducting group discussion:

1. Present a discussion topic or legitimize an appropriate student-formulated topic.
2. Establish and maintain an atmosphere of thoughtful communication without injecting teaching value judgments.
3. Make the ground rules for the discussion clear and enforce them.
4. Try to understand what students are attempting to say, but do not badger or cross-examine.

Panel discussion offers an opportunity for three to five students to investigate and report on a particular health topic. This method is similar to committee work, but it allows more give and take between the participating students. Usually 15 minutes or less is sufficient time for a panel discussion. Adjust the time allotted to the attention span and developmental level of the class. When using this method, be sure that the students who will be panel members have a precise theme to explore. A prepared outline is also necessary so that the presentation is organized.

All three of these discussion techniques allow for the exchange of information and ideas between students. In this way, children are involved in the teaching-learning process. Discussion techniques also help develop respect and understanding for the feelings and opinions of others.

As noted, to be successful discussion must be guided. Stone, O'Reilley, and Brown (1980, p. 281) note six elements that must be addressed when preparing for a discussion:

1. Choose a topic that the students can discuss and have options on.
2. Introduce the topic and motivate the class about it.
3. Prepare key questions that generate discussion.
4. Provide structure to the discussion.
5. Develop closure on the topic discussed.
6. Summarize and reinforce the key points.

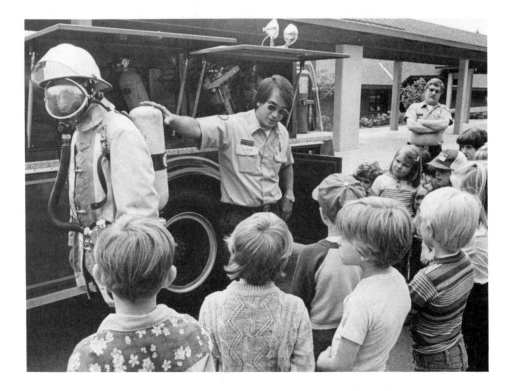

Resource speakers can be very instructive, especially if the students are properly prepared and the speaker uses visual aids to keep the students' interest.

Resource Speakers

Speakers can enrich many areas of health instruction. Possible resource speakers include doctors, nurses, police and fire department personnel, nutritionists, and health researchers. When contracting a resource speaker, be sure that you provide the person with information about your class, including grade and developmental level. In this way, a speaker is less likely to talk down to or over the heads of the children. You should also politely emphasize that the speaker stick to the specific topic to be examined, since some speakers are apt to digress to a favorite cause or concern not in keeping with your instructional objectives. Suggest that the speaker use audiovisual aids if appropriate, as this will heighten student interest. Also ask the speaker to allow time for a question and answer session.

Before the speaker addresses the class, be sure that you have provided adequate instruction so that the students are not introduced to the topic cold. Also provide information about the position and background of the resource speaker. For example, what exactly is a nutritionist? What does a nutritionist do and for whom does the person work?

ACTION-ORIENTED METHODS

A variety of action-oriented or student-centered activities can be used to enliven health instruction. These range from seatwork activities to field trips. Whenever possible, any method selected should help students to discover concepts through action-oriented means. Methods that incorporate at least two of the senses can greatly facilitate learning. Listening is fine, but listening and seeing, tasting and smelling, touching, feeling, and doing are better.

Dramatizations

Plays and skits, role playing, and puppet shows are all effective dramatization techniques. Each of these methods is an excellent way of allowing students to express their feelings. Thorough preparation and follow-up are essential, however, lest these activities be seen merely as fun, with the point of the exercise being missed.

Presenting a play involves use of a script and props. You can use a commercial script or have students write their own. A skit is much more informal. Only an outline for the story needs to be prepared, not an actual script. Each character speaks extemporaneously. Props are not requried. Nonetheless, plays and skits are both quite time-consuming.

Role playing, or sociodrama, is a technique whereby students act out roles identifed by you or by them. Each student is given a basic description of the role and the situation. The actual role playing is done with little or no rehearsal. A typical sociodrama should last from one to three minutes. It should then be followed by class discussion. Why did the person react to the situation in the particular way that the role was defined? What solutions suggest themselves from the sociodrama? Are these the only possible alternatives? If time permits, have students switch roles or allow different students to play the same role.

Puppet shows are great motivators for health behavior and attitude development. They are especially effective in the lower grades. Commercial puppets may be used or children can make their own. Puppets can be used for plays, skits, or role playing (Timmreck, 1978, p. 40).

Storytelling

As a technique, storytelling is similar to dramatization. However, as the teacher you are the active participant, while the children are onlookers. Nonetheless, this is an effective method for helping students to identify positive health habits and to shape attitudes. Using a flip chart or other visual aid can heighten the impact of storytelling, although no props are needed for many stories.

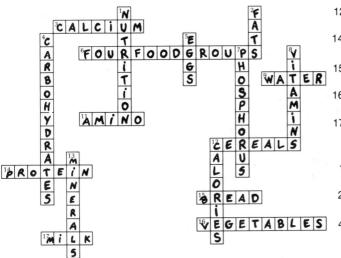

12. Foods rich in carbohydrates. Oatmeal is an example.

14. A nutrient that builds and repairs body tissue.

15. A food product rich in carbohydrates. Good for making sandwiches.

16. Lettuce, carrots, and tomatoes are examples. Can be eaten fresh or cooked.

17. Beverage from cows that is rich in protein.

Down

1. The science of food as it relates to optional health and performance.

2. Food substances that do not dissolve in water.

4. Nutrients found in many foods, especially in the Bread and Cereal Group; a source of energy.

5. Product of chickens, which are popular for breakfast. Contain plenty of protein.

7. Helps build strong bones and teeth.

8. A group of nutrients that help other nutrients do their job. Known by letter names.

12. Measure energy provided by food. Dieters count them.

13. Sometimes called the "Structural Framework" of the body.

Across

3. A mineral in milk that builds strong bones and teeth.

6. A useful guide for eating daily (three words)

9. Helps regulate body temperature.

10. Contains iodine, is low in calories, a good source of protein, and is in the meat group.

11. Parts of protein, called _____ acids.

Figure 5.2
Nutrition-related crossword puzzle developed by the Memphis Nutritional Center, Memphis Public Schools.

Flannel, Felt, and Magnetic Boards

Flannel or felt boards are made by stretching a piece of either material over a large board or easel. Objects that will cling to the fabric can be placed on the board. Such boards are quite useful as aids in telling a story of developing a concept since objects can be added or taken off during the presentation. These boards can also be used by the students in developing their own stories or presentations.

Magnetic boards serve the same purpose as flannel and felt boards. A magnetic board is simply a sheet of metal to which objects can be attached by means of small magnets. Chalk can also be used to write directly on a magnetic board.

Crossword Puzzles

Crossword puzzles are useful seatwork devices for building vocabulary and reinforcing concepts. They can be developed by you or by the students themselves. Commercial materials are also available. Crossword puzzles for younger children must be kept relatively simple. This technique is best employed with children in grade three and above. Figure 5.2 shows an example of a crossword puzzle concerning milk and milk products.

Demonstrations and Experiments

Demonstrations and experiments help make verbal explanation more meaningful to students. In a demonstration, the outcome should always be the same; in an experiment, the predicted outcome may vary. Otherwise, the two terms mean much the same. These techniques are especially good for use with elementary school children because they usually involve the senses of sight, touch, and hearing. They may involve other senses as well. Students are always interested in demonstrations and experiments because these methods help clarify what has been learned.

When considering either a demonstration or an experiment, careful planning is essential to make sure that it will actually work. All equipment should be set up ahead of time, and it is wise to have a rehearsal before the class actually views the procedure.

Appropriate areas for demonstrations and experiments include the following:

- Blood typing
- Animal feeding
- Determining the starch content of food
- Proper brushing and flossing of teeth

Introduce the procedure to the class and explain what you plan to do. All students should be able to see the activity. Encourage them to ask questions as you go, and be sure to explain what is happening at each stage. After the activity, reinforce the learning by writing important points on the chalkboard.

Exhibits

Exhibits allow students to view, examine, and touch health-related materials. Exhibits are most effective when the children help in the design and construction. Careful planning is essential, as is a central theme. Always ask yourself: What is the point of the proposed exhibit? Your answer will provide a focus question for the children, too.

Examples of appropriate exhibits include X-ray plates of broken and healed bones, safety equipment used in different types of sports, dental instruments, and samples of raw foods, such as cereal grains. If the actual objects are unavailable or impractical for classroom display, pictures can be substituted, although they are not as effective.

Everything in an exhibit should be clearly labeled. If sound and motion can be added, student interest will be increased. Use your imagination to make the exhibit as visually appealing and interest-provoking as you can.

Models and Specimens

Like exhibits, models and specimens allow students to take a multisensory approach to health-related topics. The value of models and specimens lies in their degree of accuracy. Many excellent models of body parts are available commercially. These include models of the human eye, heart, lungs, and other organs. Another useful model is Resuscitation Annie, a functional model used to teach mouth-to-mouth resuscitation.

Specimens can be obtained from biological supply houses. These include tissue samples, animal eyes, and so forth. Commercial slaughter houses can also supply some of these items. Exercise discretion in the use of specimens. For some children, such exhibits can be too grisly and models are better employed.

Field Trips

Field trips can provide rich learning experiences. This method must be used sparingly, however, because a field trip is time-consuming and often expensive. Further, parents and administrators must give their approval for any activity outside the school and liability must be considered.

A field trip should always be a culminating activity rather than an introductory one. Children should be well-prepared for the experience through prior classroom instruction. If the field trip is to be of value, the students must be able to understand what they will be seeing.

Good places for health-related field trips away from the school include the lcoal health department, a dairy farm, a food processing plant, or a sewage treatment facility. There are also many opportunities for field trips without leaving the school area. These are often quite effective as learning experiences for younger children. Although the places themselves are familiar, you can add a new dimension by explaining the structure and planning behind the situation. Examples of such on-site field trips include visits to the school cafeteria, to a crosswalk area, or to the playground. For instance, at the crosswalk area you can ask children how the crosswalk is planned for safety. Are there school speed limit signs to slow traffic during school hours? Are crosswalk lines painted on the street? Do crossing guards supervise the crossing? These and other questions will help the students see the area in a new light.

Games

Games can stimulate interest while providing a review of concepts learned through other methods. They are also sometimes a welcome relief from the normal classroom routine. In addition, games especially help younger children understand the importance of following rules and provide useful experience in socialization. Many commercially available games such as Bingo can be adapted to health-related topics, or you may wish to develop your own games if you have the time.

When using games as part of the health instruction that you provide, be sure that the fun of the activity does not overshadow the health-related content of the game. Also keep the game from becoming too competitive so that no player feels inferior.

THE USE OF MEDIA IN HEALTH INSTRUCTION

Educational media include everything from textbooks to videotape to computer-assisted instruction. For the present purposes, the term will be defined as any non-print vehicle used for instructional intent. Such media include computers, television and videotape, films, filmstrips, slides, overhead transparencies, and records and audio tapes.

Computer-Assisted Instruction

The first attempts to employ computers in the classroom were made in the 1960s. A programmed instructional format was generally used. That is, instructional information was provided by the computer in small increments. By responding to questions asked about the material by the computer, the student learned the material and received immediate reinforcement. Programmed instruction, with or without the computer as a vehicle, can be an effective educational tool, but the rigid structure and format often lead to student boredom. This is exactly what happened in the 1960s. Additionally, the computers of that time were too expensive and impractical for common classroom use.

Development of microcomputers and videodisks in the last few years has led to an increasing use of computers in the classroom. In fact, many children today come from homes where personal computers are used for a variety of purposes, from preparing business records to playing video games. In the years ahead, we shall no doubt see an increased use of computers in health instruction.

The computer holds great potential as a motivational device and also as a tool for allowing the student to apply knowledge to hypothetical problems. Gold and Duncan (1980) give two examples.

> One of the most basic ways in which the computer may serve as a motivational device is through the use of self-assessment programs. Widely used among such approaches

are the computerized dietary analysis models. These programs allow the student to input information concerning what they eat (on any single day or combination of days) and receive in return some output which identifies how well they have met some set of dietary standards. Such programs can provide an excellent introduction to the study on nutrition by developing and focusing student interest. We have made similar use of a life stress measurement program to introduce a unit on stress and a life expectancy prediction program to stimulate interest in the study of health behavior.

A great deal of software is currently available for use with computers in the classroom. There seem to be five strategies currently employed in educational software (Petosa and Gillespie, 1984).

1. Drill and Practice. Students are presented a series of questions to be answered or problems to be solved. The microcomputer immediately checks the response and provides feedback to the student. While drill and practice programs are one of the most common educational applications of computers, they can be unnec-

---

HEALTH HIGHLIGHT: WHAT IF MICROCOMPUTERS INVADED SCHOOL HEALTH EDUCATION?

The other issue addressed here is what the future of school health education could be with the microcomputer. Suggested applications of microcomputers in health education have been recognized but current efforts apparently have been minimal.

However, *when* health educators accelerate the introduction of quality "software" for various health education curriculums (primary school through college), the teaching of health will be revolutionized.

Students will be able to select health content topics from microcomputer-based programs just as they would select entrees from menus. The teaching of health by microcomputers would certainly facilitate a student's particular interests and self-pacing.

As a consequence of the capabilities of microcomputer-based programs to store footage from films of actual incidents as well as color graphics and sound, the health education teacher and student can see simulations of various "what if" situations. For example, in a CPR course, a teacher (through a microcomputer-based program) might display film footage of an individual having a heart attack. Students would be asked to respond by entering onto the microcomputer their actions. In addition to "typing" their responses on a keyboard to enter their response for the microcomputer, students could simulate CPR (if called for) by touching the place on the television screen where the heart attack victim's xiphoid process would be displayed. Or, since microcomputers could also respond to speech (e.g., Texas Instru-

ment's "Speak-and-Spell" toy), the student could also "talk" to the "victim" shown on the microcomputer-controlled television screen. The CPR microcomputer program could "talk back" to the student when appropriate.

In effect, dramatic simulations of a variety of "what if" situations that would include immediate feedback on the effects of students' responses would be produced. Other programs that could be created are only limited by our imaginations.

By 1989, 80 percent of the homes in this country will have microcomputers. They will be integrated into our lives much like the telephone and television are today. As a result, data bases and health educational "software" programs could be nearly universally accessible in the school, home and community. Just as we have "directory assistance" to provide information on telephone numbers, we could have "Health Education Operators" on call for direct inquirers to appropriate microcomputer-based health education software to answer health questions. "Health Education Operators" could identify "software" that could probably address the inquirer's questions and then the inquirers would turn toward the microcomputer-connected television for viewing the chosen "software."

Source: Chen, M.S.: When and What if Microcomputers Invaded School Health Education. *Journal of School Helath, 53,* 5, May, 1983, pp. 324–25. © 1983, American School Health Association, Kent, OH 44240.

essarily boring for students; and they tend to promote rote learning. This strategy is most often used to reinforce or review material learned elsewhere.

2. Tutorial. The microcomputer presents new information to the student and then it poses a series of questions. Based upon the responses provided by the student, the program either presents additional information or reviews the previous lesson. Users of this strategy should ensure that the software does not overwhelm the student with screen after screen of text. This repetition quickly can lead to learner fatigue.

3. Demonstration. A demonstration program allows students to observe a functioning model or situation. By observation, the student learns how systems work. For example, one commerical program demonstrates the effect of exercise on a graphic representation of a human heart and another illustrates how nerve impulses travel through the nervous system of the body.

4. Simulations. These programs imitate real or imaginary systems based on a modeler's theory of the operation of that system. Students test hypothetical courses of action by manipulating variables and observing the impact of these changes. This process allows the student to formulate realistic projections based on sound theory. Programs currently available can simulate operation of a nuclear reactor, the human circulatory system, various ecosystems, and a malaria epidemic.

5. Instructional Games. Games often utilize one or more of the strategies previously described. The instructional game differs from arcade games as it is designed to meet well-defined instructional objectives. Instructional games have explicit rules and winners, but educational concepts and information must be mastered to become successful. An example would be a commercially avaiable game which requires a knowledge of human anatomy and physiology to successfully complete a voyage through the human body. Make sure that the educational strategy employed by the instructional program is appropriate for the content area and the students' abilities. Most importantly, consider if the program being reviewed is superior to other methods of teaching the same content.

HEALTH HIGHLIGHT: SELECTING COMPUTER SOFTWARE

Compatibility

There are some technical aspects to using educational software which, if not anticipated, can lead to frustration. First, the software must be compatible with the micrcomputer. Software developed for an Atari™ microcomputer will not work in Apple™. Further, some programs designed for earlier versions of a given machine will not run in newer versions of the same machine. Software manufacturers are beginning to adapt popular programs so they will be available for the best-selling microcomputers, but any particular software package only will run on the specific machine for which it was designed. When ordering software, carefully specify the microcomputer on which it will be used.

Prospective buyers should have an opportunity to preview educational software before making a purchase. Many publishers make their software available on a 30-day approval arrangement. Currently, the quality of educational software ranges from very good to very poor. Educators can promote the future development of high quality software by conducting a careful, critical review before purchase. Software publishers also should provide technical assistance. Some publishers provide a toll-free telephone number for this purpose. Occasionally, software will contain "bugs" which prevent it from operating correctly. Being able to quickly access technical assistance in these situations can prevent needless frustration.

Evaluating a Software

A careful evaluation of educational software begins with a thorough examination of the supporting documentation. Documentation is the instructions and supportive literature that accompany each piece of educational software. These instructions will determine how quickly and effectively people can learn how to use the program. Documentation should be comprehensive and it should include clearly stated educational goals and objectives, step-by-step operating instructions, a description of how to use the program in the classroom, and a student guide with worksheets, background material, and spirit masters.

Good documentation also includes a program listing with variable definitions and directions on how to modify the program. As an educator becomes more sophisticated in the use of a program, an educator may want to tailor it to the specific needs of students. The documentation should include a bibliography of references upon which the content of the program was based. This information allows the user to judge the credibility of the content within the program. The importance of quality documentation cannot be overemphasized. Without it, determining if a piece of software can meet instructional objectives is time-consuming, difficult, and expensive.

After reading the documentation, it is important that the potential purchaser actually run the program to determine if the learning experience at the microcomputer actually matches the claims made in the documentation and promotional literature. Occasionally, the disparity between the two can be disappointing. While reviewing the program, people should ask themselves if there is an instructional medium that can teach the lesson more effectively. There are no innate capabilities of the microcomputer that make it superior to all other instructional strategies in meeting educational goals. Currently, there is a lack of educational research exploring how best to utilize the microcomputer to promote learning. The microcomputer, like all educational media, must be used judiciously if it is to be used effectively.

User-Friendly

As people go through the actual program on the microcomputer, they should notice how easy the program is to follow. The term "user-friendly" evolved to describe a constellation of factors that contribute to making the program understandable and enjoyable. A "user-friendly" program usually introduces itself by presenting a brief description of the purpose of the program and clear directions on how to run the program. These instructions should tell the user when and how to respond during the program. The program should use conversational language and a minimum of special "computer terms." Often, a "friendly" program will ask the student's name and refer to the student by name throughout the program. Ideally, the user never should feel "lost," not knowing how to respond or how to proceed to the next step in the program, and the user should be able either to exit the program or refer back to the instructions at any time. It is very important that the program be self-paced which usually is accomplished by having the student press a specially designated key when ready to proceed to the next step in the program. Programs that are not self-paced tend to progress too quickly for the novices. When a person is more familiar with the program, it will tend to move too slowly leading to boredom. Test the program to see how it handles inappropriate responses. Good programs will indicate that the response is not appropriate and ask the operator to try again. Poor programs will "crash;" the operator has confused the program's logic and it will stop functioning correctly.

Program Accuracy

Next, examine critically the educational soundness of the program. The content of the program should be accurate and the sources of information should be considered reliable. Most importantly, the content should be of educational value. The program should teach something that is worth learning. If the content is appropriate for a particular health curriculum, it should be presented in a logical, organized, and sequential fashion; it is important that the content be presented in a manner that provides an adequate cognitive challenge for students.

One of the strengths of a good microcomputer program is that it can be a tireless reinforcer. Check to see that the program reinforces correct responses and provides several attempts for a student to arrive at the correct response. If the student experiences difficulty, the program should have the capability to provide additional instruction. The computational abilities of microcomputers make it possible for good programs to provide immediate, cumulative evaluations of student performance. The program should provide a meaningful description of how well the student has learned and if there are content areas that require further study. Check to determine if these evaluations can be retained so that the classroom teachers can review student progress.

Source: Petosa, R., Gillespie, T.: Microcomputers in Health Education: Characteristics of Quality Instructional Software. *Journal of School Health,* *54,* 10, November, 1984, pp. 394–96. © 1984, American School Health Association, Kent, OH 44240.

Television and Videotape

Most school systems have access to television receivers. Many fine health-related programs, designed with the elementary school child in mind, are available. These include "Sesame Street," "Mr. Rogers' Neighborhood," and various special programs. Both the Public Broadcasting Service (PBS) and National Educational Television (NET) regularly provide programs that can be used in health education. The commerical networks also occasionally produce suitable programs.

In addition to scheduled broadcasts, public and commercial agencies also make many programs available on film or videotape. For example, *Bread and Butterflies* is a series of 15 fifteen-minute films available from the Agency for the Instructional Television (1974). The films deal with children's lives in the world of work and emphasize self-image. *Inside-Out,* available from the National Instructional Television Center (1973), is a series of 30 fifteen-minute films or videotapes that explores the feelings of youngsters between the ages of 8 and 10. Social, emotional, and physical concerns are all sympathetically examined. *Self-Incorporated,* produced by the Agency for Instructional Television (1975) is a similar series of 15 fifteen-minute programs designed for 11 to 13 years olds.

Making your own videotapes for health instruction is also a useful approach, although an expensive one because of the equipment involved. If your school has the equipment, however, you should consider using it. Record class plays, skits, and sociodramas. Also suggest that students produce their own health public service messages or "commercials" for use in conjunction with consumer health discussions.

Films

Most films used in the classroom are 16mm, although 8mm films conveniently spooled on cassettes are also available. A special projector is necessary for their use, but they have the advantage of being able to be viewed by students with limited teacher supervision. Standard 16mm films use a regular 16mm projector, a piece of equipment virtually every school has access to.

In considering films as instructional devices, keep in mind that a film should not serve as the sole basis of instruction and that every film must be carefully chosen and previewed. Mayshark and Foster (1972, pp. 288–289) suggest that teachers ask themselves the following questions when selecting films.

1. Is the film interesting and appropriate to the age and grade level?
2. Does the film convey the desired facts and concepts and is it likely to contribute to the formation of desirable attitudes?
3. Is the film accurate and up to date?
4. Can the film be correlated with and integrated into the course of study at the particular grade level?
5. Is the language well suited to the intended audience?
6. Is the film likely to be understood by students?
7. Does it meet reasonable standards of technical excellence in terms of good quality pictures, satisfactory sound, and natural acting?
8. Is the film of suitable length?
9. Are there commercial overtones that are distasteful and detract from the educational message?

Film/Filmstrip Preview

Title _____ Date Previewed _____

16mm _____ 8mm _____ Filmstrip _____ Color _____ B/W _____

Slide _____ VCR tape _____ Sound   yes _____ no _____

Producer _____ Date   _____

Length _____

Theme _____
_____

Grade level _____

Where obtained _____
_____
_____

Strengths _____
_____
_____
_____

Weaknesses _____
_____
_____

Addition points of importances _____
_____
_____

	Excellent								Poor	
Rating	10	9	8	7	6	5	4	3	2	1

Figure 5.3
Front and back of a film review card.

Keep a card file of all films that you preview. An example of a typical card entry is shown in Figure 5.3. Such recordkeeping will help you build an index of especially useful films and will warn you away from inappropriate ones.

Filmstrips

Filmstrips are continuous strips of 35mm pictures. Captions or an accompanying sound track on a tape cassette provide the narrative. Filmstrips are colorful, relatively inexpensive, easy to use, and easy to store because they take up little space. The same criteria for selecting films should be used with filmstrips.

In addition to commercially prepared filmstrips, kits are available for classroom preparation of original filmstrips. This is an activity that upper elementary school children enjoy and find highly motivating. Title and topics for original filmstrips might include *Ways of Keeping My Body Healthy, Community Health Helpers,* and *Waste Disposal in the Community.*

Slides

Another inexpensive medium is 35mm slides. These can be purchased from commercial sources or you can make them yourself if you have a 35mm camera and a bit of photographic skill. Like filmstrips, slides are colorful and easy to store. Depending upon the kind of projector system you have, one slide tray will hold from 40 to more than 100 two-by-two inch slides.

If you make your own slides, subject matter can include class activities and field trips, health fairs, environmental problems in the community, and class projects. An advantage to using slides is that you can delete or add slides to the sequence as you desire. In this way, you can keep your slide collection current.

Transparencies

Used with an overhead projector, transparencies are extremely popular as teaching tools. A transparency consists of a ten-by-ten inch sheet of transparent acetate usually mounted in a thin cardboard frame. Prepared transparencies can be purchased or you can make your own, either by using special transparency masters or by simply drawing on the acetate with felt-tipped pens. Both permanent and erasable inks are available.

One unique feature of a transparency is the ability to show progression by using a series of overlays. Overlays can also be employed to show the position of organs within the body or to add or remove captions for informal quizzes. Another advantage to using transparencies is that the classroom does not have to be entirely darkened, as in the case of films or filmstrips.

Records and Tape Recordings

Selectively used, records and tape recordings can be valuable teaching tools. Both are inexpensive and can be stopped for purposes of discussion. Finding useful records may take some work on your part, however, as not that many are available that relate directly to health instruction.

Tape recordings are in some ways more versatile. You can easily make recordings of radio and television programs, for example, or of interviews with health officials, classroom guest speakers, and so forth. Recording commercials for classroom use can be useful when teaching consumer health. Tape cassettes are even more portable than records and have the advantage of being scratchproof.

Selecting Appropriate Media

Which of the many available media should you use for a particular instructional situation? How should you prepare yourself and your students for the medium that you have chosen? These are important questions that you must ask yourself before using television, films, tape cassettes, or any other instructional medium. Kinder (1973, pp. 29–30) offers some useful guidelines:

1. Choose instructional media that fit specific objectives of the instruction. By listing your objectives first, then selecting materials that best further the attainment of those objectives, you will avoid using materials merely for the sake of using materials.

2. Prepare yourself in advance. Once you have selected the media you will use for your lesson, familiarize yourself with them and consult study guides and manuals. Further, integrate the materials you have chosen into your lesson plan, considering sequence, timing, and proper coordination of all learning materials used.

3. Prepare the class in advance. Student readiness ensures an atmosphere conducive to assimilation. Discuss with the class in advance the materials to be used, by name, type, source, and so forth. Make the students aware of the reasons for using those particular materials. Suggest things to look for and associations to consider. Introduce any new or unusual words, phrases, or symbols. Also, explain any negative features of the material beforehand.

4. Prepare the physical facilities in advance. Although students are a captive audience, they are entitled to the use of all learning materials under optimum conditions. All equipment and media should be ready before the class assembles and should be in good working order. Alternative material should be available in case of breakdown. Schedule student equipment operators, if used, and be sure that you and/or the student operator knows how to operate the equipment easily. Attend to seating arrangements, screen placement, lighting control, sound volume, and similar considerations.

5. Ensure student participation either before, during, or after the presentation. The actual degree of participation will depend on the type of material used, their purpose, and the students' age or grade levels. Audio material does not necessarily eliminate student discussion, for example.

6. Follow up the use of instructional media with related activities and an evaluation of the materials by the class. Help the students solidify associations and conclusions and encourage them to summarize the content. You might test the students on the lesson or repeat the use of the media presentation if necessary. Follow-up projects might involve individual students, committees, the entire school, or even the community.

7. Evaluate the materials that you have used. Judge how well the materials did the job they were intended to do. Consider whether the students responded positively. Then ask yourself what other materials, if any, might do a better job.

SUMMARY

A method is any activity or experience that the teacher uses to interpret, illustrate, or facilitate learning. Proper selection of methods is extremely important for developing interest and reinforcing learning. Keep the following points in mind when selecting instructional techniques. First, select methods that contribute to total learning. Second, the more complex the concept to be taught, the more methods that should be used to develop it. Third, proceed from simple methods and techniques to more complex ones. Fourth, include audiovisual aids whenever possible and appropriate. Fifth, don't overuse any one method.

Values clarification techniques are useful for helping students examine their feelings concerning health issues. The goal of values clarification is to provide the time and the setting for students to examine their own values; such activities should not be used for purposes of indoctrination. There are many kinds of values clarification activities. Among the most useful for elementary school children is the decision story. A decision story is a short, open-ended vignette that presents a real-life dilemma for the students to consider and offer possible solutions about. Decision stories offer a change of pace, promote student involvement, and stimulate creative thinking and decision-making skills.

Other effective methods used in health education include brainstorming, buzz groups, case studies, debate, storytelling, lecture, group, and panel discussion, and committee work. All these employ discussion to a greater or lesser degree. More action-oriented methods include dramatizations, crossword puzzles, demonstrations and experiments, exhibits, models and specimens, field trips, and games.

Instructional media are not methods in themselves, but they serve as valuable approaches for involving students in the learning process and for enriching the classroom. Examples of media include computers, television, films, filmstrips, transparencies, and tape recordings.

The decision to use any particular approach or method should be based on how effective you believe it will be in facilitating learning. Other relevant considerations include appropriateness, amount of time and expense involved, and practicality. Finally, the method or medium selected should be chosen because it offers some teaching advantage, not simply for the sake of novelty.

DISCUSSION QUESTIONS

1. What factors should you keep in mind when selecting methods for classroom use?
2. Discuss the strengths and weaknesses of values clarification techniques.
3. Describe the process for using decision stories in the classroom, from preparation of the stories to discussion and follow-up activities.
4. Select three types of discussion-oriented methods, such as brainstorming and debate, and discuss the strengths and weaknesses of each approach.
5. Select three types of action-oriented methods, such as dramatizations and field trips, and discuss the stregnths and weaknesses of each.
6. Why must discussion-oriented methods be structured for greatest effectiveness?
7. What are the critera for selecting films or filmstrips for the classroom?
8. Describe and discuss the considerations when selecting media for instructional use.
9. Select three types of media, such as computers and television, and discuss the strengths and weaknesses of each.

REFERENCES

Agency for Instructional Television. *Bread and butterflies: A curriculum guide for teachers.* Bloomington, Ind.: 1974.

———. *Guide to self-incorporated.* Bloomington, Ind.: 1975.

Curtis, J., & Papenfuss, R. *Health instruction: A task approach.* Minneapolis: Burgess, 1980.

Gold, S., & Duncan, D. Computers and health education. *Journal of School Health,* 1980, 50:503–505.

Hamrick, M., Anspaugh, D., & Smith, D. Decision making and the behavioral gap. *Journal of School Health,* 1980. 50:455–458.

Hochbaum, G., Rosenstock, I., & Kegeles, S. *Determinants of health behavior.* Washington, D.C.: White House Conference on Children of Yough, 1960.

Kinder, J. *Using instructional media.* New York: Van Nostrand, 1973.

Mayshark, C., & Foster, R. *Health education in secondary schools: Integrating the critical incident technique.* St Louis: C. V. Mosby, 1972.

National Instructional Television Center. *Inside-out.* Bloomington, Ind.: 1973.

Petosa, R., & Gillesppie, T. Microcomputers in health education: Characteristics of quality instructional software. *Journal of School Health,* 1984, 54:394–396.

Smith, D., Hamrick, M., & Anspaugh, D. Decision story strategy: Practical approach for teaching decision making. *Journal of School Health,* December 1981, 637–664.

Stone, D., O'Reilley, L., & Brown, J. *Elementary school health education.* Dubuque, Ia.: Wm. C. Brown, 1980.

Timmreck, T. Creative health education through puppetry. *Health Education,* January/February, 1978.

6. Evaluation of Health Education

We destroy the love of learning in children by encouraging them and compelling them to work for petty and contemptible rewards—gold stars, or papers marked 100 and tacked to the wall, or A's on report cards, or honor rolls, or dean's lists, or Phi Beta Kappa keys—in short, for the ignoble satisfaction of feeling that they are better than someone else. The fact is, whether a person gets high grades or low ones or even average ones has nothing to do with whether or not he is a good, a courageous, a loving, a beautiful or a worthy person. For too long now, you've been indoctrinated to believe that grades represent the measure of a person's value. But one day the fallacy of this premise will hit you.—Howard Kirschenbaum, Sidney Simon, and Rodney Napier, Wad-Ja-Get? The Grading Game in American Education

MEASUREMENT AND EVALUATION

Every instructional effort should be evaluated to determine how successful it has been. Both student learning and teacher effectiveness must be determined. The emphasis in recent years on teacher accountability has made evaluation more important than ever.

Measurement can be defined as the construction, administration, and scoring of tests (Stanley & Hopkins, 1981, pp. 3–4). Measurement generally results in quantitative data in numerical form. The various types of tests, rating scales, attitude scales, checklists, and observation techniques used in the elementary school are all forms of measurement. The resulting raw data, however, must be evaluated before the effectiveness of the instruction can be assessed. Data are not information; they are only the basis for information.

Evaluation is the process of interpreting, analyzing, and assessing the data obtained from measurement (Stanley & Hopkins, 1981, pp. 3–4). Evaluation can be either objective or subjective. It is a judgment of what the numerical measurement data actually mean. For example, if all the students in a class get a perfect score on a test, has the instruction been successful? Perhaps not. The test might have simply measured what was already known before any instruction. Or the test might have been so poorly constructed that the correct answers were obvious whether instruction had been provided or not.

Specifically, the purposes of measurement and evaluation are as follows:

1. *To assess the effectiveness of the learning activities.* Measurement and evaluation will help you to determine whether the learning activities that you have designed and employed have increased knowledge, helped clarify values or determine attitudes, and promoted decision-making skills. If not, the activities must be revised or replaced.
2. *To motivate the student.* Tests help students recognize how much learning has taken place. Pretests are useful for introducing the scope of a topic and making students aware of the material that will be covered. Posttests then chart actual student progress.
3. *To help develop the scope and sequence of teaching.* Measurement and evaluation can help you to determine the level of teaching and the order in which it should occur. For example, if you find that the knowledge level of your class is high, a simple review of the factual material may be all that is necessary before moving on to new subject matter. Or, if the factual material is known, you may decide to work next on developing attitudes toward this knowledge.

TEACHER SKILLS NEEDED FOR COMPETENT MEASUREMENT AND EVALUATION

Becoming competent in measurement and evaluation does not happen overnight. You are developing the skills that you will need now—in methods classes, in educational psychology classes, and during your student teaching. As you gain professional experience as a teacher, these skills will be sharpened. To be competent at measuring and evaluating, Ebel (1961, pp.67–71) notes that a teacher must know the following essentials:

1. The educational uses and limitations of tests
2. The criteria by which the quality of a test should be judged and how to secure evidence relating to those criteria
3. How to plan a test and write items
4. How to select a standardized test that will be effective in a particular situation
5. How to administer a test properly, efficiently, and fairly
6. How to interpret test scores correctly

The National Education Association (1955, p. 13) lists five other areas essential for competence in measurement and evaluation. They are as follows:

1. Knowledge of the typical behaviors of children in a given age group.
2. Knowledge of atypical behaviors in a given age group
3. A good grasp of the methodology used in teaching the subject matter
4. An ability to organize your observations so that you can recognize how your instruction is affecting the students
5. An ability to interpret your observations of student behavior

In health education, measurement and evaluation cannot be limited to the cognitive domain. You must also be vitally concerned with the forming attitudes and behavior patterns of your students. The emphasis in testing instruments is on quantitative measures, but these measures must also be employed to gain insight into qualitative areas. The remainder of this chapter will provide some guidelines for using measurement and evaluation effectively in the elementary health class.

STANDARDIZED TESTS

Tests for assessing the knowledge, attitudes, and practices of students can be grouped into two general categories—standardized tests and teacher-made tests. Each type has advantages and disadvantages, which you must weight when determining your testing needs.

One obvious advantage to using standardized tests is that they are already prepared. More importantly, such tests are usually carefully developed and refined before publication. A standardized test is developed by administering a prototype to large numbers of students. Poorly worded or misunderstood questions are then culled out, and a second, third, or fourth version of the test is again administered to a sample population of students.

The results are analyzed statistically so that a determination can be made that the test actually measures what it is supposed to measure. This is termed *validity*. The reliability of the test must also be determined. *Reliability* means that similar results will be obtained when the test is used with different groups of the target population. The higher the reliability of a test, the more likely it is that the test will provide accurate measurements of student learning.

Standardized tests are best used for pretesting and posttesting. First, the test is administered before instruction takes place to gauge present knowledge and attitudes. After instruction, the same test is administered again so that growth or change in student knowledge and attitudes can be assessed quantitatively by comparing pretest and posttest scores.

Solleder (1979) has described a number of standardized tests that can be used in elementary health education. Some have been developed by commercial testing services and others by university researchers.

The *AAHPERD Cooperative Health Education Test: Elementary Level—Preliminary Form,* published by Addison-Wesley, is designed for fifth and sixth graders. It consists of 50 four-option multiple choice questions pertaining to ten health content areas. Students are required to demonstrate and apply their knowledge and to use higher levels of analysis and evaluation. Reliability ranges from .85 to .91. The test takes approximately 45 minutes to administer.

The *Bicycle Safety Information Test,* developed by the National Safety Council, consists of 20 true/false items and is designed for use at the elementary level.

The *Health Practice Inventory,* developed by William A. Benbassat, is designed for first through third graders and measures health practices in ten areas. The format of the 63-item inventory is pictorial, and children respond in terms of what they do regarding each health practice.

The *Health Knowledge Test in Community Health,* developed by Bernadine Kussman at the University of California, Los Angeles, consists of 50 multiple choice items and is designed for fourth, fifth, and six graders. The test was based on objectives from the School Health Education Study (SHES). Reliability is .82.

TEACHER-MADE TESTS

Although standardized tests have the advantage of established validity and reliability, they also have certain disadvantages. First, such tests may not include items that you have provided instruction about, or they may include subject matter that you have not covered. Second, their readability levels may be too high or too low for your class. Third, they may have been normed with a target population different from the makeup of your class.

Teacher-made tests can be tailored to specific purposes and groups of students. This is a primary advantage. On the negative side, teacher-made tests may lack validity and reliability. However, as you gain experience, the tests that you develop should become increasingly good indicators of student learning and change.

In constructing tests, you must consider each of the following areas:

Validity. Does the test measure what it is supposed to measure? If you wish to determine changes in student attitudes, for example, a test that asks students for factual information will not fulfill your intent. A poorly constructed test, say one on which students give all correct or all incorrect answers, does not measure anything at all.

Reliability. Does the test measure accurately and consistently? As with reliability, you cannot do a statistical analysis of a test because the sample population, your class, is too small. However, you can gain an intuitive sense of how reliable the instrument is as you gain teaching experience. Comparing test results with classroom observations that you make will give you some idea about the reliability of the test.

Objectivity. Is the test fair to the students? For example, if the readability level is too high, students may be unable to supply correct answers even if they understand the concept being tested. If there is more than one possibly correct answer, students should not be penalized for providing reasonable alternatives. If some items are weighted more heavily than others, incorrect responses on these will lower the resulting total score even if most of the less weighted items are answered correctly.

Discrimination. Does the test differentiate between good and poor students? The range of scores on a properly constructed test should form a bell-shaped curve.

Comprehensiveness. Is the test long enough to cover the material? Keep in mind that a 50-item test may be no more comprehensive than a 10-item test if the items tap only certain areas while neglecting others.

Administration and Scoring. Is the test easy to give, use, and score? Keep in mind that the easiest test to administer and score may not be the best test for assessing the area. For example, an essay test, which is more difficult to score, may provide better assessment of certain concepts than an easier-to-score true/false test.

Paper and pencil tests are best suited for measuring student progress in the cognitive domain. Different types of tests for measurement in this area will be discussed next.

True/False Tests

A true/false test consists of declaratory statements that are either true or false. Students must decide about each test item and answer accordingly.

Advantages of the true/false test are

1. Because it is so widely used, the true/false test is familiar to students.
2. The true/false test is easy to construct, which is one reason it is used extensively.
3. It can be used to sample a wide range of subject matter. Because the items can be answered in a short time, a large number can be included on a simple test.
4. It is easy to score and the score is quite objective.
5. It can be used effectively as an instructional test to promote interest and introduce points for discussion.
6. It is versatile and can be employed for short quizzes, lesson reviews, end-of-chapter tests, and so forth.
7. Items can be constructed either as simple factual statements or as questions that require reasoning.
8. True/false items are especially useful when there are only two options concerning an issue.

Disadvantages of the true/false test are

1. A simple true/false item is of doubtful value for measuring achievement.
2. The true/false test encourages guessing. Even without any knowledge of the subject matter, a student can pick many correct answers by random choice.
3. Constructing items that are completely true or completely false without making the correct response choice obvious can be difficult.
4. Avoiding ambiguities, irrelevant details, and clues is difficult.
5. Unless the test consists of a large number of items, reliability is likely to be low.
6. Items that test for minor details receive as much credit as items that test for major points.
7. If the material is in any way controversial, true/false items are difficult to construct. For example, the following statement, while false, can give students a wrong perception: "Marijuana is not a harmful drug."
8. Sometimes the relative degree of truth in an item is debatable. Such items should be avoided because students will try to guess what is in the teacher's mind instead of making their own decisions.

As long as you keep the disadvantages of true/false tests in mind, such tests can be helpful for assessing student performance. Use the following guidelines when constructing true/false tests:

1. Approximately 60 percent of the items on a true/false test should be true.
2. Make the method for indicating responses as simple as possible. Usually, a blank to the left of the item is the best format.
3. Write original items. Do not lift statements directly from the textbook. (Using sample test questions from the teacher's guide is acceptable, however.)
4. True statements should not be consistently longer than false statements, as this provides an obvious clue.
5. Avoid ambiguous terms and qualifiers in the items, such as "many" and "few."
6. Use specific determiners carefully. Whenever you employ such terms as "no," "never," "always," "may," "should," "all," and "only," be sure that they do not make the correct answer obvious.
7. Avoid the use of negatively stated items. For example, "Not eating balanced meals is not good for your health" is a confusing statement at best. Further, the second "not" can easily be overlooked in a quick reading..
8. Make the items clear so that there is no doubt in the student's mind about what the item seeks to measure. One way to ensure clarity of purpose is to include the critical element of the item at the end of the statement. Underlining the crucial element is another way to achieve this end, but too much underlining can be distracting and may signal which statements are obviously true or false.
9. Avoid trick or catch questions. Such items are poor measures of achievement and are not fair to the student. They measure general intelligence and alertness, not understanding of the concept. For example, "Coffee contains a drug called codeine" is a trick question. The student may know that the substance in coffee is caffeine, but may read caffeine for codeine.

Following are examples of properly developed true/false items:

__T__	1. Drugs are harmful if they are abused.
__T__	2. Brushing your teeth regularly can help to prevent tooth decay.
__F__	3. Meat is a good source of vitamin C.
__T__	4. The heart and circulatory system move blood to all parts of the body.
__F__	5. A burn on the skin should be tightly bandaged.

Multiple Choice Tests

Items on multiple choice tests require the student to recognize which of several suggested responses is the best answer. This kind of test provides an opportunity to develop thought-provoking questions while covering a great deal of material at the same time. It is considered the best short-answer test format.

Advantages of the multiple choice test are

1. Items can be written to measure inference, discrimination, and judgment.
2. Items can be constructed to measure recall as well as recognition.
3. Guessing is minimized when there are three or four alternate choices.
4. Sampling of material covered can be extensive. Many questions can be included on a test because a response can be made quickly.

5. Scoring is objective. In a properly constructed item, only one possible response is correct.
6. Scoring is rapid.

Disadvantages of the multiple choice test are

1. Developing a multiple choice test is time consuming.
2. Items are too often factually based, unduly stressing memory.
3. More than one response may be correct or nearly correct.
4. It is difficult to exclude clues as to the correct response.
5. Incorrect but plausible alternative answers are often difficult to develop.
6. Items can take up a considerable amount of space.
7. The student must do a lot of reading.
8. The format does not allow students to express their own thoughts.

Use the following guidelines when developing multiple choice tests:

1. Express each item as clearly as possible, using words with precise meanings.
2. Make all choices plausible. When obviously incorrect options are included, the need to think is reduced accordingly.
3. Be sure that only one response option is correct.
4. Keep the choices short whenever possible.
5. The correct choice should be about the same length as the incorrect alternatives, not consistently longer or shorter.
6. For lower elementary school children, limit the choices to three. For upper elementary school children, use four choices.
7. Use parallel construction in developing the choices. Avoid confusing and ungrammatical items such as this one:

> Shock can cause a person to pass out because not enough blood goes to
> _____a. the brain.
> _____b. is being pumped to the heart.
> _____c. the lungs slow down.
> _____d. stomach.

Instead, be consistent in construction:

> Shock can cause a person to pass out because not enough blood goes to the
> _____a. stomach.
> _____b. brain.
> _____c. heart.
> _____d. lungs.

8. Scatter the position of the correct choices to avoid any set pattern.
9. Avoid negatively worded items. If you must include negatives, underline them so that they will not be missed.

Following are examples of properly developed multiple choice items:

> 1. Which of these nutrients helps to repair the body?
> _____a. carbohydrates
> _____b. fats
> _____c. proteins
> _____d. vitamins

2. A doctor's prescription
   _____a. is required to purchase all legal drugs.
   _____b. cannot be illegally obtained.
   _____c. is required only for certain drugs.
   _____d. need have only the name and quantity of the drug.
3. Which of these is <u>not</u> an inherited trait?
   _____a. shape of nose
   _____b. tooth decay
   _____c. blood type
   _____d. skin color

Matching Tests

Matching tests call for answers in one column to be paired with the correct item in another column. This kind of test is in effect a form of multiple choice test except that the number of choices is compounded.

The advantages of the matching test are

1. This type of test is adaptable to many subject areas.
2. It is especially useful for maps, charts, or pictorial representations.
3. It is fairly quick to develop.
4. The test format uses space economically.
5. It is easy to score.

The disadvantages of the matching test are

1. This type of test does not assess the extent to which meaning has been grasped.
2. It increases in difficulty as the number of items to be matched increases.
3. It tests only factual information.
4. It permits guessing.
5. It is likely to include clues to the correct answers.

Use the following guidelines when developing matching test items:

1. The test should cover only one subject area or topic.
2. For younger children, include no more than 10 items to be matched. For older children, 15 items should be the maximum.
3. Use the right-hand column for the response list.
4. Make sure there is only one possible correct response for each item.
5. Arrange the responses in random order.
6. Keep all items and responses on a single page.
7. Include more response options than terms to be matched.
8. Clearly and precisely word each response option.
9. Avoid providing clues to the correct matches.

Figure 6.1 shows an example of a properly developed matching test.

Completion Tests

Completion item or "fill-in" tests consist of a number of statements that have certain key words or phrases omitted. This type of test measures the student's ability to se-

---

Parts of the Ear

Match the definitions on the right with the terms on the left.
Write the LETTER of the correct definition in the blank next to the term.

_b_ 1. anvil
_d_ 2. auditory canal
_a_ 3. cochlea
_g_ 4. eardrum
_h_ 5. Eustachian tube
_e_ 6. semicircular canal

a. a snail-shaped organ found in the inner ear
b. a small bone in the middle ear
c. the most visible part of the human ear
d. a tunnel in the outer ear
e. part of the ear that gives you a sense of balance
f. a watery fluid
g. a thin, tight tissue
h. an opening that provides air from the throat to the middle ear
i. a nerve that carries sound to the brain

Figure 6.1.
Example of a matching test.

lect a word or phrase that is consistent in logic and style with the other elements in the statement. If students understand the implications of the sentence, they should be able to provide the answer that best fulfills the intent of the item.

Advantages of the completion test are

1. This type of test is easy to construct.
2. It has wide applications to testing situations presented in the form of charts or diagrams.
3. Guessing is minimized because the answer must come from the student.
4. Student writing ability is not a major factor.
5. Scoring is objective and fairly quick.

Disadvantages of the completion test are

1. This type of test stresses factual information. The result may be a collection of items calling for unrelated facts or isolated bits of information.
2. It places a premium on rote memory rather than on real understanding.
3. Phrasing an item so that only one correct response is elicited is often difficult. Alternative answers provided by students may be very close to correct, making scoring problematical.
4. In a poorly formatted completion test, answers may be scattered all over the page, as on a diagram, making scoring time consuming.
5. Clues within an item can allow students to respond correctly without understanding the concept being assessed.

Use the following guidelines when constructing completion test items:

1. Be sure that the items are phrased in language appropriate to the students' reading level.
2. Avoid lifting items directly from the text and simply inserting blanks for key words or phrases. Try to create original items so that students' reliance on rote memory is minimized.
3. Use blanks for significant words and phrases rather than for minor details.
4. For younger children, indicate the number of words needed for the correct response with spaces between the blanks.
5. Whenever possible, avoid "a" or "an" before a blank.
6. Don't begin an item with a blank if possible.
7. Keep a high ratio of words supplied to words called for.
8. When more than one correct answer is possible, put these alternatives in the scoring key if you are not scoring the test yourself.

Following are examples of properly developed completion test items:

1. Light enters your eyeball through a clear tissue called the _____.
2. The eyeball is filled with a fluid called _____ _____.
3. The iris controls the amount of _____ going to the lens behind it.

Essay Question Tests

The essay question test requires the student to organize information in a systematic fashion. Use of the essay question allows you to gain insight into the amount of understanding students have developed from your instruction.

Advantages of the essay question test are

1. This type of test is relatively easy to prepare.
2. Essay questions can be written on the chalkboard or even dictated, thus eliminating the expense of duplicating materials.
3. Originality and creativity on the part of the student is encouraged.
4. Essay questions stimulate students to organize their thinking.
5. Chances of cheating are minimized because of the amount of writing involved.
6. Answers to essay questions help reveal the individuality of students. Questions can invoke a variety of responses that reflect personal attitudes, values, habits, and differences.
7. Guessing at answers is reduced to a minimum.
8. Essay questions are the best-known way of evaluating the qualitative aspects of verbal expression of thought.

Disadvantages of the essay question test are

1. Determining reliability is difficult because different teachers will score essay answers in different ways.
2. Scoring is rather subjective and is unconsciously influenced by such factors as legibility, neatness, grammar, spelling, word choice, and bluffing.
3. Scoring is time-consuming.

4. Student with poor writing skills are at a disadvantage.
5. Writing essay answers is time consuming and students may feel pressured by this type of test. Slow writers are not necessarily slow thinkers, but this may be the impression given.
6. Younger children have particular difficulty in formulating and writing answers to essay questions.
7. An essay question test can sample only a limited amount of the material covered.

Use these guidelines when preparing an essay question test:

1. Develop questions that will help you assess critical thinking skills rather than retention of facts.
2. Begin with relatively easy questions. Difficult items at the beginning of the test discourage less able students.
3. Phrase the questions specifically enough so that students know what kind of a response is being asked for. However, avoid focusing too narrowly so that a mere listing of facts is called for.
4. Limit the number of questions so that students do not feel overly pressured and have adequate time to complete each answer.

Following are examples of properly developed essay questions:

1. In what ways do the eyes and hands work together as a team?
2. Why are many people against the use of nuclear power?
3. What advice would you give to a friend who has trouble getting along with a younger brother or sister?
4. How do television commercials try to get you to buy certain products? Pick one television commercial and tell how it tries to get you to buy that product.

MEASURING HEALTH ATTITUDES

The need to measure attitudes is greater in health education than in perhaps any other subject area. Remmers et al. (1965,p. 308) defines attitude as "an emotionalized tendency, organized through experience, to react positively or negatively toward a psychological object." In other words, an attitude involves feelings, values, and appreciations. An attitude can also be described as a predisposition to actions. Because one of your goals in teaching health is the development of positive health attitudes, you must assess current student attitudes.

This is no easy matter because attitudes are not within the cognitive domain and are not thus readily tapped by most kinds of tests. Even those that are designed for this purpose often lack validity, as students may respond with answers they think the teacher will favor rather than by stating their true feelings or predispositions. Thus it is important to supplement such testing instruments with other means of assessment, such as observation, informal conferences, and anecdotal record-keeping. With these limitations in mind, we will now examine some of the more common written measures for assessing student attitudes.

	Agree	Disagree
1. Brushing teeth daily is important.	_____	_____
2. Keeping my face and hands clean makes me feel better.	_____	_____
3. Smiling makes me feel good.	_____	_____
4. Smoking can lead to serious disease.	_____	_____
5. Anger can sometimes be a useful and healthy emotion.	_____	_____

Figure 6.2
Example of a forced choice attitude scale.

Attitude Scales

A scale is a testing instrument that requires the student to choose between alternatives on a continuum. Only two polar choices, such as yes-no or agree-disagree may be offered, or a range of choices between the extremes may be provided.

Figure 6.2 shows a *forced choice test,* a scale that provides only two options about each statement being considered. This kind of attitude scale is appropriate for use with younger children, who lack the developmental ability to handle more complicated attitude scales.

The major disadvantage of the forced choice test is that students can readily perceive what the "correct" response should be. They will respond accordingly even if the answer does not reflect their actual attitude toward the issue. This problem can be overcome to a certain degree by establishing an atmosphere in the classroom of warmth, trust, and rapport.

A *Likert scale* is a more sophisticated attitude scale that provides a range of choices about each attitudinal issue. The more choices that are offered, the more discrimination a student must have to complete the scale. Therefore Likert scales for younger children may offer only three choices, as in Figure 6.3, while scales for older children may offer five choices, as in Figure 6.4.

Scoring may be done in a variety of ways, depending on how the statements in the scale are phrased. For example, the continuum of responses may be weighted from 1 to 5, with the lowest score for a Strongly Disagree statement and the highest score for a Strongly Agree statement. Thus if a student checks Strongly Agree to the statement, "Being stoned all the time is no way to live," the score would be a 5. An Undecided response would rate a 3, and a Strongly Disagree would rate a 1. Note that the scoring rank must be reversed for oppositely worded statements, such as, "Experimenting with drugs is not really very risky." In this case, a Strongly Disagree response would score as a 5.

The total numerical score derived from adding the individual response scores offers a measure of how firmly opinions and attitudes are held about the issues examined in the scale. However, this measure, despite its seeming quantitative precise-

Feelings about Exercise

	Agree	Not Sure	Disagree
1. Exercise is good for a person.	_____	_____	_____
2. I like to run and jump.	_____	_____	_____
3. I would rather watch TV than play outside.	_____	_____	_____
4. I feel relaxed after exercising.	_____	_____	_____
5. Playing sports is fun.	_____	_____	_____
6. Riding my bike gives me good exercise.	_____	_____	_____
7. Playing sports and games is too much work.	_____	_____	_____
8. I would rather watch sports than play them.	_____	_____	_____
9. Exercise helps keep me healthy.	_____	_____	_____
10. Running games help make my muscles strong.	_____	_____	_____

Figure 6.3.
A Likert scale with a three-choice spread.

ness, is only a rough indicator of attitude. Bear in mind that the scoring system is arbitrary, that even with five options students are still making forced choices, and that students may respond with "correct" answers that do not actually reflect their true attitudes. Instruments used for attitude assessment should not be used for purposes of grading because this will further bias the students' responses.

Observation and Anecdotal Record-Keeping. As mentioned earlier, the use of attitude scales to assess student feelings and values has its limitations. The results of such scales are often inconclusive. Scales or other measurement devices, such as checklists or student surveys, should be augmented with other techniques, including observation and anecdotal record-keeping.

Observation is an excellent way of assessing behavior, especially when other school personnel and parents are brought into the process. Because observation can be done on an ongoing, daily basis, it can provide important clues as to attitudes and predispositions to actions. A major disadvantage of observation is that it is time-consuming. Further, you must exercise discretion so as not to violate student and parent privacy.

Anecdotal record-keeping goes hand in hand with observation. As with that technique, a disadvantage is the time that it requires. Additionally, both observation and record-keeping are subjective techniques. Your evaluation can be based on your own biases or expectations. Cultural differences can also slant your conclusions. In

Substance Abuse

	Strongly Agree	Agree	Undecided	Disagree	Strongly Disagree
1. Drug abuse can kill you.	————	————	————	————	————
2. Being stoned all the time is no way to live.	————	————	————	————	————
3. Smoking is a difficult habit to break.	————	————	————	————	————
4. Because smoking is enjoyable, it is worth the risk to good health.	————	————	————	————	————
5. Alcohol is a drug.	————	————	————	————	————
6. Using alcohol can lead to serious personal problems.	————	————	————	————	————
7. Experimenting with drugs is not really very risky.	————	————	————	————	————
8. Marijuana is a harmless drug.	————	————	————	————	————
9. Taking drugs is a copout.	————	————	————	————	————
10. Most of what you hear about drugs from teachers is not true.	————	————	————	————	————
11. Heroin use can ruin a person's life.	————	————	————	————	————
12. Drugs are a poor way of coping with problems.	————	————	————	————	————
13. Some people can use heroin without getting hooked on it.	————	————	————	————	————
14. Illegal drugs can be dangerous because you never know what is in them.	————	————	————	————	————

Figure 6.4
A Likert scale with a five-choice spread.

preparing to do anecdotal records, Mehrens and Lehmann (1984, p. 231) make the following suggestions:

1. The teacher should restrict her observations to those behaviors that cannot be evaluated by other means. Anecdotal records should be restricted to those situations from which we wish to obtain data on how the pupil behaves in a natural situation.

2. Records should be complete. There are several different styles of anecdotal records. All, however, contain the following parts: (a) identifying information—pupil's name, grade, school, and class; (b) date of the observation; (c) the setting; (d) the incident; and (e) the signature of the observer. Some contain a section for the interpretation and recommendation for action.

3. Anecdotal records should be kept by all teachers and not be restricted to only the child's homeroom teacher. The validity of the anecdotal record will be enhanced with a variety of common information gathered from different sources.

4. The behavioral incident or action should be recorded as soon as possible after it has happened. It should be remembered that any lapse of time places heavy reliance on the teacher's memory, which may become blurred if too much time elapses.

5. Keep the anecdote specific. Just as too little information does not help much in having a better understanding of a pupil's behavior, too much information can cloud the real issue.

6. Keep the recording process simple.

7. Keep the anecdote objective.

8. Anecdotal records could be compiled on slips of paper, cards, or any material readily handy. We recommend that some standard form be used for filing. Also, we recommend *against* using slips of paper, since they can be easily lost or misplaced. A large sheet of paper is preferred because it permits the teacher to write her interpretation on the same sheet as the description of the setting and incident.

9. Anecdotes should have interpretive value. A jumbled collection of anecdotes is of little value. They must be collated, summarized, and interpreted. If, for example, Ilene has only one record of aggressiveness, this is inconsequential. On the other hand, if Ilene has been observed to display aggressive behavior on 9/6, 9/14, 10/12, 10/13, and 11/21, in a variety of different settings, this behavioral pattern does become significant.

10. Anecdotal records must be available to specified school personnel. We have already indicated that we feel strongly that the anecdotal record should be shared with other teachers and especially with the school counselor if there is one. Also, this material should be incorporated in the student's folder with other test information. We also believe that a general summary should be shared with the parents, and with the pupil if he is old enough to understand it. Other than for school personnel, parents, and the students, the anecdotal record should be considered as confidential information.

11. Anecdotal records as an educational resource should be emphasized. Because anecdotal records depend so heavily on the willingness of teachers to do a good job, it is essential that teachers develop an appreciation for the value of anecdotal records in helping them obtain a better understanding of their pupils. (Indirectly, this should result in the development of better-adjusted students.)

12. Anecdotal records should not be confined to recording negative behavior patterns. In fact, the anecdotal record should record significant behaviors re-

Name _____   Date of
                                    Grade _____
Observation _____

Observer _____

Directions: Listed below are a list of characteristics related to "Respect for Others." For the student listed, check those characteristics that are appropriate.

_____ Respects views and opinions of others
_____ Is sensitive to needs of others
_____ Is sensitive to problems of others
_____ Respects the property of others
_____ Works cooperatively with others
_____ Addresses others in a respectful manner

Figure 6.5
Observation checklist for assessing respect for others.

gardless of their direction. Only in this way can the teacher obtain a valid composite picture of the student.

13. As in writing good test items, the teacher should have practice and training in making observations and writing anecdotal records.

In assessing student health attitudes, attempt to remain neutral in your observations. Variations in personal health attitudes and behaviors are not necessarily a cause for concern. Also keep in mind that children are still forming their attitudes about health-related issues. Thus you cannot expect them to have completely made up their minds about health practices. If they had, there would be far less point to your job.

Further, remember that attitude formation is a gradual process. Do not expect instant changes in behavior patterns, but do not despair. Your efforts can make a difference. With these thoughts in mind, a method you can use to help assess attitudes is the checklist. The checklist allows you, the observer, to note quickly and effectively if a trait or characteristic is present. Checklists can be useful in evaluating learning activities or some aspects of personal-social interaction. Figure 6.5 is a checklist for evaluating student behavior after a unit on respect for others.

As we have seen, measuring attitudes is difficult. Any technique used to measure and evaluate their attitudes or health practices should not be used for grading. If this is done, students will be even less likely to reveal their true feelings or their actual practices. Instead, use your evaluation to plan for future instruction and to help students understand their current level of development. The more aware they become about their own selves, the more likely it is that they will use this awareness to make conscious decisions about future behavior.

GRADING IN THE ELEMENTARY SCHOOL

Grades serve to inform students, parents, teachers, and administrators about the progress and work efficiency of the child. Ideally, grades should not be an end in themselves. Instead, they should act as motivators for students to do their best and as guides to future courses of study. For parents, student grades identify the child's strengths and weaknesses and also help clarify the goals of the school. If parents gain insight through grades as to what the school is attempting to accomplish, they will be in a better position to cooperate with the teacher in enhancing the child's education. Administrators can use grades to see how effective the curriculum is and to step in to provide extra help for students who need it by means of special programs, counseling, and so forth.

Each school district has its own approach to grading. Your task is to become familiar with the system used in your district so that you can apply the standards objectively and fairly. Two traditional grading methods widely used are the percentage method and the A to F combination method.

The Percentage Method

This grading method is based on 100%. It assumes more preciseness than can actually exist and essentially reduces the range of scores from 70 to 100. Any student falling below 70% fails. Most school districts that employ this method use a scale similar to the following one:

93–100 = A
85–92 = B
78–84 = C
70–77 = D
Below 70 = F

The A to F Combination Method

This system of grading is a combination of the percentage method and other descriptors that indicate student performance. With this method, students can be rated in relation to the group norm as well as to personal development. The A to F combination method better enables students and parents to know whether learning and work are being accomplished at peak capacity. For example, it is possible for students to make a C grade and still have them appreciate that they are working near maximum effort. A typical example of how this method is structured is as follows:

A = Doing excellent work and working at or near capacity; 95 to 100%
B = Good work and working at or near capacity; 85 to 94%
C = Average work or all that should be expected; 77 to 84%
D = Much less than should be expected; 70 to 76%
F = No noticeable progress; less than 70%
1 = Above grade level
2 = At grade level
3 = Below grade level

The numbers can be used in conjunction with the letter grades. For example, a child who receives a grade of B-2 is performing near capacity at grade level, while a child who receives a grade of B-3 is performing near capacity, but below grade level.

Other Grading Procedures

Some school districts use symbols for giving grades in health education. Most of the symbols are used to indicate a level of achievement. It is very hard for students and parents to interpret what the level of achievement indicates unless there is some information about that level (Mehrens and Lehmann, 1984). Some of the symbols used to indicate achievement are O, S, and U for outstanding, satisfactory, and unsatisfactory. The symbols P and F are also used to indicate pass or fail, while others may use E, S, N, or U (excellent, satisfactory, not satisfactory and unsatisfactory).

One of the unfortunate results is that any course using these symbols may be viewed as less important than those courses receiving the traditional A-F grades. Certainly, in the case of health education, this connotation must be avoided, because the knowledge, attitudes and behaviors developed have the potential to be life-enhancing and, in some cases, life-saving.

There are no easy answers in choosing a grading system. The best method is really a combination of systems. Each teacher and school system must weigh the advantages of each type of grading and select the one which best informs students and parents of progress.

SUMMARY

The purpose of measurement and evaluation is to assess the progress of students, to determine whether instructional objectives have been fulfilled, and to provide for planned changes in the teaching process. Measurement involves the construction, administration, and scoring of tests. Evaluation is the process of interpreting, analyzing, and assessing the data gathered during the measurement phase.

Teachers must be able to develop, administer, score, and interpret valid and reliable tests. Test instruments are best suited for measuring in the cognitive domain, but methods must also be employed to assess attitudes and actions. Either standardized or teacher-made tests can be used for measurement purposes. Both have their advantages and disadvantages, strengths, and weaknesses. The biggest advantage to using standardized tests is that they have been carefully developed and normed, ensuring a high degree of validity and reliability.

In many ways, teacher-made tests are more useful for day-to-day measurement. Among the types of teacher-made tests are true/false, matching, completion, and essay question tests. Each has its own strengths and weaknesses, which the teacher must consider beforehand. For example, true/false tests are easy to prepare, administer, and score but allow guessing and do not test critical reasoning very deeply.

Measurement and evaluation of attitudes is difficult. Attitude scales, checklists, and student surveys are of some help, but these methods should be supplemented by observation and anecdotal record-keeping. The biggest problem in using any sort of attitude scale is that students may not reveal their true attitudes, even if an atmosphere of trust and rapport has been established.

Grading can take many forms. Two traditional techniques are the percentage method and the A to F combination method. Pass-fail or satisfactory-unsatisfactory marks may also be used.

DISCUSSION QUESTIONS

1. Differentiate between measurement and evaluation.

2. Discuss the purposes of measurement and evaluation and explain how you can achieve these purposes.

3. What are some of the shortcomings of standardized tests?

4. What are some of the shortcomings of teacher-made tests? Give specific examples from various types of teacher-made tests.

5. What characteristics should a good cognitive test have?

6. Discuss some of the techniques used to assess attitude in health education. What are the shortcomings of these techniques?

7. What purposes does grading serve in health education?

8. Discuss the three most common methods of grading used in the elementary school. Explain the details of each method.

REFERENCES

Ebel, R. L. *Improving the competence of teachers in educational measurement.* Clearinghouse, 1961.

Mehrens, W. A., and Lehmann, I. J. *Measurement and Evaluation.* New York: Holt, Rinehart and Winston, 1984.

National Education Association, National Commission of Teacher Education and Professional Standards. *The improvement and use of tests by teachers: Implications for teacher education.* Washington, D.C.: The Commission, 1955.

Remmers, H. H., Gage, N. L. & Rummel, J. F. *A practical introduction to measurement and evaluation.* New York: Harper & Row, 1965.

Solleder, M. K. *Evaluation instruments in health education.* Washington, D.C.: American Alliance for Health, Physical Education and Recreation, 1979.

Stanley, J. C., & Hopkins, K. D. *Educational and psychological measurement and evaluation.* Englewood Cliffs, N. J.: Prentice-Hall, 1981.

7. Body Systems

If anything is sacred the human body is sacred, And the glory and sweet of a man is the token of manhood untainted, And in a man or woman a clean, strong, firm-fibred body is more beautiful than the most beautiful face. Have you seen the fool that corrupted his own live body? or the fool that corrupted her own live body? For they do not conceal themselves, and cannot conceal themselves.—Walt Whitman, "I Sing the Body Electric," Leaves of Grass

A UNIQUE MACHINE

The human body is a most amazing and well-organized machine. The body functions 24 hours a day, day in and day out, for an entire lifetime, with relatively few breakdowns. What other mechanism can boast of such a performance record—70 years or more of nonstop operation?

At birth, individuals are given the physical structures in which they must live. They have little control over genetic factors that program appearance and physiological functioning. For the most part, however, people begin life with sound, healthy bodies. Therefore it is ultimately up to each of us to learn ways in which to sustain and improve our physical well-being; health and health enhancement can certainly never be achieved without keeping the body and its systems in good condition.

This chapter is designed to provide you with information you can use to help children learn about their bodies. The chapter presents a brief outline and description of each of the major systems of the body and discusses how these systems function. We will examine the nervous, endocrine, respiratory, circulatory, digestive/excretory, and skeletal/muscular systems. The reproductive system will be covered in chapter 19.

THE NERVOUS SYSTEM

Because all physiological functions and many psychological ones as well are controlled in one way or another by the brain, discussion of the nervous system and its structure is a logical and appropriate beginning. The nervous system is composed of two major divisions—the central nervous system and the autonomic nervous system. The central nervous system includes the brain and the spinal cord. The autonomic nervous system includes the peripheral portions of the outlying nerves and nerve pathways not directly connected to the central nervous system.

The Central Nervous System

In conjunction with the sensory systems of the body, such as those responsible for vision and hearing, the central nervous system (CNS) plays the chief role in alerting and guiding individuals through their environments and making interaction with the world around them possible. The central nervous system allows us to perceive, interpret, and react to the various stimuli we come into contact with every day. For example, a message from the ears travels by way of the auditory nerve to the hearing center in the brain, or vice versa.

The Brain and Spinal Cord.   The brain is the "computer center" of the central nervous system. It receives messages from and sends messages to the rest of the body by way of nerves and nerve pathways that originate in the spinal cord and branch to all other organs and tissue. The general structure of the brain and spinal column is shown in figure 7.1.

The human brain, weighing about two pounds in an adult, is the center for memory, motor activity, and thinking. It contains about 13 billion brain cells. These cells have a greater need for oxygen and are more sensitive to oxygen deprivation than any other cells in the body. The soft, spongy, highly delicate, and complex brain is enveloped in three protective membranes called *meninges,* as is the spinal cord. Along with the meninges that cover it, the brain is encased and protected by the *cranium,* or skull. The spinal cord is enclosed and protected by 33 bones known as vertebrae, which are flexibly joined together to form the spinal column. The cord itself is about three-quarters of an inch in diameter and about 18 inches long in an adult. It is cylindrical and divided into two lateral halves that contain 31 pairs of ventral (front) and 31 pairs of dorsal (back) branches or roots, as shown in figure 7.2. Each ventral root contains a large number of fibers that merge with the fibers of the adjoining dorsal root to form a spinal nerve. Each of these 31 spinal nerves, in turn, divides into many more branches that serve a particular part of the body (Asimov, 1963).

Like the spinal cord, the brain is divided into parts. The major parts are the *cerebrum, cerebellum,* and *brain stem.*

The Cerebrum.   The largest part of the human brain, the cerebrum is the center for conscious mental processes. Thought and the ability to learn and reason originate in this part of the brain. In addition, all six of the sensory systems, as well as motor movement and coordination, are controlled by the cerebrum.

The cerebrum is divided into two halves called *cerebral hemispheres* in such a way that the left hemisphere controls the right side of the face and body, while the right hemisphere controls the left side of the face and body. The interior of the cerebral hemispheres is lined with white cells. These cells are covered by an exterior mantle of gray matter or *cortex.* Millions and millions of neurons are arranged in the

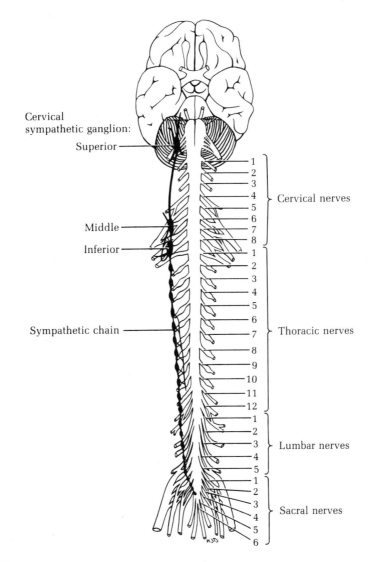

Cervical
sympathetic ganglion:
Superior

Middle

Inferior

Sympathetic chain

Cervical nerves

Thoracic nerves

Lumbar nerves

Sacral nerves

Figure 7.1
The brain and spinal column.

cortex in six layers that differ from one another in density of cell population, size, shape, distribution, and arrangement of cell processes (Campbell, 1965). At numerous points, the gray matter dips down into the brain, forming folds or convolutions that give much of the brain its wrinkled appearance. As a result of the increased surface area due to these convolutions, the amount of gray matter is greatly increased. This accounts for the much greater intellectual ability of humans as opposed to other organisms.

Since a specific area of the cerebrum controls a specific function, brain damage to a portion of the cerebral cortex may impair one sensory system to varying degrees without harming others. For example, a person's sense of taste, smell, and hearing

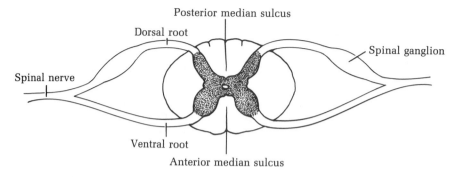

Figure 7.2
A cross section of the spinal cord.

may be damaged without motor coordination, speech, and vision being adversely affected. Or, memory may be diminished without loss of sensation to touch, and so on. The various control centers of the cerebrum are illustrated in figure 7.3. A frontal view of the brain is shown in figure 7.4.

The Cerebellum. Like the cerebrum, the cerebellum consists of two hemispheres that have an exterior of gray matter covering an interior of white fibrous cells. The cerebellum has two main functions—coordination of muscle groups, and maintenance of equilibrium. Damage to the cerebellum may result in jerky or spastic movements. A person may walk with a stagger, as if intoxicated, but memory loss and sensory impairment may not exist since these functions are mainly controlled by

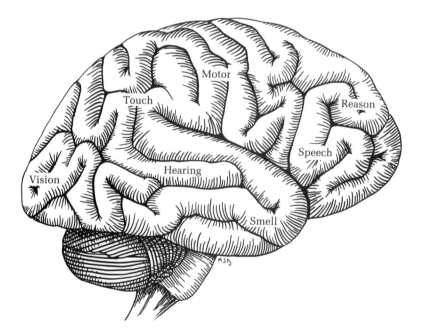

Figure 7.3
The control centers of the brain.

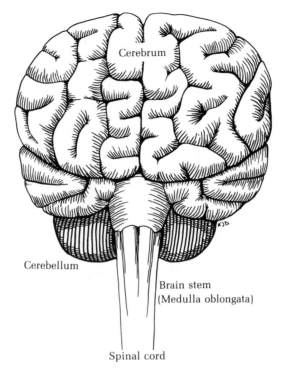

Cerebrum

Cerebellum

Brain stem
(Medulla oblongata)

Spinal cord

Figure 7.4
A frontal view of the brain.

the cerebrum. Conditions such as motion sickness and vertigo may also have some relation to cerebellum functioning (Tuttle & Schotelius, 1969).

As an example of the differing roles of the cerebrum and the cerebellum, a conscious decision to perform a task such as bicycling originates in the cerebrum, but the messages sent to the specific muscle groups that perform the task originate in the cerebellum. The directions for accomplishing the task, once it is learned, are then stored in the cerebellum until a conscious order arises from the cerebrum to initiate the task once again.

The Brain Stem.   As the name implies, the brain stem is a tubelike structure located at the base of the brain. It is the oldest or most primitive part of the human brain and is the center of physiological responses that do not require conscious thought or action in order to be performed. Circulation, respiration, and blood pressure are controlled by the brain stem, as are responses to sensory signals from the internal organs, such as hunger and thirst. In addition, fear, anger, and other emotional reactions are triggered in the brain stem.

In essence, the brain stem is a cylinder of nerve tissue that acts as a conductor between the spinal column and the cerebrum. Of the 12 pairs of cranial nerves arising from the brain, all but one do so from the brain stem itself. (The first cranial nerve, the olfactory nerve, arises from the cerebrum.) The actual connection between the spinal cord and the brain is found at the *medulla oblongata,* the very bottom of the brain stem. In fact, the spinal cord can be thought of as an long extension of the brain stem (Woodburne, 1983).

The Autonomic Nervous System

The second major division of the nervous system is the autonomic nervous system. Reflexes, as well as the physiological adaptations the body makes as a whole to its external environment, are largely controlled by skeletal muscles. These functions fall under the jurisdiction of the autonomic nervous system. In addition, the autonomic nervous system helps to regulate the internal environments of various vital organs.

THE ENDOCRINE SYSTEM

Closely associated with the nervous system is the endocrine system. The endocrine system's role is that of a regulator. Through the production and secretion of chemical substances called *hormones* from 13 tiny glands dispersed throughout the body, the endocrine system keeps the other body systems and processes in balanced operation.

The two "controller" glands of the endocrine system are the hypothalamus and the pituitary. They secrete hormones that in turn signal other endocrine glands to ac-

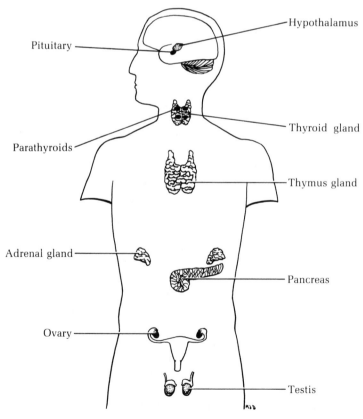

Figure 7.5
The endocrine system.

tivate. Both the hypothalamus and the pituary glands are located in the brain, thus establishing the close relationship between the endocrine system and the nervous system. Other glands of the endocrine system include the pineal, thyroid, parathyroids, thymus, adrenals, pancreas, and ovaries (in the female) or testes (in the male). The location of each of these glands is shown in figure 7.5.

The Hypothalamus

The hypothalamus is thought to be the conductor and regulator of daily operations of the body. Current research suggests that the hypothalamus is responsible for orchestrating the actions of the pituitary, which in turn triggers other endocrine glands. The hypothalamus lies in the posterior portion of the forebrain and actually consists of several separate and distinct bodies of gray matter. While scientists are still unable to explain all the actions of the hypothalamus, it is known that without signals from this master gland the pituitary would not activate, resulting in the malfunction of many normal processes.

Apart from directing the pituitary, the hypothalamus is also responsible for integrating and balancing the workings of the internal organs governed by the autonomic nervous system. The hypothalamus probably does this by exercising control over the hormonal secretions of various endocrine glands throughout the body. In addition, the hypothalamus serves as the sleep center, temperature regulating center, and appetite and hunger center for the body. Other similar centers, not clearly identified as this time, are also believed to be regulated by the hypothalamus (Ochs, 1965).

The Pituitary

Once thought to be the master gland, the pituitary is a pea-sized mass lying at the base of the brain. It is composed of three parts that, unlike the hypothalamus, are not seen spatially as separate, distinct bodies but function as separate, distinct bodies. These are the *anterior lobe,* the *posterior lobe,* and the *pars intermedia.*

Anterior Lobe. The anterior lobe is the portion of the pituitary most closely associated with the hypothalamus. It is connected to the hypothalamus through a network of specialized vessels and secretes six different hormones. With the exception of one, all other hormones produced in the anterior lobe are referred to as releasing or *trophic* hormones because they notify and affect the actions of the other endocrine glands rather than the pituitary itself.

One of the trophic hormones influences skin pigmentation and coloration by controlling chemical output of the adrenal glands. The pituitary hormone that regulates adrenal secretions in this matter is known as ACTH (adrenocorticotrophic hormone). TSH (thyroid-stimulating hormone) is another trophic hormone produced by the anterior lobe of the pituitary. It affects the thyroid by governing the rate of iodine uptake of the thyroid as well as governing the synthesis and release of thyroxin, a hormone concerned with growth and metabolism (Holmes & Ball, 1974).

The other three trophic hormones of the anterior pituitary are known as *gonadotrophins* because they trigger hormonal production from the reproductive endocrine glands. The ovaries, which are the female reproductive glands, are activated by FSH (follicle-stimulating hormone) and LH (luteinizing hormone). The testes, which are the male reproductive glands, are activated by ICSH (interstitial cell-stimulating hormone) (Turner, 1976).

The nontrophic hormone secreted by the anterior lobe of the pituitary is STH (somatotrophic hormone), sometimes referred to as HGH (human growth hormone). It is nontrophic in the sense that production does not target and trigger one endocrine gland specifically. As the name implies, somatotrophic or growth hormone is concerned with growth and development of the body as a whole and is therefore widespread in its action. Production of growth hormone is at its peak during the two periods of "growth spurt" evidenced in human development. The first spurt occurs during the first year after birth, followed by a gradual slowing until the onset of puberty. At puberty, the body once again experiences rapid development. The pubertal growth spurt for girls occurs sooner than that for boys, usually beginning between the ages of 9 to 13. For most boys, this spurt begins somewhere between ages 11 to 15. When insufficient growth hormone is produced, dwarfism may result. Excessive growth hormone may produce individuals who are abnormally large and tall (Brown & Barker, 1962).

Posterior Lobe.   The posterior lobe of the pituitary, an outgrowth of the brain stem, secretes two hormones, *oxytocin* and *vasopressin*. Oxytocin affects the smooth muscles of the uterus, particularly upon contractions during labor. It also most likely aids in conveying sperm through the uterus and into the fallopian tubes where fertilization may take place. In addition, *oxytocin* is responsible for triggering secretion of milk (not the production of milk) from the breasts during nursing (Sharrer & Sharrer, 1963).

Vasopressin has two distinct roles—one affecting circulation and the other affecting the removal of water from the body. Vasopressin causes tightening or constriction of blood vessels, producing an increase in blood pressure, which may cause problems for individuals with cardiovascular conditions. However, during hemorrhage, vasopressin probably assists in the control of bleeding by exerting pressure on vessels so as to maintain more effective circulation. Vasopression also delays urinary activity and excretion following the absorption of water (Martin, 1976).

Pars Intermedia.   The pars intermedia is the middle section of the pituitary. It does not appear to secrete hormones but rather acts as a divider between the anterior lobe and the posterior lobe.

The Pineal

Like the hypothalamus and pituitary, the pineal gland is located on the back or dorsal portion of the brain. Its function is largely unknown because it degenerates before puberty. As a result, the pineal gland in adults appears primarily as fibrous tissue. There is some evidence to suggest that the pineal gland may secrete melatonin, a substance influencing skin pigmentation, and adrenoglomerulotrophin, a substance triggering the production of aldosterone, an adrenal hormone involving kidney excretion of sodium salts (Quay, 1974).

The Thyroid

The thyroid is a butterfly-shaped gland weighing about one ounce, with each set of "wings" or lobes situated to one side of the upper trachea. It secretes two hormones, *thyrocalcitonon* and *thyroxin*. This gland also stores over half the body's iodine.

Thyrocalcitonon plays an important role in bone formation. It induces *hypercalcemia,* the production of large amounts of calcium, and is most evident and necessary in early childhood development. The importance and need for thyrocalcitonon in adults in not totally understood (Bentley, 1976).

Thyroxin has two major roles. It affects tissue differentiation during growth and development, and it influences body metabolism. The amount of thyroxin produced and secreted by the thyroid is largely influenced by the thyroid gland's ability to secure, retain, and replenish a supply of iodine.

When insufficient amounts of thyroxin are produced (hypothyroidism), growth in young children is impaired drastically, affecting skin texture, hair production, development of the reproductive organs, bone length, and mental development. Since there is also abnormal development of connective tissue, the child may appear to be extremely stocky and possibly potbellied or bowlegged along with short, thick hands and feet. The face may appear to be swollen or puffy with the tongue protruding. This condition is often referred to as cretinism. Underproduction of thyroxin in adults can cause a 30 to 45 percent reduction in the basal metabolic rate, thus producing a feeling of being cold. The heart rate is slower, blood pressure is lower than normal, and the nervous system in general becomes affected to the degree that fatigue and drowsiness are almost constant. Muscle tone also diminishes. This condition is known as myxedema. Both cretinism in children and myxedema in adults can be treated by administering thyroid extracts of thyroxin (Barrington, 1975).

Excessive secretion of thyroxin (hyperthyroidism) causes problems that produce the opposite effects. The individual becomes hyperactive and easily irritated or excited. Sleep may be difficult and restlessness persists. There is a 50 to 75 percent increase in the basal metabolic rate, producing feelings of warmth to the extent that the affected person often perspires readily. In some cases, there is protrusion of the eyeballs, with the eyelids opened widely and the pupils extremely dilated (McClintic, 1980).

The Parathyroids

Adjacent to the thyroid gland, the four parathyroids are the smallest endocrine glands in the body, each weighing about as much as a grain of rice. They govern and regulate the amount of calcium and phosphorous in the blood by manufacturing parathyroid hormone.

Insufficient amounts of parathyroid hormone (hypoparathyroidism) is most clearly evidenced in *tetany,* the jerking and twitching of muscles. Hypoparathyroidism also greatly influences the excitability of neuromuscular functioning in general (Green, 1972).

Excessive amounts of parathyroid hormone (hyperparathyroidism) can lead to bone deformities, fractures, and decalcification. Calcification of soft tissue, the kidneys in particular, can result in kidney stone, muscle weakness, nausea, loss of appetite, and constipation (Green, 1972).

The Thymus

The thymus is a short-lived gland that lies between the thyroid and the heart. It is evident at birth and is most fully developed during the early to middle teenage years.

Toward late adolescence, due to activation of the sex glands, the thymus begins to atrophy. The secretions and the functions of the thymus are not well understood, but the gland does affect in some way the manufacture of white blood cells and the production of antibodies during the immune response reactions (Villee, 1975).

The Adrenals

Set on top of the kidneys are two whitish-yellow masses, each weighing about a fifth of an ounce. These are the adrenal glands, which secrete more then 50 hormones or hormone-like substances. Anatomically, the adrenal glands consist of a deep, inner layer called the *medulla,* which is surrounded by a somewhat thinner, more rigid layer called the *cortex.* Major hormonal secretions from the medulla include epinephrine and norepinephrine. Major hormonal secretions from the cortex include glucocorticoids, mineralocorticords, and sex hormones (Eisenberg & Eisenberg, 1979).

Epinephrine (adrenalin) is the hormone responsible for the "flight or fight" response individuals display during times of great danger, anxiety, or stress. Increased production of epinephrine causes a surge in the force and rate of the heartbeat, elevation in blood pressure, heightening of sensory awareness of the environment, an increase in metabolism, and an increase in muscle strength and endurance (Friedan & Lipner, 1971).

Norepinephrine (arterenol) acts to constrict blood vessels. This hormone is thought to be solely concerned with the regulation of normal circulation (Villee, 1985).

Glucocorticords are necessary for the metabolism of fats, carbohydrates, and proteins into substances usuable by the body. The major glucocorticoid in humans is cortisol, commonly referred to as hydrocortisone (Bentley, 1976).

Mineralocorticoids primarily regulate mineral balance (especially sodium and potassium) and water balance. As a result, excretory processes of the kidneys are kept fairly constant and proper water retention is maintained in order to prevent dehydration. The major mineralocorticoid in humans is aldosterone (Best & Taylor, 1973).

Hormones like adrenosterone are chemically and functionally like the sex hormones produced by the sex glands. They activate the rise of secondary sex characteristics in both males and females. The male cortical sex hormones are predominant among both sexes even though there are both male and female cortical hormones (Kraus, 1984).

The Pancreas

The pancreas, located between the stomach and the small intestine, aids in regulating the blood sugar level through the manufacture of insulin. This hormone is produced specifically by groups of cells on the pancreas called the islets of Langerhans. When food, especially that high in carbohydrate content, is digested, the blood sugar level is elevated. Insulin is then secreted in order to lower the blood sugar by helping metabolize glucose (sugar). As glucose is used by the body for energy, the secretion of insulin subsides.

If an insufficient amount of insulin is produced by the islets of Langerhans, a chronic condition known as diabetes mellitus results. Individuals suffering from this condition must modify their diets by restricting the amount of carbohydrates they ingest daily. In addition, depending upon the severity of the insufficiency, some diabetics have to take artificial doses of insulin, either orally or by injections, so that a balanced blood sugar level can be maintained. If the blood sugar level of a diabetic remains below normal, insulin shock, characterized by extreme dizziness and weakness, will occur and death results quickly unless carbohydrates, such as juice or candy, are administered immediately. If the blood sugar level remains above normal, diabetic coma, characterized by a gradual loss of coherence over several days, will occur and death may result unless insulin is administered.

Reproductive Organs

The ovaries in the female and the testes in the male are reproductive organs that are also considered to be endocrine glands because they secrete hormones that determine sexual characteristics. A more detailed description of the reproductive system can be found in chapter 19.

THE RESPIRATORY SYSTEM

To the elementary school child, many body systems, such as the endocrine system, may appear somewhat abstract since these systems' functions take place largely unnoticed to a young observer. Nevertheless, all children at an early age can appreciate the important role that breathing plays in their lives. As a result, the respiratory system is more easily grasped at the elementary school level. Components of the respiratory system include the lungs, nose, throat or pharynx, epiglottis, esophagus, trachea, bronchi, alveoli, diaphragm, and rib cage. These components are illustrated in figure 7.6.

The Nose

The only visible part of the respiratory system is the nose. Through the nose air is inhaled into and exhaled from the body. Additionally, the nose, in which the sense of smell originates, signals olfactory nerves and can thus warn of harmful gases, and it allows drainage of secretions from the sinus cavities within the skull. However, its main function is to filter the air before it passes into the rest of the respiratory tract. The narrow passages of the nasal cavity are lined with fine hairs called *cilia* that sift bacteria and dust and carry these impurities to lymph tissue. Mucous secretions help trap bacteria and dust and also moisten the air being inhaled. The nose helps warm incoming air as well.

The Pharynx

From the nose, air moves down into the throat or pharynx. The pharynx is a funnel-like structure that begins at the base of the skull and extends to the base of the neck (Woodburne, 1983). It plays an important role in the digestive system as well as the respiratory system. The lower portion of the pharynx ends in two tubes, the esophagus and the trachea.

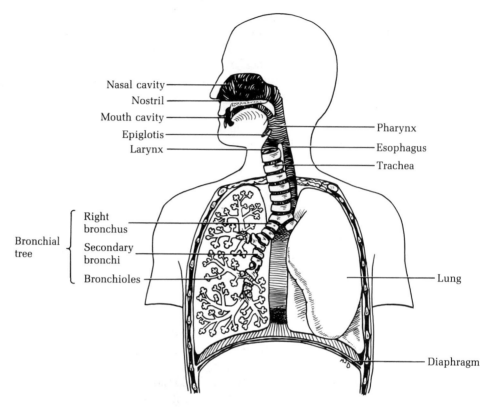

Figure 7.6
The respiratory system.

The Esophagus and Epiglottis

While the esophagus and epiglottis are primarily associated with the digestive system, they also have respiratory functions. The esophagus is the tunnel through which food is transported to the stomach. The epiglottis is a small flap of fibrous cartilage positioned just above the esophagus near the base of the tongue. When food enters the mouth and swallowing begins, the epiglottis covers the entrance to the trachea, the other tubular division of the pharynx, so that food is channeled through the esophagus, preventing choking.

The Trachea, Bronchi, and Alveoli

Inhaled air is conducted from the pharynx to the trachea, a long narrow pipe often referred to as the windpipe. Like the pharynx, the trachea branches into two smaller pipes, called *bronchi.* One bronchus extends toward the right side of the chest cavity into the right lung; the other extends toward the left side of the chest cavity into the left lung. Each bronchus continues to split into smaller and smaller tubules, called *bronchioles,* which penetrate inner lung tissue. The tiny, terminal branches of the bronchioles form enlarged air pockets called alveolar sacs that expand into various-

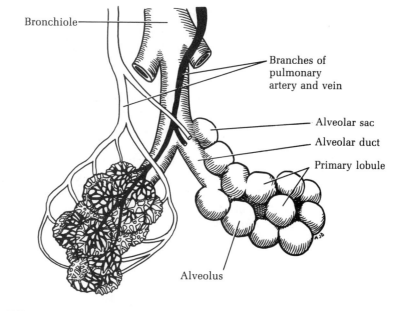

Bronchiole

Branches of
pulmonary
artery and vein

Alveolar sac

Alveolar duct

Primary lobule

Alveolus

Figure 7.7
Branching of bronchioles, alveolar sacs and alveoli into lungs.

sized *alveoli*. The alveoli are the functional units of lung tissue. Filling with air, they
inflate the lungs upon inhalation. Expelling air and carbon dioxide upon exhalation,
they deflate the lungs. (Nilsson & Lindberg, 1973). The bronchioles, alveolar sacs,
and alveoli are shown in figure 7.7.

The Lungs

The lungs, two fan-shaped structures found on each side of the chest cavity, are gas
exchange organs for the entire body. Oxygen, which makes up about 20 percent of
the air we breathe, is trapped in the alveoli and transported in the blood via the pulmonary vein back to the heart, where the oxygen-enriched blood is pumped to the
rest of the body. Conversely, blood coming from body tissue is rich in waste products,
particularly carbon dioxide. Blood from this direction is pumped from the heart into
the lung cavity via the pulmonary artery. From the lungs, carbon dioxide is then expelled from the body during exhalation by being forced back out through the respiratory tract and finally released from the nose.

Each lung is enclosed in a protective double membrane known as the *pleura*.
Sometimes the pluera, because of infection, become inflamed, causing a painful
condition called pluerisy. Other infections of the lungs and respiratory passages can
result in communicable diseases such as influenza, colds, pneumonia, or tuberculosis. Irritants of the bronchial and lung tissue like pollen, cigarette tar and gases, asbestos, coal dust, or industrial pollutants can also affect or cause a variety of respiratory ailments that vary in degree from bronchitis and allergies to emphysema and
lung cancer.

The Diaphragm and Rib Cage

Air is mechanically forced in and out of the lung cavity by means of muscular actions of the diaphragm and the rib cage. The diaphragm, a domelike sheet of muscle, separates the *thorax* or chest cavity from the abdominal cavity and is attached to the chest wall. Air is inhaled into the lungs when the rib muscles pull the rib cage upward and outward causing the diaphragm lying below it to contract and flatten. As a result, air is forced into the chest cavity so that the volume of the chest cavity increases and the lungs expand or inflate. Then, as the diaphragm moves upward, relaxing its contraction, and the rib muscles loosen, moving the rib cage downward and inward, the volume of the chest cavity decreases and the lungs deflate (Strand, 1983). This cyclical action of inhalation and exhalation is what we commonly call breathing. Breathing, or *respiration,* occurs involuntarily about 12 times a minute for adults and about 15 times a minute for children. If breathing stops because of injury, death will occur in four to six minutes. Even if breathing is resumed within a few minutes, brain damage may occur due to oxygen deprivation to the brain cells.

THE CIRCULATORY SYSTEM

Life-sustaining oxygen, provided by the respiratory system, is made available to all parts of the body through the circulatory system. The heart pumps oxygen-rich blood to all body tissue. The oxygen is exchanged for carbon dioxide and other waste products of cell functioning. Not only is blood the vehicle for gas exchange, it also aids in stabilizing body temperature, supplying nutrients, furnishing disease-fighting antibodies, transporting hormones, delivering waste products to the kidneys, and regulating the body's acid balance. Besides the heart and blood, other components of the circulatory system include the various blood vessels that carry blood from the heart to the body tissue and vice versa. An overall view of the circulatory system is shown in figure 7.8.

The Heart

The heart, positioned between the *sternum* or breastbone and spinal column, is in essence a hollow muscle about the size of a fist. By its rhythmic muscular contractions and relaxations, the heart continuously pumps blood through vessels that circulate the blood from the heart to the rest of the body and then back again. The anatomy of the human heart is illustrated in figure 7.9.

The heart lies in a pouch called the *pericardium* and is made of three layers—the *epicardium, myocardium,* and *endocardium.* The epicardium is the outermost layer. It forms the pericardium in which the heart lies and surrounds the middle heart layer, the myocardium. The myocardium composes the bulk of the muscular heart wall and is often the site for cardiac damage normally labeled "heart attack" but technically referred to as myocardial infarction. The inner wall of the heart muscle is the endocardium. It consists of a thin layer of connective tissue and smooth muscle covered by a scalelike tissue. The valves of the heart are covered by the endocardium (Best & Taylor, 1963).

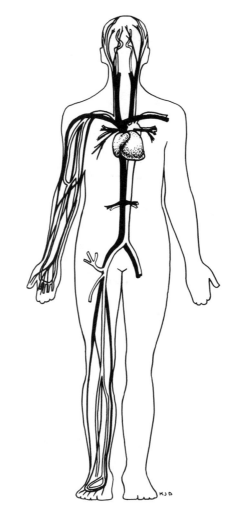

Figure 7.8
The circulatory system.

A wall of muscle also runs through the middle of the heart, separating it into two sides or chambers. The right side of the heart receives incoming blood from the body tissue and channels this blood into the lungs where it deposits carbon dioxide and picks up oxygen. The left side of the heart receives oxygen-rich blood from the lungs and pumps it to the rest of the body.

There is an upper division and a lower division of each chamber. The upper division of each chamber, called the *atrium*, is a thin-walled section that merely receives blood. The lower division of each chamber, called the *ventricle*, is a thick-walled section that exerts a strong contraction or pumping action on the blood. This contraction is associated with heartbeat or pulse.

Valves between each atrium and ventricle allow for the flow of blood from the upper section to the lower section. The tricuspid valve, composed of three flaps, is in

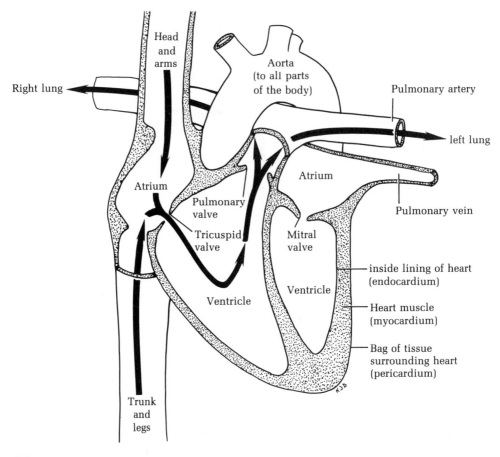

Figure 7.9
Components of the heart.

the right chamber of the heart, and the biscuspid or mitral valve, composed of two flaps, is in the left chamber of the heart. After opening to permit the flow of blood from the atrium to the ventricle, the valves close during the contraction of the ventricles so that blood cannot flow backwards into the atrium (Hole, 1986). Sometimes a malfunction of the opening and closing mechanism of the valves may occur as a result of a birth defect or illness. When this happens, some backflow can be heard with the use of stethoscope. This condition is called a heart murmur. Heart murmurs can vary in their degree of severity.

The Blood

Blood carries oxygen and nutrients to tissue and absorbs tissue waste products, transporting them to the lungs or kidneys. Heat, hormones, and antibodies are also all delivered to cells and tissue by the blood. Additionally, the blood provides the body with the proper ratio of buffer systems referred to as acid balance or pH.

Blood is made up of two major components—blood corpuscles and plasma. Corpuscles constitute about 45 percent of the total blood volume and include red blood cells or *erythrocytes,* white blood cells or *leukocytes,* and blood platelets or *thrombocytes.* Plasma, which resembles egg white, constitutes about 55 percent of the total blood volume and is 90 percent water. The remaining 10 percent is composed of blood proteins, cellular supplies such as glucose, amino acids, fats, and salts, cellular products such as hormones, antibodies, and enzymes, cellular waste products such as urea and uric acid, and gases such as oxygen, carbon dioxide, and nitrogen (Johnson, Delanney, & Cole, 1985). Because plasma is 90 percent water, many of the properties most people associate with blood, bleeding, and circulation arise mainly from functions of the blood corpuscles. In consequence, a more detailed discussion of the properties of blood corpuscles follows.

Red Blood Cells. Red blood cells, or *erythrocytes,* are the component that gives blood its color. A main function of these cells is to transport oxygen and carbon dioxide. Oxygen and carbon dioxide combine with *hemoglobin,* a protein substance that is the most important constituent of red blood cells. Since erythrocytes are the only cells in the human body that do not have a nucleus, they age rapidly, having an average life span of about four months. New red blood cells are constantly being manufactured from old, fragmented erythrocytes in the red bone marrow found in spongy bones like those of the skull, arms, ribs, and thighs (Kraus, 1984).

If either an insufficient amount of red blood cells is produced or an insufficient amount of hemoglobin is contained in the red blood cells, anemia results. People suffering from anemia have less physical strength, tire quickly both physically and mentally, have less general body resistance, and are thus more prone to illness. Several specific types of anemia exist. Sickle cell anemia, a potentially fatal inherited condition found mainly in blacks, results from the destruction of abnormally shaped (sickle-shaped) erythrocytes because of the presence of an abnormal type of hemoglobin. Pernicious anemia arises when the red blood cells that are manufactured are not only insufficient in numbers but mature abnormally and are much larger and more fragile than normal. This condition can often be alleviated by providing the anemic person with large quantities of liver and vitamin B_{12} (Keele & Neil, 1971). Nutritional anemia occurs when there is an iron deficiency in the diet. Iron deficiency anemia can be treated by increasing the ingestion of iron-rich foods.

White Blood Corpuscles. White blood cells, or *leukocytes,* are specialized blood cells that protect the body by either engulfing foreign substances that enter the bloodstream and tissue or by producing *antibodies,* specific chemical substances used to fight specific infectious diseases. The white blood cells that engulf foreign substances are called *phagocytes;* the white blood cells that produce antibodies are called *lymphocytes.* Phagocytes make up about 65 percent of all leukocytes, while lymphocytes make up the remaining 35 percent (Green, 1972). Lymphocytes are a chief component of lymph, a fluid much like blood but lacking erythrocytes that also helps fight infection. Lymph has its own separate circulation throughout the body called the *lymphatic system,* which is characterized by specialized clusters of tissue called lymph nodes located in specific body regions like the neck and under the arms.

Blood Platelets. Blood platelets, or *thrombocytes,* are tiny oval or spherical cells that are probably produced in red bone marrow. Thrombocytes are essential for the coagulation of blood. Coagulation is a complex chemical process making use of more than 35 compounds. Simply stated, upon hemorrhage platelets quickly disintegrate and release or in some way affect the release of many of the chemicals needed for coagulation. In addition, thrombocytes easily clump together to form a sticky lump that entraps white blood cells to form a clot (Milne, 1965).

The Blood Vessels

Blood being pumped from the heart to the rest of the body and back again is circulated through a meshlike group of tubes or vessels that can be classified either as *arteries, capillaries,* or *veins.* Arteries originate from the heart ventricles and carry oxygenated blood to other parts of the body. The right ventricle gives rise to the pulmonary artery, which transports blood rich in carbon dioxide to the lungs where it deposits carbon dioxide and receives oxygen. Oxygenated blood is then circulated back to the left atrium via the pulmonary vein and finally to the left ventricle. The left ventricle gives rise to the main coronary artery, the *aorta,* which channels blood into smaller and smaller arteries that eventually branch throughout the body into even smaller vessels called *arterioles.* The semilunar valves, positioned at the opening between the pulmonary artery and the aorta, open only into arteries, thus prohibiting backflow of blood into the atria upon relaxation of the ventricles (Villee, 1983).

The arterioles, the smallest arterial branches, give rise to countless microscopic tubules called capillaries, which reach every cell of the body. It is here, at the capillary level, that oxygen and nutrients are delivered and carbon dioxide and other cellular waste products are absorbed. The capillaries merge to form larger vessels called *venuoles,* which in turn unite to form veins. Veins then transport blood rich in carbon dioxide back to the heart through the right atrium, the right ventricle, and into the lungs where gas exchange takes place and oxygenated blood is ready once again to be pumped from the left chamber of the heart to the rest of the body.

THE DIGESTIVE/EXCRETORY SYSTEM

The digestive system, as shown in figure 7.10, converts the food that we eat into usable substances that can enter the bloodstream and supply the energy needed for fueling all other bodily systems. The excretory system removes nonusable food substances and wastes that are byproducts of the body's various chemical processes by eliminating them as feces from the rectum or as urine from the kidneys.

When food is swallowed, it travels from the pharynx to the esophagus and into the stomach, where digestive juices chemically act upon it. From the stomach, food is channeled into the upper section of the small intestine and further metabolized by enzymes from the pancreas and liver bile stored in the gall bladder. It then moves through the remaining portions of the small intestine, whose walls absorb the nutrients and pass them into the bloodstream. Food substances not absorbed by the alimentary canal (digestive tract) constitute nondigestible matter, which is funneled into the large intestine where bacteria decomposes it. Additional water in the mate-

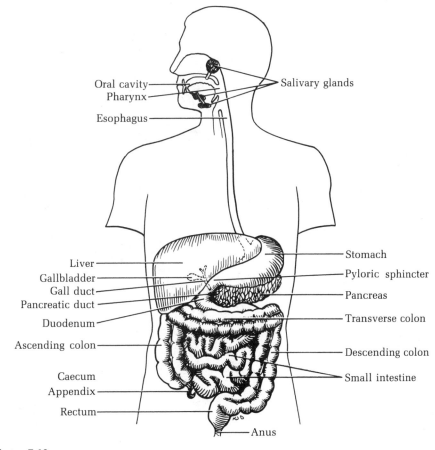

Oral cavity
Pharynx
Esophagus
Salivary glands

Liver
Gallbladder
Gall duct
Pancreatic duct
Duodenum
Ascending colon
Caecum
Appendix
Rectum

Stomach
Pyloric sphincter
Pancreas
Transverse colon
Descending colon
Small intestine
Anus

Figure 7.10
The digestive system.

rial is also absorbed. Then the remaining material moves into the rectum where it is eliminated from the body as feces through the anus.

Toxic or waste substances in the plasma as well as bacteria entering the bloodstream are filtered by the kidneys. Chemical reactions that yield the by-products water, urea, uric acid, and various salts are also filtered by the kidneys, channeled to the bladder, and excreted from the body as urine through the urethra. The excretory system is illustrated in figure 7.11.

The Stomach

Before entering the stomach, each mouthful of food is mechanically broken into a smaller, moister mass called a *bolus* by the chewing action of the jaw and teeth accompanied by enzymatic secretions from the salivary glands in the mouth. As noted,

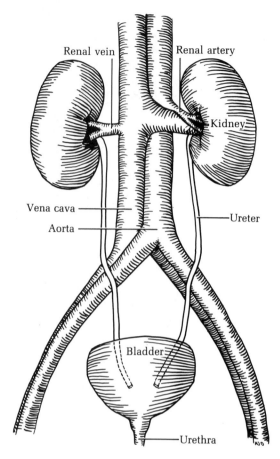

Figure 7.11
The excretory system.

the epiglottis blocks the trachea during swallowing so that food is automatically channeled from the pharynx to the esophagus where involuntary peristaltic (wavelike) muscular contractions push it into the stomach.

A special ring of muscle called a *sphincter* joins the esophagus and stomach. The sphincter muscle is signaled by peristalsis of the esophagus to open and allow the passage of food into the stomach. When the sphincter muscle tightens or contracts, it closes the entrance to the stomach. The sphincter generally remains contracted to prevent backflow of stomach contents into the esophagus during digestion (Best & Taylor, 1973).

The stomach is a muscular, saclike organ lying in the upper left portion of the abdominal cavity just below the ribs. It is the only structure in the alimentary canal that can expand. The stomach functions as a storage area for food and as a secretory organ. When completely empty, the stomach cavity is quite small, but when full an adult stomach can hold just in excess of a quart. At the rate of about three per minute, gentle peristaltic waves are triggered a few minutes after food enters the stomach. This churning action mixes the food with gastric secretions such as hydrochloric acid and pepsin until the food becomes a gellike mixture called *chyme*. Food remains in the stomach from a half hour to four hours before being forced through the pyloric sphincter into the small intestine (Nilsson & Lindberg, 1973).

The Small Intestine

The most important component of the digestive tract is the small intestine. It is here that the vast majority of food, which leaves the stomach as a soupy mixture, is digested and absorbed. The small intestine is a tightly coiled tube about 22 feet long and is made up of three sections—the *duodenum, jejunum,* and *ileum.* The duodenum, the first section, is joined by the stomach and is a much shorter segment (one foot) than either the jejunum or the ileum, which are both comparable in length (Keeton, 1986).

The inside of the small intestine contains numerous ridges and folds that are covered by tiny fingerlike projections called *villi.* The ridges and villi greatly increase the surface area of the small intestine. Covering the lining and villi are countless, tightly packed cylindrical cells called *microvilli.* The chyme is pushed through the small intestine by peristaltic action (McClintic, 1980).

As food is being propelled through the upper portion of the small intestine, ducts from the pancreas and gall bladder open into the duodenum in order to deliver both pancreatic enzymes and liver bile. The pancreatic enzymes present in the small intestine—amylase, lipase, and trypsin, and chymotrypsin—are each capable of digesting one of the three major classes of food—carbohydrates, fats, and proteins. Bile, produced in the liver and stored in the gall bladder, is not an enzyme but rather a complex compound of bile salts and cholesterol. It breaks up fats into smaller droplets by acting much like an emulsifying agent (Hole, 1986.)

In the small intestine, food substances are broken down into their simplest chemical form and are absorbed through the walls of the jejunum and ileum into the bloodstream (Hole, 1986). The remaining non-nutritive chyme in the small intestine is then propelled to the *cecum,* a functionally unimportant projection of the large intestine in the lower right portion of the abdominal cavity, from which the large intestine or colon begins to ascend or move upward. (The appendix lies at the tip of the cecum.)

The Large Intestine

There are three components of the large intestine—the *ascending colon, transverse colon,* and *descending colon*—which in essence surround the small intestine and lead into the rectum and anus, also considered parts of the large intestine. The ascending colon is a tubelike structure that moves upward on the right side of the abdominal cavity in the direction of the liver to the mid-abdomen, where it crosses over to the left, giving rise to the transverse colon. In turn, the transverse colon joins with the descending colon, which moves downward along the left side of the abdominal cavity. One of the main functions of the colon is the reabsorption of water used in the chemical processes of digestion so that it is channeled back into the body. The large intestine is also responsible for secretion of salts, including iron and calcium, that are too high in blood-level concentration. These salts are mixed with the remaining chyme decomposed by bacteria, and converted into feces. Feces are stored in the rectum, in the final portion of the large intestine adjoining the descending colon, until distension triggers rising pressure in the rectum followed by muscular movement. The feces are then expelled from the body through the rectum and its opening, the anus (Ruch & Fulton, 1969).

The Kidneys

While solid waste products are eliminated from the body through the colon, liquid waste products are chiefly excreted as a result of the action of the kidneys in the form of urine. The kidneys, bean-shaped organs about four inches long, are located on either side of the lower back region of the spinal column. Microscopic tubules called *nephrons* are the kidneys' functional units. If the nephrons could be unraveled and attached to one another, they would be about 75 miles long (Tuttle & Schotelius, 1969).

The nephrons collect waste products, such as urea and uric acid, that have been delivered by the circulatory system and filtered in the kidneys. Waste products are transported to the kidneys in the blood through the renal artery, a major artery leading directly from the aorta to the kidneys. As the renal artery penetrates the kidney and its nephrons, it branches into smaller arterioles that form a closed pouch or bulb formation at the end of each nephron. This pouchlike formation is called *Bowman's capsule,* and it gives rise to a long coiled tubule which empties into other nephron tubules that in turn empty into specialized collecting tubules that run to the central cavity of the kidney. The arterioles that reach the Bowman's capsule branch further into a small network of capillaries lying within the capsule itself. This capillary network is called the *glomerulus* and is the site where filtration of waste products takes place and urine is formed. Molecules in the blood that are small enough to pass through the membranes of the glomerulus will be filtered into the collecting tubules of the nephrons and transported to the central cavity of the kidney. A duct from each kidney called the ureter conveys urine to the urinary bladder where it is stored and then excreted through another duct, the urethra, to the outside of the body (Strand, 1983).

THE SKELETAL/MUSCULAR SYSTEM

The body and all its organs and systems are given support, protection, and mobility by the skeletal/muscular system. More than 200 bones make up the human skeleton and over 600 muscles attached to these bones allow body movement and act as a protective covering for the trunk or thoracic area. The bones are connected by joints, often containing a lubricating fluid to enhance flexibility. Some joints, such as the hip or shoulder, are extremely movable, allowing a rotation motion. These are called ball-and-socket joints. Other joints, such as the elbow or knee, allow movement in only one direction. These are called hinge joints. Many others, like those of the spinal column, provide rather restricted movement. These are called fixed joints.

Bones are composed of a porous, inner layer of spongy tissue surrounded by hardened outer compact bone material. The ends of the long bones of the body con-

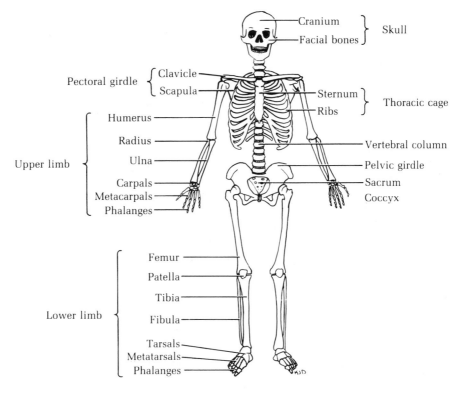

Figure 7.12
The skeletal system.

tain red marrow essential for manufacturing red blood cells. In infancy, bones are elastic, flexible, and soft. Through the maturation process, with the ingestion of minerals like calcium and phosphorous as well as vitamin D, bones become more rigid and also grow thicker and longer.

The skeletal/muscular system gives form and shape to the human body. The most characteristic skeletal feature in humans is the vertebral or spinal column, which gives the support needed for walking upright. Other major human bone structures and their attached muscles of particular importance are the skull, sternum and rib cage, pelvis, bones of the legs and feet, and bones of the arms and hands. The human skeletal structure is illustrated in figure 7.12.

The Spinal Column

Composed of 33 bones called vertebrae, the spinal column or backbone, as shown in figure 7.13, extends from the base of the head down to the hip region and allows for bending, twisting, and turning motions of the upper body. Because the spinal vertebrae encase the delicate spinal cord that conducts all body messages to the brain, any injury along the spinal column is extremely serious and could lead to paralysis or death.

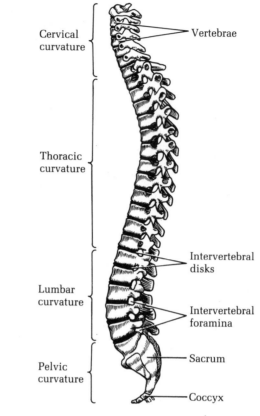

Cervical curvature

Vertebrae

Thoracic curvature

Lumbar curvature

Intervertebral disks

Intervertebral foramina

Pelvic curvature

Sacrum

Coccyx

Figure 7.13
The spinal column.

There are five divisions or groupings of bones in the spinal column. The first seven vertebrae are called the *cervical* vertebrae and comprise the neck. These are followed by 12 other bones known as the *thoracic* vertebrae, which support the upper trunk region. The five *lumbar* vertebrae extend to the waist and are followed by five fused *sacral* vertebrae in the lower back. The *coccyx,* four relatively small bones, marks the end of the spinal column and is commonly referred to as the tailbone. The upper 24 bones of the spine, the cervical, thoracic, and lumbar vertebrae, are more flexible structures than the sacral and coccyx vertebrae because they are joined by separate pieces or disks of cartilage that cushion the impact of walking, running, jumping, and similar movements.

The Skull

The human skull, situated above the spinal column, includes the cranium and the bones of the face. The cranium is a group of 16 large, flat, hard bones that form a domelike structure surrounding and protecting the brain. The bones of the face form protective coverings for the eyes, nasal passages, and the inner face or cheeks.

These bones also make up the hinged upper and lower jawbones, the maxilla and the mandible respectively, that give shape to the oral cavity and support the teeth (Woodburne, 1983).

The Sternum and Rib Cage

The sternum is a flat, elongated, rigid bone that is very thick because it protects the heart. Attached to both the sternum with cartilage in the front and to the thoracic vertebrae in the back are ten pairs of ribs that form a cagelike structure called the rib cage. Two other pairs of ribs are attached to the thoracic vertebrae but are not attached to the sternum and are thus referred to as floating ribs. The rib cage protects the lung cavity.

The Pelvis

The pelvis is formed by connections of the sacral and coccyx vertebrae of the back with the hipbones in the side and front portions of the body. When joined together, these bones form a large, bowllike structure. The pelvis helps to protect some of the organs of the reproductive system and the excretory system as well as supporting the upper part of the body. The pelvis, with its ability to rotate, also aids in twisting, turning, and sitting motions.

Bones of the Legs and Feet

Extending from each side of the hip is the upper leg bone or *femur*. It is the largest bone in the body. The femur is attached to the shin or *tibia*, the largest bone in the lower leg, at the knee or *patella*. To the outward side of the tibia lies the *fibula*, the other lower leg bone. Since the leg bones are porous, they are especially adapted for supporting body weight and providing mobility. Heavier, thicker bones would not be suitable for these functions.

The tibia and fibula are joined to the bones of the feet at the ankles or *tarsals*. Seven tarsal bones form the posterior part of the foot, the largest being the *calcaneus* or heel bone (Woodburne, 1983). Extending from the tarsals are the five long bones of the upper foot called the *metatarsals*, which are arched and joined to the 14 bones of the toes, the *phalanges*. Because these bones are arched, they provide further support and stability for maintaining the body in an upright position. The bones of the legs and feet are shown in figure 7.14.

Bones of the Arms and Hands

The bones of the arms and hands are illustrated in figure 7.15. Hinged to the flat, triangular *scapula* or shoulder blade is the upper arm bone or *humerus*, which hangs below the collarbone or *clavicle*. The humerus is attached at the elbow to both the *ulna*, the longer lower arm bone, and the *radius*, the shorter inner arm bone. These bones in turn connect with the eight wrist or *carpal* bones that provide flexibility and rotation for the hands. Attached to the carpals are the five *metacarpals* that form the

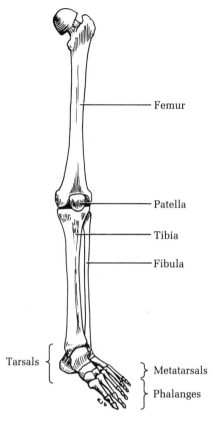

Figure 7.14
Bones of the legs and feet.

palm of the hand. These are then joined to the 14 *phalanges,* the bones of the fingers. Because of the multiple joints in the fingers, the hands are ideal for performing clutching and grasping motions.

The Muscles

The 600 muscles responsible for moving the skeletal structures at will are called voluntary muscles because their movements are triggered by conscious thoughts and actions. Many other muscles that act upon body systems and internal organs do so without messages from the individual and are therefore referred to as involuntary muscles. Each voluntary and involuntary muscle is composed of thousands of threadlike fibers joined together in bundles, which may be thickened and strengthened as a result of exercise. Because the fibers of voluntary muscles display a striated pattern under the microscope, voluntary muscles are sometimes called striated muscles. The involuntary muscle fibers of the body systems and internal organs appear smooth and are thus sometimes called smooth muscles. The cardiac muscle, although functioning like a smooth or involuntary muscle, has its own characteristic fiber appearance (Keeton, 1986).

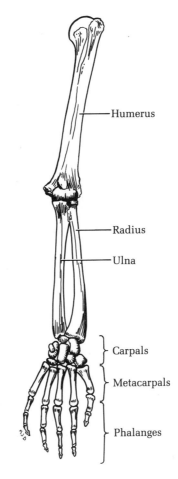

Humerus

Radius

Ulna

Carpals

Metacarpals

Phalanges

Figure 7.15
Bones of the arms and hands.

The muscles of the body are organized and operate in groups rather than as isolated structures so that a single action, such as lifting the leg, is dependent upon the contraction of certain muscles accompanied by the simultaneous relaxation of others. The most important groups of skeletal muscles are those that move the shoulders, arms, chest, back, and legs.

Although numerous muscles cover the scapula, the major ones are the *trapezius* in the back of the shoulder blades and the *deltoid* connected to the front, rounded portion of the shoulder. The *triceps* on the outer upper arm bone and the *biceps* on the inner upper arm bone are the chief muscles covering the humerus, while the *brachioradialis* of the radius and the *aconeus* and *flexor* group of the ulna are the major muscles in the lower arm. The chest is supported by a large muscle group called the *pectorals,* the *pectoralis minor* covering the sides of the ribs and the *pectoralis major* covering the chest, while the *lattisimus dorsi* covers the back and the ribs attached to the thoracic vertebrae. The major muscles of the thigh are commonly called the hamstring muscles and include the *biceps femoris* on the outer

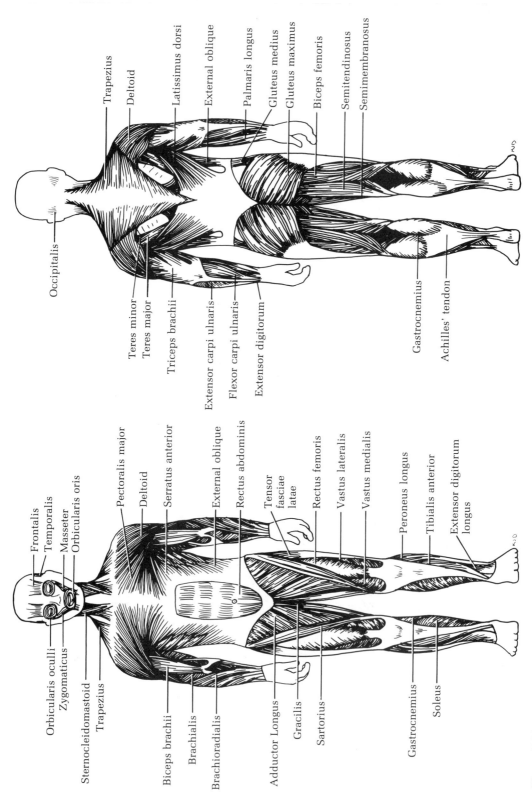

Figure 7.16
The major muscles of the human body.

thigh and the *semimembranesus* and the *semitendinosis* on the inner thigh, all of which flex at the knee and aid in the extension of the hip. The major muscles of the leg include the *gastrocnemius* or calf muscle and the *soleus* or ankle muscle (Shaver, 1983). The major muscles of the human body are shown in figure 7.16.

SUMMARY

Almost every individual begins life with a sound, healthy body, but one that requires care and maintenance. Knowledge of the body systems and how they interact with one another is important in building and promoting personal health and well-being. Each body system has special roles and functions that directly or indirectly affect all other body systems. The brain and nervous system receive messages from all other parts of the body and act to keep both an internal and external balance. This internal balance is greatly dependent upon the release and regulation of hormones from the endocrine system, which strongly influences growth, development, and reproduction. Oxygen, essential to all cells, is channeled into the body by the respiratory system and delivered to all tissue through the actions of the circulatory system. Other chemicals and nutrients are ingested, broken down, and made useable to cells and tissue by the digestive/excretory system so that vital processes can take place. Finally, the skeletal/muscular system provides physical shape and structure for the body, also assisting in protection and movement.

DISCUSSION QUESTIONS

1. What are the two major divisions of the nervous system? Describe and differentiate each.
2. Describe the functions of the cerebrum, cerebellum, and brain stem.
3. What are the overall functions of the endocrine system?
4. Explain why the hypothalamus is considered to be the master gland.
5. Briefly describe the functions of each of these glands: pituitary, pineal, thyroid, parathyroid, thymus, ardenal, and pancreas.
6. Explain how oxygen is transported by means of the respiratory system from the nose, into the lungs, and finally to body tissue. Also explain how the respiratory system expels waste gases.
7. Describe in detail how the blood circulates from the heart to all parts of the body and then back to the heart.
8. Discuss the pumping action of the heart, explaining how the atrium and ventricle in each heart chamber function.
9. Differentiate between red blood cells, white blood corpuscles, and blood platelets.
10. Describe how food moves through the digestive system, from the mouth to the stomach and intestines, and to the rectum.
11. Explain how liquid waste products are filtered and removed from the body by the excretory system.

12. What are the main functions of the skeletal/muscular system?
13. Discuss the importance of the spinal column.
14. Differentiate between voluntary and involuntary muscles.

REFERENCES

Asimov, I. *The human brain: Its capacities and functions.* Boston: Houghton Mifflin, 1963.

Barrington, E. *An introduction to general and comparative endocrinology.* London: Oxford University Press, 1975.

Bentley, P. *Comparative vertebrate endocrinology.* London: Cambridge University Press, 1976.

Best, C., & Taylor, B. *Endocrine control systems.* In *Physiological basis of medical practice.* Baltimore: Williams and Wilkins, 1973.

Best, C., & Taylor B. *The human body: Its anatomy and physiology.* New York: Holt, Rinehart, & Winston, 1963.

Brown, J., & Barker, B. *Basic endocrinology.* Philadelphia: F. A. Davis, 1962.

Campbell, H. *Correlative physiology of the nervous system.* London: Academic Press, 1965.

Combs, B., Hales, D., & Williams, B. *An invitation to health: Your personal responsibility.* Menlo Park, Calif: Benjamin/Cummings, 1983.

Eisenberg, A., & Eisenberg, H. *Alive and well: Decisions in health.* New York: McGraw-Hill, 1979.

Friedan, E., & Lipner, H. *Biochemical endocrinology of the vertebrates.* Englewood Cliffs, N.J.: Prentice-Hall, 1971.

Fulton, J. (Ed.) *Textbook of physiology.* Philadelphia: W. B. Saunders, 1949.

Green, J. *An introduction to human physiology.* London: Oxford University Press, 1972.

Hole, J. *Human anatomy and physiology.* Dubuque, Iowa: Wm. C. Brown, 1986.

Holmes, R. & Ball, J. *The pituitary gland.* London: Cambridge University Press, 1974.

Johnson, W., Delanney, L., & Cole, T. *Essentials of biology.* New York: Holt, Rinehart, & Winston, 1985.

Keele, C., & Neil, L. *Samson Wright's applied physiology.* London: Oxford University Press, 1971.

Keeton, W. *Essentials of biological science.* New York: W.W. Norton, 1986.

Kraus, D. *Concepts in modern biology.* New York: Cambridge Book, 1984.

Martin, C. *Textbook of endocrine physiology.* London: Oxford University Press, 1976.

McClintic, J. *Physiology of the human body.* New York: John Wiley, 1980.

Milne, L. *The biotic world and man.* Englewood Cliffs, N.J.: Prentice-Hall, 1965.

Nilsson, L., & Lindberg, J. *Behold man: A photographic journey of discovery inside the body.* Boston: Little, Brown, 1973.

Ochs, S. *Elements of neurophysiology.* New York: John Wiley, 1965.

Quay, W. *Pineal chemistry.* Springfield, Ill.: Charles C. Thomas, 1974.

Ruch, T., & Fulton, J. (Eds.). *Medical physiology and biophysics.* Philadelphia: W. B. Saunders, 1969.

Sharrer, E., & Sharrer, B. *Neuroendrocrinology.* New York: Columbia University Press, 1963.

Shaver, L. *Essentials of exercise physiology.* Minneapolis: Burgess, 1983.

Strand, F. *Modern physiology: The chemical and structural basis of function.* New York: MacMillan, 1983.

Turner, C. *General endocrinology.* Philadelphia: W. B. Saunders, 1976.

Tuttle, W., & Schotelius, B. *Textbook of physiology.* St. Louis: C. V. Mosby, 1969.

Villee, C. *Biology.* Philadelphia: W. B. Saunders, 1985.

Villee, D. *Human endocrinology: A developmental approach.* Philadelphia: W. B. Saunders, 1975.

Woodburne, L. *The neural basis of behavior.* Columbus: Merrill, 1967.

Woodburne, R. *Essentials of human anatomy.* New York: Oxford University Press, 1983.

8. Techniques for Teaching Body Systems

Thus to the artist the human body is often a thing of beauty and always a subject of interest; to the scientist it is the end product of 500 million years of evolutionary refinement, the highest form of life known; to the theologian it is the image of God and the temple of the spirit; to the average child it is simply me, my person. In any case it is something very worthy of study and appreciation—Walter Greene, Frank Jenne, and Patricia Legos, *Health Education in the Elementary Schools.*

PLANNING LEARNING ACTIVITIES

A sound, healthy body is the basis for optimal personal health and well-being. From the instant of birth and throughout life an individual strives first to meet basic physiological needs. As a result, instruction about the function and care of the human body and its interacting systems is of the utmost importance to children, especially at the elementary school level. Learning opportunities should demonstrate and emphasize health practices that ensure maintenance of body systems so that children develop positive health habits that will enhance their physiological growth and development.

Because children generally enjoy and are interested in participating in physical activity and discovering the unseen "mysteries" of their own body actions, teaching about body systems should be an exhilarating and challenging experience for you. Throughout instruction, children should be made aware of the interrelationships between all body systems and should develop a sense of "ownership" in regard to the body so that personal commitment to its upkeep is fostered.

Concepts to be Taught

- The human body is a highly organized and well-developed "machine."
- The human body is made up of seven major systems, each of which has special functions that interact with all other body systems.

- Daily care and maintenance of the human body and an understanding of how its systems operate serve as the foundation for personal health and well-being.

- The nervous system acts as the body's computer by receiving, interpreting, and sending messages that help to direct and guide all other body systems so that the individual can make both internal and external adjustments to the environment.

- The endocrine system helps to maintain balance between all body systems through the secretion from various glands of chemical substances called hormones that influence the actions of body organs and structures.

- The reproductive system becomes activated in adolescence and is designed for creating and perpetuating human life.

- The respiratory system provides the pathway and mechanics for oxygen to enter the body.

- The circulatory system, through the pumping of blood by the heart, delivers oxygen and other essential chemicals to all cells and tissue of the body.

- The digestive/excretory system is responsible for mechanically and chemically breaking down food so that it can be used for energy to fuel the operation of all body processes. Substances that cannot be used to provide energy are eliminated from the body as waste products.

- The skeletal/muscular system provides the body and its parts with shape, support, protection, and movement.

- Although body systems operate in standard ways, personal differences in structure and physical functioning affect individual growth and development.

Cycle Plan for Teaching Topics

Topic	Grade Level						
	K	1	2	3	4	5	6
Nervous System	**	**	***	**	***	***	**
Endocrine System	**	**	*	**	***	***	**
Respiratory System	***	***	*	**	***	***	**
Circulatory System	***	***	*	**	***	***	**
Digestive/Excretory System	***	***	*	**	**	***	**
Skeletal/Muscular System	***	**	***	***	*	***	**

Key: *** = major emphasis, ** = emphasis, * = review.

VALUE-BASED ACTIVITIES

Being Good to Me

Divide students into small groups and ask each group to list five *routine* things they do for themselves that they consider beneficial. Compare group listings to see how many listings relate to care of the body. Then write each listing relating to care of the body on the board and ask the groups to rank order them in terms of importance in maintaining body functioning. Follow with general discussion.

Body Drawings

Provide each student with paper long enough to fit body length. In pairs, have students trace each other's body outlines. Each student then draws and labels the internal body systems. On the reverse side, under each body system heading, have the student list at least two reasons why he or she feels the system is important. Tack the completed body drawings to the wall, interspersing the body parts side of some with the written side of others.

Rank Ordering Health Practices

Prepare a handout that lists each body system and three health practices that affect it. Ask students to rank order the practices according to the positive influence each practice has on that system, "1" being the most positive. Examples:

Digestive/Excretory System	Skeletal/Muscular System
_____Eating fresh fruits and vegetables	_____Sitting and standing straight
_____Eating foods high in fiber	_____Getting plenty of exercise
_____Limiting sweet snacks	_____Relaxing during the day

In the class discussion that follows, indicate that all the practices are important but that some more directly influence specific body systems than others.

Body Systems Position Statement

Divide the class into six groups, each representing a different body system, with the exception of the reproductive system. Have each group be responsible for developing and presenting a five-minute statement that argues for the position that their system "is 1." After all the positions have been presented, have the students vote to determine a "winner." Follow with a discussion of why students voted the way they did.

Body Care Collage

Provide students with poster board and ask the students to make a collage of people with diverse body types and habits that may influence body functioning. Collages should be made from magazine pictures and newspaper clippings and should depict the varying health status of the people depicted. Accompanying each collage should be a brief written description that summarizes the student's attitudes and opinions regarding how care of the body can influence growth and development.

Body Image Sentence Completion

Provide students with handouts containing incomplete statements such as the following:

My body is _____

I like my body because _____

I take good care of my body by _____

The bones of my body are _____

I help my muscles by _____

When I breathe I _____

When I eat _____

My brain _____

Encourage values-related rather than mere factual statements. However, accept all statements without being judgmental.

Body Songfest

Divide students into small groups and assign each a different, but familiar tune such as "Mary Had a Little Lamb," or "Old MacDonald Had a Farm." Using the tune, each group writes a song about the body and its systems and performs the song for all other classmates. If possible, it might be fun to record the songs on a cassette recorder.

Decision Stories

Present decision stories such as the following to the class. Follow the procedure discussed in chapter 5 for using the stories as a values-clarification activity.

Rita's Dilemma

Rita comes from a large, loving family. She has three brothers and four sisters. Her family is poor, but her parents do the best that they can. After studying about body systems in class, Rita is aware that it is important to have a physical exam regularly in order to make sure that the body is functioning properly. She is now in the fifth grade but hasn't seen a doctor since kindergarten. Rita knows that her parents are having a hard time taking care of all the children. There never seems to be enough money to live on. Rita is feeling fine and has only missed one day of school this year, because of a cold.

Focus question: Should she mention anything to her parents about getting a checkup?

Pamphlets

John's parents are very overweight and don't exercise much. In school, John learned that these factors can be unhealthy for the heart and lungs. He is also a bit overweight and is sensitive about his weight. John would like to say something to his parents but he feels that he has no room to talk since he's not a very good example. He has thought about leaving some pamphlets around the house that he got from class speakers on how to take care of your circulatory and respiratory systems.

Focus question: How should John handle this problem?

DRAMATIZATION

Have students dramatize different body systems as if they actually were the body system in question. Use your creativity in outlining this activity. The following examples may be helpful:

The Nervous System

Tell students that they are going to act like the parts of the nervous system that send and receive information or signals. Form the class into a circle with each student standing arm's length apart. Have the students cup their hands in front of them to form a pouch or "mailbox." Drop a message in one student's pouch and have that student pass the message along to the student to his or her right, and so on. Explain that the students are acting as the nerve pathways. Stop the message by tapping a student on the head. This student represents the brain. The student then reads the message, which gives a command such as to touch your toes or stand on one leg. Everyone follows the directions. Send additional messages, indicating that the class is functioning like the nerve pathways and brain of the nervous system.

The Endocrine System

In order to demonstrate that hormones are chemical substances produced by certain organs and carried by the bloodstream to other organs, divide the class into the following groups: one student to represent the brain; six students to represent the bloodstream; 12 students to represent various organs; four students to represent hormones. Three students who are representing the bloodstream lie down on the floor, face up and head-to-toe, and the remaining three students lie parallel, leaving about three feet between them, forming a path. The student representing the brain stands at one end of the path. The 12 students who represent organs stand at the other end of the path in groups of three facing each other with their hands joined and raised in an arch. They are labeled as either the pancreas, kidneys, bones, or thyroid (or any other grouping that you like). The arrangement is illustrated in figure 8.1. The

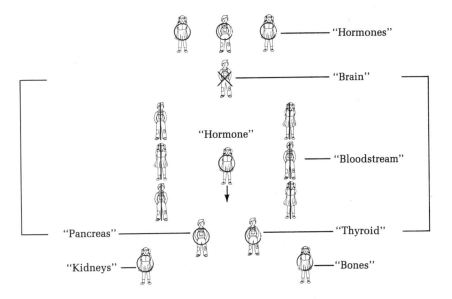

Figure 8.1
Dramatizing the endocrine system.

"brain" then takes one student representing a hormone and starts him or her down a walk through the path or "bloodstream." At the end of the "bloodstream" the "hormone" stands under the arch of the "target organ" and tells the message, such as pancreas should help with breaking down sugar; bones should grow; kidneys should produce a substance that gives the body a spurt of energy; thyroid should make iodine. Then the "brain" takes another "hormone" and so on until all the "hormones" have traveled through the "bloodstream." Reverse roles if desired.

The Digestive System

With chalk, draw the basic organs of the digestive system (mouth, esophagus, stomach, and intestines) on the floor. Assign students a spot to stand on within one of the organs and have each group join hands. You represent food and walk first into the "mouth." The students in this area stomp around as you weave in and out. Then progress toward the "throat" and "esophagus." Students unclasp their hands and twirl you down the "esophagus" into the "stomach." When you are in the stomach area, the students enclose you and walk around in a circle. After several rotations, say "ready" and go into the area of the "intestines." After holding steady for a brief period of time, students unclasp their hands and you leave the digestive system.

As We Age

Place the students in groups of four and assign each group member a specific age range—childhood, early adulthood, middle adulthood, and late adulthood. Give each group one activity to act out that highlights one body system. Walking upstairs, for example, could represent an activity that emphasizes the skeletal/muscular system. Group by group, students enact the example as if they were the age selected, going from youngest to oldest. Before enactment, encourage students to observe people at the given age to see how they function. Follow the activity with a discussion about how people of different ages perform various physical activities. Avoid stereotyping age groups.

Inside-Out

Divide the students into groups of five and ask each group to write a fantasy play about a girl or boy who is able to travel through a human body, meeting different body systems along the way. You should serve as a resource, but avoid giving too much direction, thus stifling creativity. Have the students perform their plays, with one acting as the traveler, while the others represent body systems or specific organs.

DISCUSSION AND REPORT TECHNIQUES

Presentation from the School Nurse

Ask the school nurse to prepare a brief presentation of his or her duties and how he or she assists students in helping them care for their bodies. The nurse should also

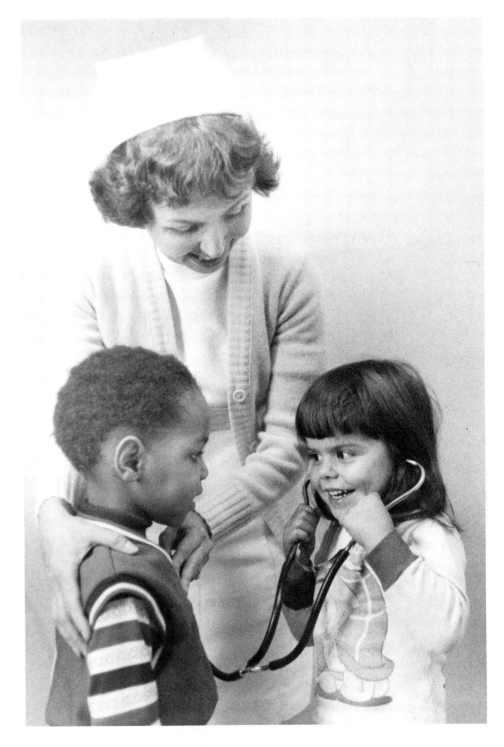

The school nurse is always a valuable resource.

outline the basic procedures of a physical examination, indicating which measures are used to assess specific body systems. Allow time for a question and answer session and follow the presentation with class discussion.

Body Part Pointers

Assign each student a different body part and have the student write a short report about it, including its functions, body system affiliation, and ways to care for it. A cover sheet with an illustration of the body part should be made as well. Collect the reports, organize them in sequence according to body system categories, and collate the reports into one body systems booklet that can be used by the class as a resource.

Body Part Breakdown

After completing the preceding lesson, assign students a condition or illness that can disturb the functioning of their given body part. Have them make a brief oral presentation to the class describing the condition and its effects.

Voluntary Health Organization Panel

Invite representatives from several voluntary health organizations that deal with a specific organ or body system, such as the Heart Association, Kidney Association, and Lung Association, to address the class. Their presentations should be geared to the age of the students and should include facts about each organization's founding, purpose, and projects. Use a panel discussion format.

Donation Debate

Following the presentation by voluntary health organization representatives, divide the students into groups and have each group present an oral argument for convincing people to donate money to their respective causes. This should be handled in a debate format where each group first makes a statement without reference to other groups' comments. Then a rebuttal period is allowed. Following the debate, each student is given the imaginary sum of $100 and a checklist that solicits contributions. Tell students that they may divide their money among one, some, or all of the organizations as they wish. Collect the donation checklists and report the results to the class.

Replacement of Body Parts

For older elementary school students, provide information regarding various surgical procedures available to replace body parts that either malfunction or become injured or amputated. In this teacher-led discussion, you could also provide information about various organ donation programs and some of the medical, ethical, and social problems associated with organ transplants.

Body Systems Practices

Assign students to a body systems group and ask them to read about and compile a list of five daily measures that can be taken to enhance the functioning of that system. List the five measures on large pieces of posterboard that bear the body system heading and tack them on the walls of the classroom. Each day for a week, call attention to one of the posters in order to reemphasize specific health practices.

EXPERIMENTS AND DEMONSTRATIONS

Doll Dimensions

In order to familiarize students with their own bodies, ask them to bring in a doll. Let them measure the doll's height and then their own to find the ratio. For example, if the doll's height is 8 inches and the student's is 40 inches, the ratio of body proportions is 40/8 or 5 to 1. For every inch the doll measures, the student's proportions should be five times greater. Have students measure various doll dimensions, such as arm length, leg length, and neck circumference, and then calculate what their own respective measurements would be using the ratio if the doll was proportioned like a real human. Follow this by taking accurate body measurements to determine which students' dolls are best proportioned.

Brain Viewing

Obtain the brain of a sheep or cow. Have students compare the parts of the animal brain to those of a human brain, using a model of the human brain for the comparison.

Skeletal System Model

For demonstration purposes, obtain an anatomical model of the human skeleton. Discuss the skeleton, its major bones, and the role of the skeleton.

How We Breathe

Saw off the bottom of a clear glass gallon jug or obtain a similar demonstration bottle. As shown in figure 8.2, attach a balloon to each end of a Y-shaped tube and insert the tube in the jug using a one-hole stopper. Place a thin rubber sheet over the open mouth of the jug and tie a marble in the center of the sheet to act as a handle. Pull down on the sheet and let it go back to its original position. Repeat several times so that the balloons inflate and deflate. Explain that the balloons represent the lungs. The rubber sheet acts as the diaphragm. The jug is the rib cage and lung cavity. The Y-shaped tube represents the respiratory passages from the nose to the lungs. Provide an appropriate physical explanation for the phenomenon, depending on the age and science ability of your students. The balloons inflate and deflate because of a difference in air pressure inside the jug (lung cavity) and outside the jug (the body).

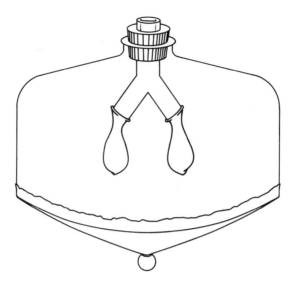

Figure 8.2
Lung-action model.

Breathing Rate

Have students relax by reading a story, resting, or a similar approach. Then ask them, while sitting, to count the number of times they breathe in a minute as you clock them. Next, have students run in place beside their desks for a minute. Then immediately time their respiration rates. Compare resting and active breathing rates.

Heart Rate

Perform the same procedure, but have students count the number of times their hearts beat in a minute. Have them do this by counting the pulse in their wrists. Compare resting and active heart rates.

Heart Action

Use an eye dropper to represent the heart and some red colored water to represent blood. Draw the water in and out by squeezing and releasing the eye dropper bulb. This mimics the beat-relax-beat-relax action of the heart.

Pair students and ask them to listen to the heart sounds of a partner by placing an ear on the partner's chest.

Obtain a stethoscope, explain its function, and demonstrate its use.

Properties of Blood

Prepare several slides of your own blood in front of the class and let students observe the slides with microscope. In order to demonstrate coagulation, run a clean needle through these slides at about 30-second intervals until the needle picks up a fine

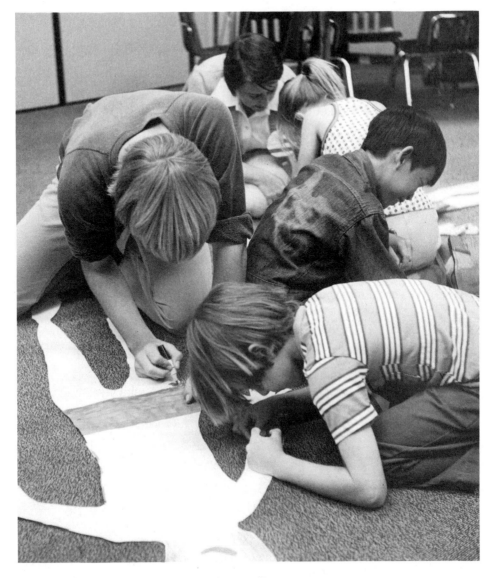

Body drawing is a good way to teach systems values.

thread of blood (fibrin). Record the time it took to pick up fibrin. This means the blood has begun to clot in that time interval.

Eating Away

Place a small amount of the white of a hard-boiled egg in a test tube or beaker. Add a little bit of pepsin and a few drops of hydrochloric acid. Nothing much should happen. Then add a few drops of water and observe the egg white. The corrosive action is similar to the action of digestive enzymes on food in the stomach. In this demonstration be especially careful with the acid so that you or the children are not burned. Lock all chemicals away after the demonstration.

The Small Intestine

In order to demonstrate the size of the small intestine, obtain a 22-foot rope and show it to the class. Explain that this is the length of the adult small intestine. Then coil the rope in a box to demonstrate its configuration in the body.

Muscle Workout

To demonstrate the fatigue factor on muscles, have students do the following three activities while you time them with a stopwatch. Have the students follow these directions:

Grasp a clothespin end between your right thumb and index finger. Count the number of times you can open and close the pin in 20 seconds. Record your score. Repeat the procedure two more times.

Put your left hand, palm up, on your thigh and count the number of times you can curl and extend your fingers, making a fist, in 20 seconds. Record your score. Repeat the procedure two more times.

Hold a book in your hand with your arm hanging straight down. Count the number of times you can raise and lower your arm above your head in 20 seconds. Repeat the procedure two more times.

Them Bones

To demonstrate the necessity of calcium for adding strength to bones, place the leg bones of a chicken in a jar of vinegar. After about a week, the vinegar will dissolve some of the calcium and the bones will feel quite soft. If left in the jar for a few weeks, the bone will become soft enough to tie into a knot!

PUZZLES AND GAMES

Body Parts Puzzle

Divide the students into groups. Provide each group with a sealed package containing body parts made of construction paper. Each packet should contain identical parts. Separate the groups and provide each with a large piece of paper that has the outline of the human body on it. At your signal, groups open their packets and place the body parts where they should be on the paper. The group to finish first wins. Time each group so that a few days later the same game can be played, with teams trying to improve their previous time score so that they are competing against the clock rather than against each other.

Skeleton Puzzle

Using the same procedure, provide each group with a packet containing bone parts made of cardboard or construction paper. The first group to place all bone parts correctly wins.

Brain Says

Play this game following the same rules as those for "Simon Says" in order to emphasize that the brain is the body's conductor or director. Give commands and eliminate students who act without saying "Brain says" preceding a command, until one student is the winner.

Bean Bag Toss

Cut several holes in the bottom of a very large cardboard box. Label each hole so that it represents a different endocrine gland and secure the box against the wall. Let each student have three chances at tossing a bean bag into the holes. Score one point for getting the bag into the hole and two points if the student can name one function of the gland or one of the hormones it secretes, just so long as that function or hormone has not already been named by another student. Tally scores and announce the winners. Repeat this game periodically, being sure to change the order, so that students who were first during the previous game have to go last, and vice versa.

Pin the Heart on the Clown

This game aids in teaching the location of the heart. Make a poster or large picture of a clown and a cutout of a heart. Blindfold students one at a time. Twirl them around three times. Now, they are to try to place the heart in the right location. The student who pins the heart closest to the correct spot wins.

Yarn Pass

This game illustrates that the circulatory system has many veins, arteries, and capillaries that transport blood to all parts of the body. Assign each student to be a certain body part. Two students are assigned the same part and stand beside one another. Assign two students to be "leaders." The rest of the students are paired, with each pair of students playing the role of one specific body part, such as the stomach, toes, brain, and intestine. Have the pairs of students stand in rows, across from each other. One leader walks with red yarn by each of the left-hand side body parts while another leader walks with blue yarn to the right-hand side body parts. Hold the ends of the balls of yarn as they are passed around from part to part, making a web-type mesh.

Hokey-Pokey

To emphasize the importance of bones and muscle development for active movement, play Hokey-Pokey. Have everyone form a circle and sing along as you lead them in the Hokey-Pokey lyrics:

> Put your right arm in
> Take your right arm out
> Put your right arm in

And shake it all about
Do the Hokey-Pokey
And turn yourself around
That's what it's all about

Continue, naming all parts of the body. For older students, you can use medical names for bones. For example:

Put your right ulna in
Take your right ulna out. . . .

Body Systems Scramble

Give each student a prepared sheet as shown in figure 8.3.

Body Systems Crossword Puzzle

Give each student a prepared crossword puzzle sheet as shown in figure 8.4. This activity will help teach vocabulary and reinforce concepts about body functions. In the figure, the answers have been supplied.

BULLETIN BOARDS

Our Magnificent Machine

To highlight the theme of the human body as a magnificent machine, use several body systems, each for a separate bulletin board, and compare the system to an analogous machine. For example, the nervous system could be illustrated as "Our Human Telephone System," where incoming trunk lines of outlying phones convey messages to the main switchboard. The trunk lines represent the nerve pathways to the spinal cord and the switchboard represents the brain. The digestive system could be illustrated in terms of the automobile and its need for fuel—particularly the correct fuel in order to keep it running in top shape. The regulating mechanisms that exist in examples like home thermostats for heating and air conditioning or smoke alarms that signal potential danger could be used as analogies for the endocrine sys-

1. Licurlrctoy ___ ___ ___ ___ ___ ___ ___ ___ ___ ___ ___
2. Gesditevi ___ ___ ___ ___ ___ ___ ___ ___ ___ ___ ___
3. Ersonuv ___ ___ ___ ___ ___ ___ ___ ___ ___ ___ ___
4. Tiresoprary ___ ___ ___ ___ ___ ___ ___ ___ ___ ___
5. Lesekalt ___ ___ ___ ___ ___ ___ ___ ___ ___ ___
6. Ridonecne ___ ___ ___ ___ ___ ___ ___ ___ ___ ___

Figure 8.3
Scrambled body systems terms worksheet.

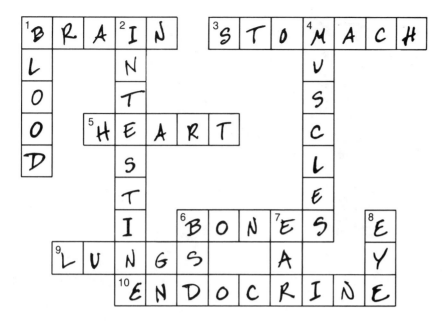

Across

1. Main organ of the nervous system.
3. Organ of the digestive system that acts as a receptacle for food.
5. Main organ of the circulatory system.
6. These make up the skeletal system.
9. Main organs of the respiratory system.
10. System that acts as a body regulator by its secretion of homones.

Down

1. Fluid that carries oxygen and nutrients to all cells.
2. Organ of the digestive system that allows for absorption of nutrients into body.
4. Essential for all body movement.
7. Main organ of hearing.
8. Main organ of seeing.

Figure 8.4
Crossword puzzle for body parts.

tem. Use your imagination—or let your students use theirs—in devising illustrations for other body systems.

Body Systems of Animals Compared to Human Systems

Compare human body systems or their major organs with those of lower animals. Let students decide which animals they would like to investigate in learning about comparisons. Students should be assigned to a specific group dealing with a specific body system. It may be helpful to compare using two or three animals for a given body system. To many children, especially younger ones, the only "animals" are mammals. But as the body systems of many mammals are evolutionarily close to human body systems, suggest that nonmammal species also be included in the comparisons. Suggest that students investigate the body systems and organs of birds, reptiles, and insects—all of which are animals.

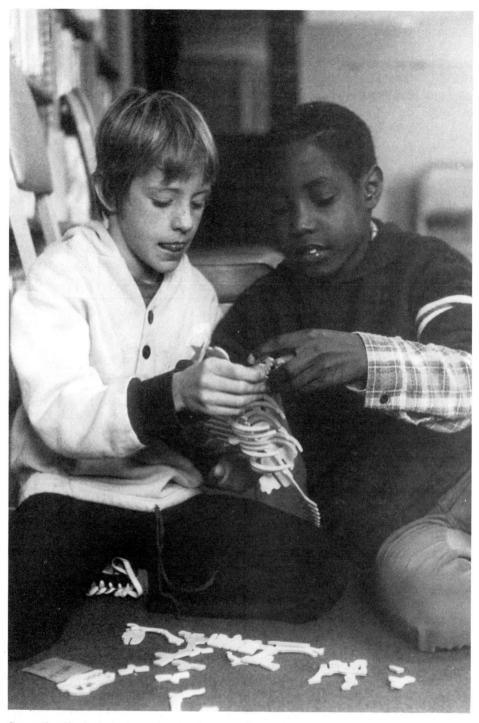

Comparing the body systems of animals—even dinosaurs—to humans is helpful in understanding their function.

OTHER IDEAS

Chain Reaction

To demonstrate how the nerves transfer messages from the brain to all parts of the body, set up dominoes in any formation. Have the students gather around. Let one student start the action by tipping the first domino. The students will note with interest that the dominoes fall one after another. Repeat the demonstration several times using various domino configurations.

Endocrine Energy

This activity will convey the information to younger elementary school students that at certain times a person can get a spurt of energy when frightened or excited due to an increase in adrenaline (epinephrine) secreted by the adrenal glands. A good analogy of this process is a comparison with Popeye. When Popeye is in danger, he eats spinach and his muscles strengthen. He can then handle anything. The parallel can be made by reading a Popeye story or showing a Popeye cartoon.

Breathing Safety

Emphasize that it is essential for a person to breathe to obtain oxygen. Note that children have a tendency to play in places or with things that might result in suffocation. Review rules related to breathing safety and illustrate each rule by a poster or display in the classroom.

Plants, Air, and Us

This activity helps illustrate that humans and plants work together to stay alive. People breathe in oxygen and give off carbon dioxide; plants take in carbon dioxide and give off oxygen. To demonstrate the concept, obtain two plants. Place one in an airtight container. Place the other in a nice airy spot. Observe what happens in a few days. This activity is also appropriate for teaching environmental health.

Respiratory System Travelogue

Draw a diagram of the respiratory system on a chart or overhead transparency. Take the class on an imaginary trip through the respiratory system. You are the tour guide. Use props and tour guide dialogue. This activity can be used for any body system.

Circulation Chart

To aid the students in understanding the circulation of the blood from the heart to the body and back to the heart, prepare a large diagram of the circulatory system. Explain the functions of the arteries, capillaries, and veins. Then prepare and issue individual handouts of the diagram. Have the students color-code the arteries (red), capillaries (gray), and veins (blue).

Eating by the Rules

This activity will help demonstrate that proper digestion involves following certain rules of eating. "Make believe" eating allows practice in the correct way of eating. Instruct the class to pretend they are holding an apple. Talk through each step: First, bite the apple. Second, chew the apple carefully. Third, swallow a little at a time. Include sound effects with each step.

Body Builders

Craft time with Popsicle sticks, yarn, and cloth scraps will allow each student to make a character with "bones," "muscles," and "skin." Popsicle sticks provide the frame. Yarn wrapped around sticks represents muscles. Cloth scraps serve as skin. Additional features can be added to give each model some unique characteristics.

9. Personal Health: Problems and Diseases

In addition to the ethical, intelligent role that a person should take in his or her own health care, it will soon be evident that from a monetary viewpoint, a person will have to practice preventive health care at its best.—Fay R. Biles, Ph.D., Past President, American Alliance for Health, Physical Education, Recreation, and Dance.

DEVELOPING GOOD HABITS EARLY

The human body must be given daily attention in order to ensure its continued performance. This attention is the responsibility of the individual. Thus it is essential that personal health habits be learned at an early age. The body can put up with only so much inattention and abuse. Eventually, the result is a deterioration of good health. Inattention to personal health practices in childhood will have its consequences in later life. Without a solid foundation from which to begin, personal health in adolescence and adulthood is threatened.

This chapter focuses on the areas of personal health that are considered the most crucial for the elementary school child. These areas include personal appearance, care of the senses, dental health, exercise, relaxation, and sleep, and disease control and prevention, and chronic illness in children.

PERSONAL APPEARANCE

Interest in personal appearance seems to apply to all age groups. A multitude of factors can influence personal appearance, including genetics, socioeconomic status, illness, and so forth. However, in this section of the chapter, only care of the skin, care of the nails, care of the hair, and the importance of posture will be discussed. Care of the senses, dental health, exercise, relaxation and sleep, and disease control and prevention will be considered as separate topics. In addition, because of its far-reaching effects on almost all other areas of health, nutrition will be presented in a separate chapter.

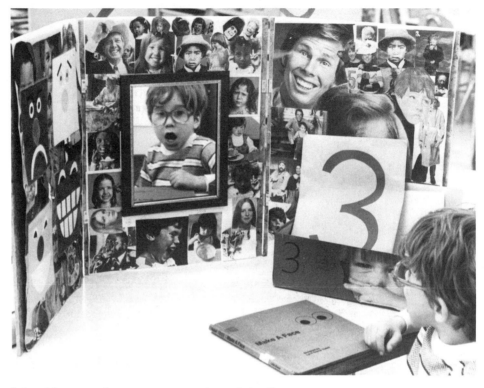

Interest in personal appearance seems to apply to all age groups.

THE SKIN

The skin is the largest organ of the body, and is composed of three layers—the outer skin (epidermis), the "true" skin (dermis), and the subcutaneous layer (fat tissue). Skin is certainly one of the most observable features of any individual. Personal appearance is affected by skin cleanliness, general complexion, and any irregularities or infestations present. The skin is also highly functional. These functions include the following:

- Protection against foreign matter trying to enter the body.
- Regulation of body temperature both through delivery of blood (heat) to body surfaces and the secretion of sweat, which produces a cooling effect.
- Elimination of minute amounts of waste products through perspiration.
- Absorption of electromagnetic radiation, including ultraviolet, infrared, visible light, and X rays, thus prohibiting passage to underlying structures.
- Conversion of ultraviolet light to vitamin D.
- Storage of fat and water in subcutaneous tissue for use as needed.

The skin can be damaged in many ways. Common injuries include cuts, abrasions, and burns. Chemical irritants, insect bites, and rashes are also responsible for skin damage, usually temporary and dealt with by the regenerative processes of the skin itself. A variety of skin conditions may require medical attention, however.

Skin Conditions

Since skin conditions are numerous and vary in degree of severity from sunburn and dandruff to psoriasis and exzema, only those that are most frequently seen in school-age children will be discussed. These include acne, athlete's foot, boils and carbuncles, impetigo, pediculosis, ringworm, scabies, warts, and sunburn.

Acne. This condition, characterized by blemishes on the face, neck, shoulders, and back, in the form of pimples, whiteheads, and blackheads, arises when oil glands become overly active in their secretions, thus blocking skin surface ducts. Pimples are small, pus-filled inflammations, whiteheads are oil blockages that lie beneath the skin, and blackheads are hardened, dried plugs of oil at the skin surface. Acne is generally considered a problem for pre-teens and teenagers but may affect people in their twenties, thirties, and forties as well. The condition is not contagious. There is no known cure, but a variety of cleansing treatments coupled, if necessary, with the administration of either surface (local) or oral antibiotics can control the condition. Persons with acne should avoid makeup and skin creams with an oil base as these applications will further block the pores of the skin. Most affected individuals usually "outgrow" the conditions as their oil glands provide a more balanced output.

Athlete's Foot. This condition is a superficial, contagious fungal infection that produces red, cracked, itchy, scaly skin between the toes. Infected areas are sometimes also accompanied by an unpleasant odor. Athlete's foot can affect any age group, but it is more prevalent among teenagers and adults, with some individuals more susceptible to the infection than others. The condition is believed by many physicians to be more likely contracted in damp environments, such as showers and swimming pools. Athlete's foot can be prevented by complete drying of the skin between the toes after bathing or swimming. Skin infections such as ringworm and athlete's foot are frequently very difficult to treat or cure (Jones, Shainberg, & Byer, 1985).

Boils and Carbuncles. Boils and clusters of boils called carbuncles result from blockage of a hair follicle usually in the head, neck, arm, buttocks, or leg, producing a hardened core (or cores in the case of carbuncles) of staphylococcus bacteria just below the skin surface. These hardened lumps cause swelling, redness, and pain. Because it is teeming with infectious bacteria, the pus that exudes from a boil or carbuncle when it ruptures must be disposed of carefully. Boils and carbuncles should be continually cleaned and covered with a compress but never squeezed. Washcloths and towels should be laundered immediately. Because boils or carbuncles may indicate the presence of other infections or illness, they require medical attention.

Impetigo. This highly contagious skin infection, caused by both streptococcus and staphylococcus bacteria, is characterized by lesions or breaks in the skin usually around the hands and mouth. Initially the lesions appear as wet-looking red sores. The sores then fill with pus and develop a crusted-over appearance. Since impetigo can be spread quickly, any afflicted child should be excluded from school and directed to a physician. Application of either ammoniated mercury ointment or sulfa ointment is generally prescribed (Creswell, Newman, & Anderson, 1985).

Pediculosis. Lice infestation, or pediculosis, arises when head or body lice—extremely small, parasitic insects—attach to hair shafts. They are passed from infested persons either through direct contact or contact with an article of clothing or object used by the infested individual. Itching results and a secondary infection may occur. Application of an appropriate insecticide can destroy the lice. To prevent widespread outbreaks, school children should be thoroughly inspected for lice.

Ringworm. This condition is caused by the same fungal infection that causes athlete's foot. The term ringworm is applied when areas of the body other than the feet are affected. Ringworm is often characterized by circular lesions that are clear in the center but exhibit fluid on the edges. Personal cleanliness as well as avoiding dampening the skin without completely drying it may help. Oddly enough, ringworm is more prevalent in young children than in older children and adults, whereas the reverse is true for athlete's foot. It is believed that adults may be more resistant to ringworm because of increased secretions from oil glands, which appear to contain a natural antifungal compound (Creswell, Newman, & Anderson, 1985).

Scabies. This condition is typified by almost unbearable itching and possible lesions, especially on the face, armpit, arm, waist, and groin areas. Scabies is caused by the hatching of parasitic mite larvae deposited into the inner epidermal layers by burrowing female mites. The resulting infection is usually mild but may produce severe fever, headaches, and other general disease symptoms. Exclusion from school is necessary, and the application of a 5 percent sulfur ointment produces successful results (Stone, O'Reilly, & Brown, 1980, p. 124).

Warts. Warts are clustered, bumplike, horny outgrowths usually appearing on the hands and fingers. They are more frequent among children than adults. Growths that appear on the soles of the feet are called plantar warts and may be more painful since they are pushed back into the skin. Warts are produced by a viral infection and can be transmitted from individual to individual or from place to place on the same person through picking and scratching. Although they may disappear without attention, self-treatment may be harmful. As a result, warts should be treated by a dermatologist, who may use an acid solution, freezing, or surgery to remove them.

Sunburn. Individuals with fair or light complexions should not stay in the sun for extended periods of time because they are more vulnerable to sunburn than others. If fair-complexioned people must be in the sun for a long time, they should cover the exposed areas of the skin with a good sunscreen (Taking Care, 1984).

Care of the Skin

Daily personal cleanliness is the best means of caring for the skin. Washing the hands, feet, and face a few times each day with warm water and soap helps to remove dirt, bacteria, and oil. Although a daily shower or bath is not necessary, it is a good practice to encourage. Also, emphasize the need to wear proper clothing to suit temperature variations in order to protect the skin. This is especially necessary for individuals who are exposed to the sun for long periods of time. Different skin types may require different kinds of daily care. For example, persons with oily skin may need to clean their faces more often than people with dry skin. Allergic skin reactions to certain soaps, lotions, or creams may result, so that nonallergenic preparations may be necessary. Therefore be sure to provide instruction concerning general skin care principles as well as information about special needs. Additionally, children need to know that a dermatologist is a physician who specializes in care of the skin and skin disorders in the event a problem arises.

THE FINGERNAILS AND TOENAILS

Fingernails and toenails are outgrowths of the skin itself that originate from the inner epidermal layers. The nails arise from live roots within these inner layers and die as they grow out from the roots. As a result, fingernails and toenails are hard, horny cells that develop into keratin tissue that can be cut painlessly. Cuticles, softer but nevertheless hardened skin tissue, surround fingernails and toenails and sometimes break or crack because little oil reaches them. Both the nails and cuticles protect the fingers and toes.

Care of the Nails

Nails should be kept long enough to allow them to fulfill their protective function but should be trimmed or cut periodically in order to avoid both breakage and the collection of bacteria underneath them. When trimming the nails, a straight-across cut rather than a rounded one is recommended so that the fleshy part of the skin is not damaged. If this happens, ingrown toenails may result because the new growth of skin will then overlap the nail, causing the nail itself to dig into inner skin layers.

Nails should be cleaned daily and the fingers especially should be kept free of dirt and bacteria when eating or handling food. Cuticles should be kept soft and continually pushed away from the nail. If cuticles are not softened or kept pushed back, rough edges can develop that may tear nearby skin, causing hangnails.

Changes in the normal appearance and growth of nails and cuticles may indicate underlying health problems. For example, nails that become excessively brittle or begin to show ridges may be the result of some form of dietary deficiency or hormonal imbalance (Hamrick, Anspaugh, & Ezell, 1986).

THE HAIR

Hair grows in all regions of our bodies. Males and females have the same amount of hair in the concentrated areas (e.g., under the arm and on the scalp), but they differ in the amount of hair on various parts of the body (e.g., face). Hair growth, color, and coarseness is determined by heredity and pigment.

Like the nails, hair is an outgrowth of the skin itself. It originates from hair follicles in the dermis. The hair root within the follicle is composed of living cells that are nourished by blood vessels. As a result, removal of hair by its roots produces painful sensation. However, as is the case with nails, the visible hair shafts themselves are deadened keratin tissue that can be cut painlessly. Hair shafts on the head grow from about two to six inches before they begin to fall out naturally upon being combed or brushed. Except in cases of inherited male pattern baldness, rare illness, or as a result of some forms of chemotherapy, hair that falls out is continually being replaced.

Hair serves a protective role. Hair on the head guards against excessive exposure of the underlying scalp to solar radiation, as does body hair to some degree. Body hair also acts as a skin covering that assists in the regulation of body temperature. In addition, the eyelashes shield the eyes from dust and other irritants.

Care of the Hair

Hair need not be washed or shampooed daily. However, it should be cleaned often and brushed or combed neatly several times a day. Unnecessary combing, teasing, bleaching, and heat exposure should be avoided. Since dull, brittle appearing hair, like the nails, may be a signal of underlying health problems, close attention should be paid to changes in its growth patterns and texture.

POSTURE

Posture is more than just standing or sitting straight up. Posture refers to graceful, efficient movement of the body, whether walking, standing, or performing any type of motion. All parts of the body should be used correctly to maintain balance. When a person has poor posture, the muscles bear the burden of the off-center weight, and the person becomes fatigued much quicker.

Poor posture may be caused by a number of problems, including weak muscles, bone deformities, and careless habits of walking, sitting, and standing. Because students spend so much time during the school day sitting at a desk, it is important to encourage the students to sit properly. Each desk should be at an appropriate height for the individual to allow both feet to touch the floor without straining. The seat of the desk should allow the knees to be higher than the hips to remove stress from the lower back. The back of the chair should encourage the proper spinal curve when the child is seated. The tray of the desk should be slanted sufficiently so the student does not have to lean forward to write and read.

Posture can be positively influenced through proper nutrition for proper bone growth, exercise to tone the muscles, properly fitting clothing and shoes, well-designed furniture (including desks, chairs and beds), lifting and carrying objects properly, and proper education.

Poor posture is most often seen in junior high and senior high school students who are self-conscious about height. However, some posture defects are skeletal in nature. For example, *scoliosis*, or curvature of the spine, may produce posture defects. In addition, sometimes after an illness, injury, or infection, poor muscle tone may cause slouching or slumping. In most instances, however, these types of posture defects can be corrected under the care of an orthopedic surgeon either through surgery, various exercises, or a combination of surgery and exercises.

THE SENSES

By conveying a myriad of messages to the brain each day, the sensory organs keep us in touch with our physical and emotional environments. Five major senses keep us informed about the world around us. These are vision, hearing, touching, tasting, and smelling.

THE SENSE OF VISION

The ability to see is probably the most important sense of all. Information about images and patterns is recorded in the eyes, the sensory organs for sight, and conveyed to the brain. This information cannot be detected by the eye in the absence of light because light provides the basis for perceiving light and dark gradation, color distinction, and form or shape differentiation.

Proper vision is a key to a child's educational development. Eye problems frequently are found in children who are slow in learning to read. It is the teacher more than anyone else who sees students when they are trying to achieve. For this reason, you should observe the students for possible indications of vision problems. Some of the signs of eye trouble in your students are

- eyes crossed, in or out
- reddened, itching, or watering eyes
- frequent sties
- short attention span
- turning the head to use only one eye
- frowning or placing head close to a book when reading or writing
- sloppy handwriting
- excessive blinking or rubbing of eyes
- losing place while reading
- confusion of similar words
- unusual awkwardness while walking and poor eye-hand coordination
- frequent headaches or dizziness
- blurring of vision
- good performance on oral work, but poor written work

Visual Defects

Problems associated with the eyes and vision are numerous. Visual defects most frequent among school children include amblyopia, astigmatism, hyperopia, myopia, strabismus, and wall-eye.

Amblyopia. This condition results in dimness of vision without changes in the eye structure. One eye, the "lazy eye," allows the stronger eye to dominate and therefore becomes weakened. Amblyopia occurs without any known trauma, injury, illness, or physiological impairment necessarily preceding it. Exposure to certain chemical toxins may bring on amblyopia, or a disturbance of the optic nerve may be the cause. Sometimes amblyopia originates with a "blind spot" that grows increas-

Health Highlight: Modern Eye Problems

Although computers are commonly used in schools to enhance instruction, this progress could come with a price. Many optometrists believe the computer display terminals can aggravate existing eye problems, as well as cause pain and discomfort. The continual focusing on the terminal is what puts stress on the eyes. Those who work with computers complain of headaches, blurred vision, itching and burning eyes, eye fatigue, flickering sensations, and double vision.

A key factor contributing to eye problems among computer operators is the physical environment. Most rooms in which computer work is done are over-lighted, inadequately ventilated, and visually ill suited to properly viewing the computer screen. Lightly tinted polarized lenses can help reduce some eye problems. Further, some computer screens now have tinted screens to reduce glare.

Source: *Medical Update*. Volume VIII, Number 10, April, 1985, p. 5.

ingly larger. Amblyopia can be detected by a thorough eye examination. It is desirable to detect and treat amblyopia at an early age. Remediation includes the use of corrective lenses and vision training to teach the amblyopic eye to function normally. The "lazy eye" is often patched as part of the vision training.

Astigmatism. This condition results from abnormal curvature of the lens and cornea, which inhibits proper focusing. Images appear blurred and, because of strain in attempting to accommodate, discomfort in the form of headaches may result. Astigmatism can be corrected by wearing prescription eyeglasses or hard contact lenses.

Hyperopia. This condition is also called farsightedness because people with hyperopia have no difficulty in seeing objects at a distance. However, because the eyeball is shortened and the image falls behind the retina, the hyperopic individual has trouble focusing on objects close at hand. Severe eye strain and crossing of the eyes may result. Wearing prescription eyeglasses with convex lenses can alleviate this condition (Wiseman, 1982).

Myopia. Nearsightedness, or myopia, is the opposite of hyperopia. It occurs when images fall in front of the retina because of an elongation of the eyeball. As a result, the myopic individual can focus on objects close at hand but not those farther away. Concave lenses can compensate for eye elongation when properly prescribed. Depending upon the degree of the condition, nearsighted students may not necessarily show reading difficulty if the task is done at their desks, but they may have difficulty in reading from the board if they are sitting toward the back of the classroom (Wiseman, 1982).

Strabismus. The crossing of the eye inward due to a shortening of the outer muscles surrounding the eye is called strabismus. Depending upon the muscular defect, strabismus may be helped by means of eyeglasses, wearing a patch on the normal eye, surgery, or a combination of procedures. If strabismus is left untreated, visual acuity as well as visual accommodation may be impaired (Stone, O'Reilly, & Brown, 1980).

Wall-Eye. Wall-eye is the opposite of strabismus. With this condition, the eye turns outward instead of inward. The same treatments as those for strabismus apply.

Care of the Eyes

The eyes are among the most sensitive and delicate organs in the body. Because they work in conjunction with each other, an injury, infection, or impairment to one eye may result in damage to the other. Therefore, any visual abnormality should be dealt with either by an optometrist or an opthamologist. Optometrists are health professionals who specialize in the examination of the eyes and the determination of visual abnormalities. Opthamologists are physicians who are licensed not only to examine the eyes but also to treat eye diseases and perform surgery.

In your instruction, emphasize individual responsibility for protecting the eyes from harmful chemicals like dyes, bleaches, cleansing products, insecticides, and cosmetic irritants. Also stress the potential danger of playing with objects that could penetrate or damage the eye, such as air rifles, fireworks, and slingshots. Teach children to keep dirty hands, fingers, and soiled materials away from the eyes and to alert adults to any eye discomfort or visual problem. They should never self-medicate the eyes with drops, ointments, or creams.

Eye examinations should be given at birth, followed by additional testing around the age of 5, during adolescence, and every two years thereafter. More frequent eye examinations may be needed after the age of 40 because the aging process usually affects vision. In addition, eye examinations often uncover many underlying health problems such as diabetes, glaucoma, high blood pressure, and systemic infections.

The teacher should make adjustments in the classroom to help remediate some of the problems of students with poor vision. Have the students sit toward the front of the class so they can see the board more clearly. Some students might need a written handout if they have tremendous difficulty in seeing the board.

THE SENSE OF HEARING

The sense of hearing greatly assists communication with others. It also provides information about the environment in the form of sounds, noises, and danger signals. Additionally, the ears help an individual to maintain a sense of balance and equilibrium.

Hearing Impairments

The inability to hear can arise from a variety of causes, including congenital defects, illness and injury. Hearing disabilities may be classified as either *central, conductive,* or *sensorineural.*

Central. Central hearing loss is thought to be caused either by a malfunction in the transport of sound impulses from the cochlear nerve to the brain or by the brain's inability to interpret the sound. Although sounds are hard to differentiate, speech can sometimes be heard. Treatment is difficult (Auxter & Pyfer, 1985).

Conduction. Conductive hearing loss can occur for a variety of reasons and is characterized by some sort of blockage or structural defects in the auditory canal or middle ear that warps or muffles the vibrations. Some conditions of conduction deafness can be corrected, and most are amenable to treatment (French and Jansma, 1982).

Sensorineural. Sensorineural hearing loss results from nerve damage and is therefore not treatable. Since sound is not effectively converted by the auditory nerve into electrical signals, the brain does not receive sound impulses and hearing is greatly distorted or absent (Auxter and Pyfer, 1985).

Care of the Ears

The ears should be protected from loud noises, blasts, or other environmental hazards that can cause damage to the eardrum or affect frequency detection. Teach children to recognize the dangers of inserting anything into their ears as well as the importance of informing an adult of any ear discomfort. Children who continually pull on their ears or seem to have trouble with balance and equilibrium should be referred either to an otologist or an otolaryngologist, physicians specializing in care of the ears. Hearing tests should be administered at the preschool level as well as periodically throughout the school years.

Pay close attention to children who seem inattentive or unresponsive; these behaviors may signal hearing impairment rather than intellectual or emotional difficulties. The teacher should watch students for the following indications of hearing problems:

- chronic nose and throat trouble
- runny ear
- complaints of pressure, ringing, or buzzing in the ear
- frowning when trying to listen
- leaning forward or turning the head while listening
- good written work, but poor oral work

The best thing to do for a child with hearing loss is to detect the condition early and get medical attention. In the classroom, the teacher should place the child near the front of the room, look directly at the student, and speak clearly and slowly. Provide the student with a written handout to help the student keep up with any lesson that is presented orally.

THE SENSE OF TOUCH

Numerous sensory receptor cells in the skin provide the body with the sensations of pain, heat, cold, and touch (pressure). There is a different type of sensory receptor cell for stimuli causing each of these sensations. Heat receptors obviously trigger sensations very different from those triggered by touch receptors, for example, even though all skin sensory cells send comparable signals through the central nervous system. The difference in sensations occurs because the message from each of the four types of receptor cells is sent by a special nerve ending and is received in a particular region of the brain. That is, heat receptors send electrical impulses through specialized nerve endings to the heat centers in the brain, while touch receptors send their messages to the touch centers of the brain. Different areas of the skin vary in their degree of sensitivity, with the fingers being among the most sensitive.

The sense of touch arises when unequal pressure occurs between the skin and an object or material in contact with it. This unequal pressure produces a depression in the skin and touch is perceived (Seaman and DePauw, 1982).

Care of the Sense of Touch

Problems associated with loss of sensation are neurological in nature and are as a result complex and varied. Therefore very little can be done by the individual to affect the sense of touch. However, children should be aware of diminished sensation in any part of the body and report such an occurrence.

THE SENSES OF TASTE AND SMELL

The senses of taste and smell are closely aligned since they each enhance and are enhanced by the other. These senses can affect health in many ways, for example, influencing choices of food.

Taste buds are the sensory receptor cells within the visible *papillae*, or bumps on the tongue. Hairlike projections on the taste buds are stimulated by food entering into the mouth and send impulses to the brain from connecting nerves. There are about 9000 taste buds altogether. The large papillae at the back of the tongue contain as many as 200 taste buds each.

The tongue itself contains taste centers, each of which is more sensitive to a particular taste. The tip of the tongue is receptive to food that is sweet, whereas the rear of the tongue keys into bitter-tasting food. Salty foods are more easily tasted on the sides toward the front of the tongue, while sour foods are more easily tasted on the sides toward the back. In addition, the tongue differentiates temperature as well as texture of foods, adding greater variety to the sense of taste.

Food is not easily tasted if nasal passages are blocked in some way, as in the case of a head cold. Food in the mouth produces odors in the form of vapors that travel through the nasal passages where they stimulate receptor cells in the upper nose region. If the passages are blocked, the odors do not reach these cells, and the sense of taste/smell is diminished accordingly. Many other substances, such as perfume, give off vapors that are carried to the nasal passage and stimulate receptor cells there. Nerve endings attached to these cells join to form the olfactory nerve (first cranial nerve), the nerve that sends messages concerning smell to the cerebral cortex.

Care of the Senses of Taste and Smell

As with the sense of touch, not much can be done personally to maintain the senses of taste and smell. Impairment because of blockages of the nasal cavity due to colds or infection is temporary and will abate. Impairment due to nerve damage, although a rare occurrence, cannot be reversed so that loss of taste and smell may be permanent.

DENTAL HEALTH

Clean, polished-looking teeth and a bright, glowing smile can do much to enhance self-confidence and project a positive image in the minds of others. These emotional benefits are certainly important, but strong, healthy teeth are also essential to overall physical health. Without adequate dental care and upkeep, certain food may not be digested properly or even eaten at all in later life, jaw and facial deformities can result, affecting speech patterns, and personal health in general may suffer. All but a very few school children experience problems with teeth and gums, such as dental caries and gingivitis. (Pollock & Middleton, 1984).

It is imperative that children at an early age learn to follow effective practices that will help ensure the lifelong health of their teeth and oral cavity. They must understand how these habits contribute to good dental health and why teeth are important to preserve and maintain.

A baby's first set of teeth begin to surface at about the age of 6 to 8 months. All of these teeth are normally in place by age 2. They begin falling out around age 5 or 6, as they are replaced with permanent teeth. There are 32 permanent teeth—8 incisors, 4 cuspids, 8 bicuspids, and 12 molars. A tooth has running through its interior core a pulp canal or cavity that serves as the tooth's blood supply. This is surrounded by a bonelike material called *dentin*. Outside the dentin lie roots that fit into sockets of the jawbone. The roots are covered by a material similar to dentin called *cementum*. The visible portion of the tooth surfacing through the gums is called the crown and is covered with a substance called *enamel*.

Dental Problems

By far, the most frequent dental problem among children is dental caries—cavities produced within the teeth due to decay of tooth enamel that, if untreated, may extend into the dentin and pulp canal. Other common dental conditions among children include abscess, gingivitis, halitosis, and malocclusion.

Dental Caries. Tooth decay leads to the loss of many or all of the permanent teeth. Although false teeth can be fitted, they are generally not as effective, comfortable, or satisfactory as permanent teeth. Tooth decay results from a buildup of *plaque*, an invisible, sticky film of harmful bacteria whose continual growth in the mouth seems to be enhanced by the presence of foods containing processed sugars. Proper and frequent flossing and brushing of the teeth with a fluoride toothpaste seems to inhibit the buildup of plaque.

Abscess. Abscess is an infection of either the tooth root or gums that produces localized pus. This condition may result for a variety of reasons. Release of toxins from the oral abscess to other parts of the body can cause harm not only to the teeth and gums, but to health in general. As a result, medical attention is imperative.

Gingivitis. This term refers to inflammation of the gums but is often used to denote a specific infection called Vincent's disease (trench mouth), which is characterized by pain, bleeding from the gums, possible ulceration of the gums, and excessive salivation. Gingivitis can be caused in part by poor nutrition, use of tobacco products, and poor brushing and flossing habits. Fortunately, many advances have been made recently in the care of the teeth and gums that assist in the care of gingivitis, such as public water fluoridation and mouth rinses (Consumer Reports, 1984).

Care of Your Teeth

Floss your teeth before you brush them. Flossing helps remove plaque from between the teeth. What is plaque?

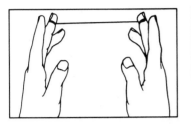
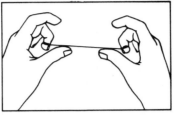

To floss the teeth, break off about one-half meter of floss. Wind most of it around one of your middle fingers. Wind the rest around your other middle finger.

Now hold the floss between each thumb and forefinger. Allow about three centimeters between them, to guide the floss between the teeth.

Hold the floss tightly. Move it back and forth to ease it between the teeth. Band the floss toward the tooth as you do this. Gently slide it into the space between gum and tooth.

Now scrape the floss up and down against the side of the tooth. Do the same thing for each pair of teeth. Use a new piece of floss each time.

Brushing

Be sure to use a flat, soft-bristled toothbrush.

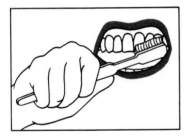
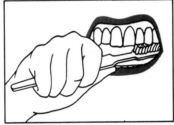
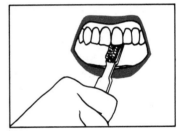

Place the ends of the bristles against the outside of your teeth. Angle the brush against the gums.

Move the brush back and forth. Use short, gentle strokes. Do this to the outside of all your teeth and gums.

Brush the insides of your teeth and gums the same way you brushed the outsides, moving the brush back and forth. Brush the tops of your teeth too.

Brush the insides of your front teeth and gums up and down with the front end of your brush.

Figure 9.1
Proper flossing and brushing techniques.
Source: Adapted from *Health* by Hamrick, Anspaugh, & Ezell (Columbus: Merrill, 1986).

Halitosis. This is another term for bad breath. Continued halitosis is usually indicative of poor oral and dental health practices. Referral to a dentist may be necessary.

Malocclusion. Maloccusion refers to improper alignment of the upper and lower teeth when the jaw is closed, thus producing either an overbite or an underbite. Through the use of braces fitted by an orthodontist, a dentist who specializes in these problems, malocclusion can be corrected.

Care of the Teeth

Daily flossing and brushing of the teeth, preferably after each meal but at least once, is the best way to maintain good dental health. Flossing should be done first since it removes plaque from between teeth. Flossing should be done using about 18 inches of floss wound around the middle fingers until only a few inches are left. The ends of the remaining floss section are then grasped between each thumb and forefinger and eased between the gum and tooth so that a scraping motion against the side of the tooth can occur. This procedure should be repeated with each tooth, using a new section of floss each time. Brushing removes plaque from tooth surfaces and is best accomplished by angling the brush against the gumline so that a back and forth (side to side) motion using gentle strokes can be done on the outside, inside, and biting surfaces of the teeth. A fluoridated toothpaste is recommended. Proper flossing and brushing techniques are illustrated in figure 9.1.

In addition to daily flossing and brushing, particular attention should be paid to diet. Avoidance of sweets is recommended, and the intake of food high in vitamin D during childhood will help develop strong teeth. Regular dental examinations, preferably twice a year, from childhood through adulthood will also do much to ensure good dental health.

EXERCISE, RELAXATION, AND SLEEP

Exercise, done according to sound physiological principles in a routine or scheduled regimen, is necessary for the maintenance and enhancement of personal health. The body also requires relaxation and sleep in order to renew its energy and strength resources. Body systems that are not allowed to recharge and rejuvenate themselves will ultimately demonstrate various malfunctions that can have drastic effects on the general health and well-being of the individual. Both short- and long-term personal health can be greatly enhanced by appropriate periods of exercise, relaxation, and sleep.

Exercise

Exercise, when it is an integral component of a person's lifestyle, can be of value in a variety of ways. Fitness not only builds up the strength and resistance to injury of the muscles themselves, it is also beneficial to the entire body. Individuals engaging in planned exercise programs that include not only conditioning or calisthenics but also extended exercise such as jogging, swimming, or bicycling show more resistance to chronic ailments, including fatigue, backaches, headaches, anxiety, muscular weakness and atrophy, high blood pressure, and some cardiovascular conditions associated with heart disease.

Cardiorespiratory Fitness. To carry out bodily processes, the body requires energy. This energy, which is supplied in the form of oxygen, is extracted from a specially stored, energy-rich compound called ATP (adenosinetriphosphate). Through a complex chemical chain reaction, ATP breaks down to release oxygen and make it available to the body. This process is termed an *aerobic* release of energy, that is, one that takes place in the presence of oxygen. The oxygen released by the ATP is replenished through the breathing process.

If the task is particularly demanding or strenuous, not enough oxygen may be immediately available to meet the energy demands of the activity, no matter how rapidly the person breathes. When this happens, additional energy is provided *without* further initiation of ATP breakdown and the release of additional oxygen. This latter process is therefore considered *anaerobic*, or taking place without sufficient oxygen replenishment. However, the anaerobic mechanism for supplying energy is short-lived and produces fatigue associated with muscle soreness due to a buildup of lactic acid in the muscles as a waste product of anaerobic energy release.

A chief aim of any exercise program should be to develop and improve an individual's aerobic capacity so that intense physical activities can be maintained for longer periods without running short of sufficient oxygen. To do this, exercises that require the heart and lungs to do more work should be stressed, such as running, jogging, and swimming, so that both of these organs become more efficient at delivering oxygen to the cells. Since the heart is a muscular organ, the more strenuously it is taxed with the appropriate type and duration of activity, the larger and stronger its muscle fibers become. Thus a gradual increase in stroke volume will occur with fewer beats per minute. *Stroke volume* refers to the amount of blood the heart is able to pump with each contraction or beat. More and more blood (oxygen) is therefore being delivered to tissue by the heart, which in turn is beating or working less. Aerobic exercises also improve the muscles of the ribs and diaphragm so that the rib cage is lifted higher, allowing greater expansion of the lungs. Breathing is made easier and exercise can continue for a longer period of time without adverse effects.

Aerobic exercises that improve cardiorespiratory fitness are not generally lacking in the routine of most elementary school children's lifestyles. However, it is essential that planned, prescribed exercise programs be provided by specialists, such as physical educators and exercise physiologists, to meet individual needs, particularly as the individual grows older.

Skeletal and Muscular Fitness. Although cardiorespiratory fitness should be the foundation for any exercise program because it increases the body's ability to perform strenuous activity, emphasis on muscular strength and skeletal support is also important. Along with aerobic exercises, calisthenics and *isotonic exercises* (exercise with little or no body movement, such as pushing against a wall) can develop muscular strength and power. Muscle fibers become thicker as a result of regular exerise and therefore stronger. In addition, coordination between muscle groups is improved as well as coordination between muscles and nerves. Static stretching in particular can help produce flexibility of muscles, which enhances skeletal support and fitness.

Relaxation

Relaxation is one of the body's most useful tools in combating fatigue, either physical, mental, or both. By learning how to relax during the day so that alert and conscious functioning continues, a person can reduce feelings of listlessness, tiredness, apathy, tension, and aches and pains.

Fatigue may be due solely to physical overexertion or to a drain of mental capabilities after engaging in such chores as reading, writing, problem-solving, or studying in general. Fatigue can also be produced by adverse environmental conditions, such as improper ventilation or lighting, or by emotional stress.

Relaxation involves the releasing of physical and mental tension through varied and diverse means that can include doing nothing, meditating, watching television, listening to music, taking a hot bath, or relaxing the muscles with a massage. The ways in which an individual chooses to relax should be based on personal interests, environment, or setting, and comfort with the procedure or technique. Regardless of how achieved, relaxation needs to be incorporated into every individual's lifestyle, just as exercise does, so that stress reaction can be minimized and personal health and well-being can be maximized.

Sleep

The body's need for sleep must be met consistently in order to maintain good personal health. Unlike exercise and relaxation, sleep is an involuntary process that does not require a planned or prescribed regimen that must be purposely enacted by the individual. In fact, scientists still cannot fully explain all the mysteries associated with sleep, including its cause and why it is needed.

The amount of sleep needed varies from individual to individual. Most adults need about eight hours sleep in order to awaken easily and without fatigue. The amount of sleep needed decreases as age increases. Newborn infants spend a majority of their time sleeping, while most older adults sleep less than eight hours at night but may require short naps during the day. Elementary school children need eight to nine hours of sleep a night (Payne & Hahn, 1986).

DISEASE CONTROL AND PREVENTION

Despite all the measures that an individual takes to maintain personal health, from time to time *pathogens*, or disease-causing microbes, invade the body and either escape or inhibit its natural disease-fighting mechanisms. However, if an individual has fostered personal health, susceptibility to infectious diseases will be lessened. Such individuals are also more likely to recuperate more quickly when disease does strike. Nevertheless, children and adults come into contact with pathogens daily and need to know about the nature of pathogens, how they can enter the body, how they are dealt with by the body, and what means are available to prevent the spread of disease.

The Body's Defense Against Pathogens

The body employs three lines of defense against disease. The first line of defense consists of the skin and mucous membranes. If pathogens penetrate this line (e.g., through broken skin), the second line of defense starts into action. The second line of defense consists of phagocytes (white blood cells) which attack and engulf the pathogen. When pathogens begin to reproduce in the body, the body develops antibodies to fight off infection—the third line of defense.

In the early stage of infection, called the *incubation period*, there are still too few pathogens in the body to cause symptoms of the disease. The incubation period varies in length from a few days to a few weeks, depending on the specific pathogen.

When the pathogen has reproduced in abundance, the infected individual is then in the *prodrome period* of the illness. General symptoms such as chills, fever, or headache are now present. In this stage, the disease is highly contagious. Because the symptoms are still general ones, however, a specific diagnosis cannot be made. During this time, the circulatory system begins to deliver to localized cells increased levels of phagocytes. The body also manufactures other disease-fighting chemicals such as interferon and lysozyme. An increased delivery of blood to sites of localized infection may produce swelling, inflammation, aching, heat, and body temperature rise associated with general disease symptoms of the prodrome stage.

Next, *clinical disease symptoms* begin to appear. These are the specific and characteristic signs of a given illness, such as the red blotches or eruptions of measles. In reaction to the disease, *antibodies* are produced in the blood to act as the body's major defense against the continued reproduction and spread of pathogens. Since a particular pathogen triggers the manufacture and release of a particular antibody, a diagnosis can be made at this stage of illness. In addition to the natural chemical defenses produced by the body, antibiotics and other drugs will probably be prescribed by a physician.

After the antibodies and prescribed drugs have become effective in destroying large numbers of pathogens, severe disease symptoms begin to subside and antibody manufacturing begins to diminish. The infected individual enters the *convalescent period* of illness. At this stage, the person shows signs of recovery but may nevertheless be prone to relapse and may still be contagious. Finally, however, full recovery should occur, and manifestations of the disease or disease-fighting chemicals will no longer be present. It is important to realize that during convalescence general body resistance has been lowered in warding off infection and full recuperation is not likely to be immediate. As a result, a child returning to school after illness, even though free of disease, should not be expected to immediately perform at an optimum level.

Contributions of Epidemiology and Immunology

Advances in the fields of epidemiology and immunology have done much to control and prevent infectious and communicable diseases. *Epidemiology*, the study of the nature and spread of disease within populations, provides answers to questions concerning the identification of pathogens themselves and the ways in which these pathogens are transmitted to people. *Immunology* supplies procedures that can be used to prevent many of these diseases from occurring or to treat the diseases when they do occur.

Epidemiology has made clear that personal hygiene and clean and sanitary environment are crucial in controlling infectious illness. Improved sanitary measures, such as ensuring a safe water supply, have had great impact on minimizing the spread of many diseases that once killed people throughout the world in epidemic proportions. Also, thanks to artificial immunization methods, individuals no longer have to risk exposure to infection in order to develop natural immunity but are now able to acquire immunity by being vaccinated or injected with a weakened strain of the pathogen itself. "Childhood" vaccinations cause the triggering of antibody production without forcing the body to experience severe disease symptoms or fight a full-fledged infection. Illnesses such as diphtheria, tetanus, whooping cough, smallpox, and polio, which once threatened the lives of children and adults, are now controllable. For this reason, immunizing all children is essential and should be promoted by parents, teachers, and school officials, as well as by the medical community.

Chronic Illness in Children

Although the vast majority of children suffer from infectious illness only occasionally, without long-lasting disability, some children are afflicted with chronic conditions that need special understanding and attention, especially by the teacher and other school personnel. You should be aware of these conditions so that you will be more sensitive to the needs of students who suffer from them. Chronic illnesses in children include allergies, cancer, congenital heart abnormalities, and cystic fibrosis.

Allergies. Allergies are the most common disorder of the immune system. One of the most severe allergies is asthma. Like all allergies, asthma results from a hypersensitivity to a specific allergen such as certain kinds of food (milk, eggs), animal hair, pollen, pollution, or grass. Asthma, which manifests itself by a swelling of the bronchial tubes, is characterized by violent attacks of wheezing and respiratory difficulty. These attacks may be triggered by stress. As a result, a child who is asthmatic or suffers from other allergies may be more "nervous" or "high-strung" than other children (Insel & Roth, 1985). More than 1.5 million children, mostly boys, suffer from asthma (Seaman & DePauw, 1982). Unlike asthma, other allergies such as hay fever may be seasonally occurring conditions.

Cancer. The number of new cancer cases in children 6 to 17 is 12 per 100,000. The most common type of cancer in this age group is leukemia, a blood disorder in which white blood cells are manufactured uncontrollably. Leukemia in children tends to be more acute than leukemia in adults. The disease is characterized by internal bleeding, weakness, anemia, and fatigue. Whenever possible, a child with cancer should be allowed to participate in normal classroom activities, particularly when the child is in a state of remission, a state of temporary "normalcy" of unpredictable length.

Real progress in treating childhood cancer has been made during the past three decades, according to the National Center for Health Statistics. Since the 1950s, deaths from leukemia have fallen 50 percent, from lymphoma 32 percent, from Hodgkin's disease 80 percent, from bone cancer 50 percent, and from kidney cancer 68 percent. The dramatic reduction in deaths is due almost entirely to improved forms of treatment (*Harvard Medical School Health Letter*, 1984).

Congenital Heart Abnormalities. Each year, about 40,000 children are born with some type of cardiac condition that affects either the heart muscle itself or the vessels or valves of the heart. *Septal defects*, one of the most common abnormalities, occur when holes exist between either the right and left atria or between the right and left ventricles. Sometimes septal defects and constriction of the valve between the right ventricle and the pulmonary artery, the vessel carrying deoxygenated blood to the lungs, produce a more severe congenital condition that restricts the amount of blood that can be channeled to the lungs to receive oxygen. This condition is referred to as *pulmonary stenosis*. The most serious congenital cardiac disorder, *tetralogy of Fallot*, results from four defects that usually involve a ventricle defect accompanied by pulmonary stenosis and thickening of the right ventricle. This causes a change in position of the aorta, the major heart artery. As in the case of a child with cancer, a student with a congenital heart condition should be included in as many routine classroom activities as possible (Fait & Dunn, 1984).

Cystic Fibrosis. This is an inherited disorder that results from a deficiency of pancreatic enzyme. It affects about 2000 children born each year. Because of lack of pancreatic enzyme, both digestion and respiration are impaired. Early treatment with a special diet including an enzyme preparation can usually prevent extremely severe symptoms in early childhood. However, even with proper medical treatment, there is only a 50 percent survival rate. Teachers should understand the nature of cystic fibrosis and the effects of medication. The students with cystic fibrosis should be encouraged to participate in all appropriate activities (French and Jansma, 1982).

SUMMARY

Personal health, a most desired and cherished possession, is of concern to everyone, for without good health, the quality of life is diminished considerably and day-to-day existence becomes a burden instead of a joy. To ensure good personal health, each individual must assume responsibility for taking care of his or her own body so that it is kept in good condition. Learning to maintain and enhance one's health and well-being in early childhood through sound health practices is crucial for sustaining high levels of personal health in later life. Therefore it is important to teach children the elements of personal health, including an appreciation for personal appearance, the senses that allow them to relate to their environments, and good dental health. In addition, children must be taught to exert purposeful, conscious action in incorporating and integrating regular intervals of exercise, relaxation, and sleep into their living patterns. While all people come under attack from disease-producing pathogens and have to ward off infection from time to time, individuals who engage in effective personal health practices are less susceptible to illness and tend to recuperate more quickly with less drastic results. Even those individuals who are plagued by a chronic condition can better sustain and enhance their total health status by learning and following sound health practices.

DISCUSSION QUESTIONS

1. Describe the three layers of the skin.
2. Why should persons with acne avoid skin creams with an oil base?
3. Discuss the hazards for overexposure to the sun by fair-skinned individuals.
4. Discuss the similarities and differences in hair growth between males and females.
5. Describe proper posture while sitting at a desk.
6. List the possible behavioral indications of vision problems.

7. Discuss the remediation of amblyopia.

8. Discuss the classroom adjustments a teacher should make for a student with poor vision.

9. List the possible behavioral indications of hearing problems.

10. Discuss the negative influences on gingivitis.

REFERENCES

Auxter, D., & Pyfer, J. *Principles and methods of adapted physical education and recreation.* St. Louis: Times Mirror/Mosby, 1985.

"Tooth decay: The early problem." *Consumer Reports*, March, 1984.

Consumer Reports, March, 1984.

Creswell, W., Newman, I., & Anderson, C. *School health practice*, eighth edition. St. Louis: Times Mirror/Mosby, 1985.

Fait, H., & Dunn, J. *Special physical education*, fifth edition. Philadelphia: Saunders, 1984.

French, R., & Jansma, P. *Special physical education.* Columbus: Merrill, 1982.

Hamrick, M., Anspaugh, D., & Ezell, G. *Health.* Columbus: Merrill, 1986.

Harvard Medical School Health Letter. July, 1984.

Insel, P., & Roth, W. *Core concepts in health*, fourth edition. Palo Alto, Calif.: Mayfield Publishing Company, 1985.

Jones, K., Shainberg, L., & Byer, C. *Health science*, fifth edition. New York: Harper & Row, 1985.

Medical Update, VIII, *10*, April, 1985.

Payne, W., & Hahn, D. *Understanding your health.* St. Louis: Times Mirror/Mosby, 1986.

Pollock, M., & Middleton, K. *Elementary school health instruction.* St. Louis: Times Mirror/Mosby, 1984.

Seaman, J., & DePauw, K. *The new adapted physical education: A developmental approach.* Palo Alto, Calif.: Mayfield Publishing Company, 1982.

Stone, D., O'Reilly, L., & Brown, J. *Elementary school health education: Ecological perspectives.* Dubuque, Iowa: Wm. C. Brown, 1980.

Taking Care. 6, *7*, July, 1984.

Wiseman, D. *A practical approach to adapted physical education.* Reading, Mass: Addison-Wesley, 1982.

10. Techniques for Teaching Personal Health

It is a distortion, with something profoundly disloyal about it, to picture the human being as a teetering, fallible contraption, always needing watching and patching, always on the verge of flapping to pieces; this is the doctrine that people hear most often, and most eloquently, on all our information media. We ought to be developing a much better system for general education about human health, with more curricular time for acknowledgment, and even some celebration, of the absolute marvel of good health that is the real lot of most of us, most of the time.—Lewis Thomas, *The Lives of a Cell*

THE CONCEPT OF PERSONAL HEALTH

Health education was formerly limited to hygeinic practices. Since those days, health education has branched out to include concepts from sociology, psychology, and other disciplines; however, we must not overlook the importance of teaching children about taking care of their bodies. In teaching personal health, emphasize to your students that enhancing well-being is largely an individual responsibility. The concept of personal health is an abstract idea that young children need to be familiarized with, yet many of the practices associated with health maintenance are already familiar to them and can be used as a base for building understanding of the concept. To do this, relate daily health practices to overall well-being. In this way, children will begin to see that discrete practices, such as face washing or tooth brushing, are components of an overall approach to optimum health. That is, a person does not wash simply to clean a part of the body, and tooth brushing and flossing are not simply done to help prevent tooth decay. Rather, these and other personal health practices are parts of an overall maintenance and health enhancement program. To bring this point home, note that personal body cleanliness plays an important role in the prevention of disease, just as proper dental care contributes to overall health.

The techniques described in this chapter are designed to teach not only specific health practices but to foster good personal health habits. Knowing how to brush one's teeth properly is of little value unless tooth brushing and allied dental care are attended to on a regular basis. For this to occur, children must personalize the information that you present and make decisions to develop good habits. Continually emphasize that personal health is a matter of personal accountability.

Concepts to be Taught

- Personal health maintenance and enhancement are essential to one's well-being.
- The attainment of personal health and well-being is an individual responsibility, but one that can be facilitated by school, community, and social resources.
- Personal health is influenced by choices made and actions taken based on individual values, attitudes, beliefs, and knowledge.
- Daily care and upkeep of one's personal appearance is an important component of personal health.
- Personal appearance is influenced by health habits concerning care of the skin, nails, hair, and posture.
- Preservation of the five major body senses—vision, hearing, touch, taste, and smell—is essential to personal health because the senses keep us in touch with our physical and emotional environments.
- Adequate dental care may help to prevent jaw and facial deformities, speech abnormalities, and malnourishment in later life, thus safeguarding personal health.
- Consistent, routinely scheduled, prescribed exercise programs promote personal health and well-being by strengthening cardiorespiratory and muscular fitness.
- Relaxation and sleep allow bodily processes and functions to renew their energy sources, thus helping to combat physical and mental fatigue.
- Personal health is sometimes adversely affected by the contraction of an infection or communicable disease.
- The implementation of daily health practices will lower the potential for contraction of an infection or communicable disease.
- Chronic illnesses can occur in people of all ages, causing them to alter or modify certain practices of behavior in order to maintain personal health.

Cycle Plan for Teaching Topics

Topic	K	1	2	3	4	5	6
				Grade Level			
Personal Appearance	**	**	**	***	**	***	**
The Senses	**	**	***	*	***	***	*
Dental Health	***	***	***	***	***	**	*
Exercise and Fitness	***	**	**	***	*	*	**
Relaxation and Sleep	***	**	**	***	**	*	**
Disease Control and Prevention	***	**	**	***	***	**	***
Chronic Illness in Children	**	**	**	**	***	*	**

Key: *** = major emphasis, ** = emphasis, * = review.

VALUE-BASED ACTIVITIES

Before and After

Have students either draw or cut out pictures illustrating facets of personal appearance that need improvement. These are the "Before" pictures. Each student describes how he or she believes personal appearance could be improved and then draws an "After" picture to illustrate these opinions and ideas.

What Sleep Means to Me

Have students sketch or paint a picture showing their interpretation of the value of sleep. Have them write a statement about their picture, such as

> I smile more when I get enough sleep.
> I can run faster when I get my sleep regularly.
> I am always tired but I hate to go to bed.
> I get sleepy in school when I stay up too late.

Pretty Face

Provide the class with six to eight pictures of smiling, well-groomed children of varying ethnic backgrounds. Number the pictures and ask each student to rank order them from the most desirable personal appearance to the least desirable. Group students so that they can compare their rankings. Note to the class that attraction to a certain type of personal appearance is based on individual preference, not that other types of personal appearances are necessarily less desirable. Emphasize that there is lots of room for individual expression in personal appearance but that neatness and good grooming provide the foundation.

Self-Portrait

Provide large pieces of paper and crayons to each student. Ask the students to draw a picture of themselves. (This may best be done at home where a mirror is available and time constraints are removed.) On the reverse side, have students list what they perceive to be their positive attributes. Also have them describe the measures they take to promote personal health.

Health Products Awareness

Assign care of a body part, such as hair, skin, teeth, or nails, to a specific day of the week and ask students to bring to class a health product that they or someone in their family uses for the care of that body part. For example, on a day that hair is assigned, products may include shampoo, hairbrushes, conditioners, and combs. Group students who have similar products together so that each group can explain the benefits of using the particular product. Discuss the differences between those products that are purely cosmetic and those that enhance health. (You may want to bring in additional health products that students may not initially think of to use in caring for the body.)

Relaxation Ranking

Prepare a list of ten ways people can relax during the day. Ask each student to rank order the measures from most effective to least effective. Divide students into small groups and indicate that each group must come to a *consensus* ranking. Record each group's ranking on the board and allow for explanations, questions, and summarization.

Values

The purpose of this activity is to explore personal health behavior and relate personal values to that behavior. Give students a handout on which is presented a statement for their consideration. After they read the statement, have them answer the questions below it. An example:*

> Each of us has habits which can be considered healthy; and each of us has habits that are unhealthy. Considering your physical health: What three personal habits of yours can you think of that are unhealthy?
> 1.
> 2.
> 3.
> Why do you do these things?
> 1.
> 2.
> 3.
> What are the consequences of continuing these unhealthy behaviors?
> 1.
> 2.
> 3.

Values Continuum

For each of the questions below, ask students to place themselves on the continuum.*

Always   Never

1. I brush my teeth daily.
2. I floss my teeth daily.
3. Physical health is more important than mental health.
4. Appearance is more important than health.
5. Schools are concerned with students' health.
6. My teacher is healthy.
7. It is as important to smell good as to be healthy.
8. I use a deodorant.
9. I use hair spray.
10. I wash my hands before eating anything.

---

*Source: Greenberg, Jerrold S. *Student-Centered Health Instruction.* Reading, Mass.: Addison-Wesley Publishing Company, 1978.

11. Candy machines should be allowed in school buildings.
12. I listen to my stereo turned up as loud as it will go.
13. I go to bed whenever I feel like it.
14. You should shampoo your hair every day.
15. Everybody needs eight hours of sleep every night.
16. I am healthy.
17. I should visit my dentist two times a year.
18. Makeup is important for a girl to look her best.
19. I do not have any unhealthy behaviors.
20. Regular physical examinations are very important.

Body Senses Position Statement

Assign students to one of five body senses groups. Have each group prepare a brief argument or position statement in which they try to convince others that their sense (vision, hearing, touch, taste, or smell) is the most important for general health and safety. After each position is presented, each student votes by secret ballot, tallies are reported, and then summarized.

Personal Health Sentence Completion

Have students provide endings to statements such as the following:

I like the way I look because _____
Sleep is _____
I take care of my eyes by _____
If I lost my sense of hearing, _____
Sitting, standing, and walking straight helps to _____
Lack of exercise makes me _____

Decision Stories

Present decision stories such as the following, using the procedures outlined in chapter 5.

Clean Up Your Act

Jimmy Jay was a friendly boy who was fun to be with. He was smart and a very good student, so both his teacher and his classmates admired him. When someone needed a helping hand, Jimmy Jay was always there to offer assistance. There was only one problem with him. Jimmy Jay didn't take a bath very often so he smelled bad and his hair always seemed dirty. Sometimes this made it hard to be around him.

Focus Question: What would you do if you had to sit next to him in class?

Vision Problems

Kathy was the youngest member in her family. She had two older brothers. Both her parents and her brothers wore eyeglasses. Kathy felt sorry for them because she thought that glasses made people look funny and they seemed to be such a nuisance. You couldn't run or play games as easily because they were always falling off. Kathy has just found out that she is going to have to wear glasses, too, and she is having trouble getting used to the idea. You are a good friend of Kathy's. You have perfect vision and don't wear eyeglasses. You sense that Kathy is feeling sorry for herself—and feeling jealous of your good vision.

Focus Question: What would you say to Kathy?

Teeth and Truth

It's been over a year since Danny has been to the dentist. Danny knows that his mother forgot about his regularly scheduled dental appointment because he answered the phone when the hygenist called to remind them about the appointment. He didn't tell his mother because he didn't want to go back. But for the last few weeks, one area of Danny's mouth has been feeling funny every time he eats. Danny hates going to the dentist. He is also afraid that he will be punished if he tells his mother what he did.

Focus Questions: What should Danny do? Why?

Left Out

Sally has just moved to town in the middle of the year and has entered your class. She is a nice person but rather shy. It seems as though she has trouble making friends easily because of her quiet nature. The problem is made even worse because Sally does not take part in group games during recess. Your guess is that Sally has some condition or illness that keeps her from playing with everyone else, but you're not sure. Since she is new in town and has no friends, there is no one you can ask about Sally's problem. Or maybe it's none of your business.

Focus Question: What should you do?

The Crooked Teeth

Some people do not think it is important to have their crooked teeth straightened. They may feel this way because their crooked teeth do not bother them, because treatment is expensive, or because they do not want to worry with wearing braces.

Mary's teeth are very crooked. The boys at school are constantly making fun of her at school. Mary has discussed this problem with her parents and would very much like to have her teeth straightened. But, her parents say that they did not have their teeth straightened when they were young and cannot understand why it is so important to Mary. Also, they really cannot afford the expense of braces.

Focus Question: Mary is very upset over the situation. What can she do?

The Christmas Party

Elizabeth's teacher has asked her to be in charge of the 6th grade Christmas Party in her room this year. This is really an honor for Elizabeth, and she wants to do everything just right. But, Elizabeth cannot eat sugar and most of the holiday treats are loaded with sugar. Elizabeth thought of maybe having a "Sugarless Christmas Party" with lots of vegetables and dips and other foods without sugar. But, Elizabeth is really worried that the other students would turn up their nose at this idea. She certainly doesn't want the party to be a flop.

Focus Question: What do you think she should do?

Source: Fodor, Glass, & Gmur. *Good Health for You.* River Forest, Illinois: Laidlaw Brothers Publishers, 1983.

All Alone

Charlie is in your class. Nobody plays with him because he wears sloppy and dirty clothes. Charlie does not have parachute pants or Levi's like the other guys in the class. Charlie is usually left all alone because he doesn't fit in with the group. After working with Charlie on an assigned science project, you really like Charlie. In fact, he is one of the nicest and sincere people that you have ever met. After meeting Charlie's parents, you realize that they cannot afford to buy Charlie many clothes. You really want to be Charlie's friend but everyone at school will laugh at you if they know you are his friend.

Focus Question: What should you do?

Careless Coughing

Katie is your very best friend. Everytime somebody sees one of you, the other is always close by. Katie is very nice and clean. She is mannerly and she is a perfectionist, except in one area—her health. She always has a cold, because she never wears her coat when it is cold. Katie never thinks anything about coughing in your face without covering her mouth. She coughs freely wherever she wishes. You try to remind her as often as possible but it doesn't help. You usually end up getting her cold.

Focus Question: How can you convince Katie to cover her mouth when coughing so she won't spread germs?

DRAMATIZATION

Grooming Guidelines

Divide the class into several groups. Assign each group a certain grooming practice. Meet with each group to explain the important rules to follow for each practice. The group then coordinates a pantomime to illustrate the rules. As each group performs, other groups must guess what practice is being demonstrated. After each group finishes, go over the rules with the class, pointing out correct methods.

Bedtime Battles

Divide students into small groups and present them with the same dilemma: Parents are trying to get their two children, ages 5 and 8, to go to sleep. The children are resistant but the parents try to use logic and information about the need for sleep. Let each group act out how they perceive this dilemma can be solved.

Sense Loss Scenarios

Divide students into five groups, assigning one of the body senses to each. Each group writes and performs a scenario of what one morning's activities would be like if they did not have that sense.

Keeping It Under Control

Divide students into small groups and assign the following roles: child, doctor, mother, father, child's sibling, teacher, classmates. Have each group dramatize the various reactions and behaviors that might be exhibited by the assigned characters if the child had been diagnosed as having a serious contagious illness such as hepatitis, mononucleosis, or tuberculosis. Follow the dramatizations with a lengthy discussion period.

DISCUSSION AND REPORT TECHNIQUES

Presentation by Health Professionals

Invite various health professionals, such as dentist, orthodontist, optometrist, opthamologist, or audiologist, to address the class and describe their activities and to inform students about sound personal health practices in their field.

Grooming: Role Playing

By assuming the roles of paper dolls, students will be able to make decisions concerning their own personal appearance. The materials you will need are girl and boy paper dolls, dressed to represent Neat Ned, Clean Cathy, Wrinkled Winnie, and Unkempt Karl. Have the students assume the role of the particular paper doll they receive. They can create conversations about why Ned and Cathy are more pleasant and attractive dolls. The teacher may offer suggestions throughout the role playing if needed. Let the students take turns so that everyone will have a chance to participate. As an additional activity, provide a simple paper doll outline pattern so the children can create their own dolls and dress them as they wish.

Screening Procedures

Prepare an outline of the various screening procedures that are commonly used in school systems. Include screening measures that may not necessarily be available in your school but are used widely. Ask each student to choose one procedure and write a report about it. Collect the reports and collate them into a screening procedure booklet that can be used as a resource.

Safeguarding the Senses Report

Divide students into groups representing each of the five senses. On following days, have each give an oral presentation of at least five health practices that safeguard that sense. Each group should list practices on posterboard, which can be tacked to walls around the room for special emphasis.

Infectious Disease Prevention

Engage in a teacher-led discussion of infectious or communicable disease prevention. In this discussion, be sure to include the following points:

- Infections are caused by invisible organisms.

- Disease-producing organisms can be spread by direct contact, indirect contact, or vector transmission.

- Immunizations that one receives in childhood guard against many illnesses.

- Sound health habits will help to guard against those infections not covered by immunizations.

- General disease symptoms include chills, fever, headaches, and stomach upset.

- Children should report general symptoms to parents or their teacher.

Voluntary Health Organization Panel

Follow the same procedure as outlined in chapter 8 but contact representatives of organizations that focus on chronic conditions.

A Really Relaxing Time

Ask each student to write about or describe an event, time, or situation that was particularly relaxing. Students should discuss the factors they think contributed to relaxation in the situation and factors that contribute to relaxation in general.

EXPERIMENTS AND DEMONSTRATIONS

Frown-Free

Ask each student to bring a mirror to class. As the students look at themselves in the mirror, tell them to smile and notice any wrinkles or indentations. Then tell them to frown as if they were sad or made. They should notice more wrinkles when they frown than when they smile. Discuss how a nice smile enhances personal appearance.

Tooth Anatomy

- Obtain a large model of the teeth or make your own. Have students make smaller models from clay or soap.

- Obtain a chart showing a cross section of a tooth and have students make similar drawings.

- Obtain X-ray plates of a child's teeth so that the position of permanent teeth beneath the baby teeth can be clearly seen. If you cannot obtain X-ray plates, substitute drawings from a text.

Teeth and Digestion

Give each student a graham cracker, vanilla wafer, animal cookie, or saltine. Have them chew it without swallowing and note what takes place. Explain that the teeth grind the food. At the same time, saliva and digestive enzymes in the mouth act on the food. Children should note how the taste of the cracker sweetens as this happens. The chewed cracker is being changed to a moist bolus so that it can be swallowed easily.

Care of the Teeth

After a milk break or lunch, give each student a disclosing tablet to chew. (These can be purchased at any drugstore or pharmacy.) Let them examine their teeth in a mirror to note the darkened regions indicating plaque buildup. Then, give each student a few pieces of apple to chew, which acts as an abrasive, much like toothpaste. Have them look in the mirror to note any disappearance of plaque.

Posture Perfect

Demonstrate incorrect and correct ways of sitting, standing, and walking. Then, give the following commands to the class:

Everybody sit wrong.
Everybody sit right.
Everybody stand wrong.
Everybody stand right.
Everybody walk wrong.
Everybody walk right.

Repeat several times and mix the order of commands.

Shadow Play

The purpose is to gain an understanding of various postural defects and practice posture improvement. The materials you will need are a shadow screen (a bed sheet may be used), lights, and equipment necessary for the demonstration. This is an excellent way for children to compare and dramatize good and bad posture. A narrator, chosen by the group, discusses various aspects of maintaining good posture while standing, sitting, walking, and reading. As the narrator discusses each posture, a pupil standing behind the screen will demonstrate poor posture; and at the same time another will demonstrate proper posture. The positions of narrator and shadow-casters can be changed so that all children participate.

Properties of Skin

Ask each student to take off a shoe and sock so that one foot is bare. Have the students feel the difference between their skin and the sock covering the other foot. Let them notice the cooling reaction and ask them why one foot feels cooler than the other. Then, dab the foot with alcohol, demonstrating the evaporation principle. Ask the students how perspiration relates to this principle. Also have students pull on the skin covering their foot. Ask them if some places are tighter than others on the foot. Why does this matter? Ask them if some places are more sensitive than others. What does this tell us about skin?

Skin Examination

Have each child examine the skin on the back of his or her hand with a magnifying glass. They will notice the creases and folds when the hand is relaxed, and also the dirt, which will disappear after washing. Have the class note the pores and tiny hairs. Discuss perspiration and body odors. Tell the class to note the oil and hair glands and tell them what they do for the skin and one's appearance. To show how "hidden dirt" stays on the skin, even when a pupil thinks she is clean, rub the back of the hand with a small piece of cloth dipped in alcohol. Let the class see the cloth before and after rubbing the skin.

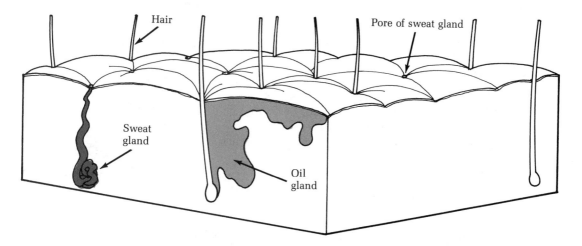

Fingerprints

Provide students with white paper and a stamp pad. Have them place their fingertips on the pad and then make an impression on the paper. Ask students to label the prints with their names. Then, let them compare each other's prints to see that no two patterns are exactly the same. Discuss the anatomy of the skin ridges that form fingerprints (and footprints).

Manicure Demonstration

Obtain small bowls, soap, and emery boards for all students. (For older students, scissors may be used in place of emery boards.) Demonstrate the proper way to clean and cut nails, as well as ways to care for the cuticles. Let students give themselves a manicure.

Eye Anatomy

If possible, obtain a model of the eye and explain its major components. If one is unavailable, make your own or use a large chart showing the anatomy of the human eye.

Ear Anatomy

Follow the same procedure with a model of the human ear.

Pupil Dilation and Constriction

Pair students and have them face one another so they can see their partner's eyes. Tell them to look at the partner's pupils for a few seconds and observe their size. Then, at your signal, ask all students to close their eyes and not to reopen them until you tell them. Explain that upon your signal, they are to open their eyes and look quickly at their partner's pupils. Give the signal after about 45 seconds and have the students note the constriction of the pupils upon being exposed to light.

Focusing Properties of the Eye

Take white paper, preferably with a glossy finish, and mount it on a large piece of folded cardboard that can be set on a desk top. This setup represents the retina. Then, darken the room, light a candle, and move a magnifying glass representing the lens back and forth between the candle and cardboard screen until a clear image of the candle can be seen on the screen. It will be upside down, just like images that focus on the retina.

Sound Conduction and the Ear

To demonstrate the relationship between vibrations and sound, stretch a rubber band between your thumbs and have students pluck it. They should note the movement (vibration) of the rubber band as it is plucked and the resulting sound. Then have students feel the movement (vibrations) of their throats as they talk.

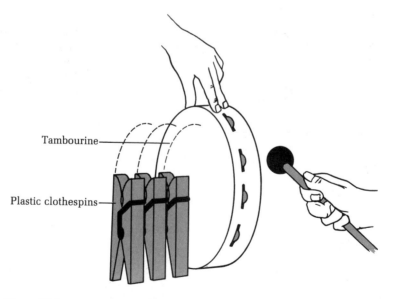

Figure 10.1
Sound conduction demonstration setup.

Explain that vibrations produce invisible waves in the air called sound waves, which conduct sound. To demonstrate wave properties, have students take turns gently tossing pennies or pebbles in a large pan of water. These waves move out concentrically, as do sound waves.

Explain that the ear is designed to receive and transmit sound waves to the brain. If the signal does not reach the brain, then sound is not heard. To demonstrate this, set up a tambourine and place three plastic clothespins next to the outer face, as shown in figure 10.1. The tambourine represents the eardrum and the clothespins represent the three bones in the middle ear that carry vibrations to the inner ear where they are changed to electrical impulses and sent to the brain. Begin beating on the tambourine so that its vibrations knock over the first clothespin, setting up a chain reaction. Explain that the eardrum and the bones of the middle ear transmit vibrations in a similar way. Remove the first clothespin and repeat the demonstration. This time, the vibrating tambourine face does not transmit sound energy to the remaining clothespins because one pin has been removed. This is analogous to a malfunction in the middle ear, a conductive hearing impairment.

Sound Localization

Pair students. One student is blindfolded, sitting in a chair. The other student, who acts as the "tester," stands nearby and taps a pencil against a glass. The blindfolded student points to the direction he or she believes the sound is coming from. Have the tester move to several locations throughout the room, sometimes holding the glass high above the floor and sometimes holding it low. Repeat this with several other students to note differences. Also do the experiment with several blindfolded students who have one ear plugged to note differences in sound localization ability.

Taste Localization

Use a tasting kit with students to demonstrate the various taste centers of the tongue. These kits can be ordered from most scientific supply houses.

Taste and Sight

Blindfold students. Have them taste several foods and guess what they have eaten. Ask how closely aligned the senses of vision and taste seem to be.

Taste and Smell

While still blindfolded from the previous activity, have students hold their noses as they taste several foods. Have them note their diminished ability to distinguish differences.

Microscopic Organisms

To demonstrate that many organisms cannot be seen without a microscope, take a sample of water from a classroom aquarium or from a local pond and prepare microscope slides. Allow each student to examine the slides under a microscope. Indicate that although most microscopic organisms are not disease-causing, almost all disease-causing organisms are microscopic.

Need for Exercise

Obtain two mice or hamsters and place them in separate cages. Provide one with an exercise wheel and a large amount of space. Limit the size of the other cage and do not provide an exercise wheel. Allow a few weeks to pass and then observe the differences in behavior and appearance between the two animals. Do not carry on the experiment any longer than necessary so as not to cause the experimental animals undue suffering.

PUZZLES AND GAMES

This Is The Way We . . .

To emphasize daily grooming practices for younger children, for a few days, begin the school day by leading the class in the following song while they mimic the activity.

> This is the way we wash our face
> Wash our face, wash our face
> This is the way we wash our face
> So early in the morning.
> This is the way we brush our hair
> Brush our hair, brush our hair
> This is the way we brush our hair
> So early in the morning.

And so on.

Personal Health Bowl Game

Divide the class into six groups. Three groups are in the A division and three groups are in the B division. One of the groups in each division is responsible for writing ten short questions concerning personal health practices, either in general or in one specific category, depending on your preference. This group will also serve as master of ceremonies or MC for each division. The other two groups in each division compete against one another for point totals by accumulating points if they answer the question correctly or by subtracting points if they miss the question. Questions are asked of teams on a rotating basis and the entire team may confer for 45 seconds if needed. At the end of the match, the A division champs meet the B division and compete using new questions—five of which are written by A division MCs and five of which are written by B division MCs. Also, A division runners-up compete against B division runners-up.

Aerobic Games and Dancing

Divide the class into teams or groups and conduct various aerobic games such as relay races, three-legged races, and jump-rope-athon or synchronized movements to music that enhance cardiovascular fitness. Discuss the effect of each activity on the heart and lungs with the class both before and after the activity. You may wish to plan aerobic games and dancing with a physical education specialist.

Exercises

Here are some exercises for your students.

Turtle/Rabbit Run. Have children run 50 steps in place slowly, then 50 steps very fast. Repeat twice.

Gorilla Walk. Children spread their feet apart, bend at the waist, and grab their ankles. Have them walk stiff-legged holding their ankles.

Inchworm. Children get into pushup position with body and arms straight and hands on floor. Keeping hands still, children walk feet up as close to hands as possible.

Bear Walk. Keeping legs and arms straight, children bend, put their hands on the floor, and walk.

Frog Stand. Have students get into a squatting position with hands on floor. Then they pull up their knees to rest on their elbows.

Frog Leap. Children stoop down with both hands on the floor in front of them. They lean forward and stand on tiptoe, and then leap forward, resuming the original position. Repeat several times.

Labeling Game

On large sheets of posterboard draw or have the students draw the following: hand, eye, ear, nose, and tongue. Tack the posters to the wall. Use pieces of paper to make large labels of the various parts or functions of the body parts depicted. Divide students into two teams that each form a line, pairing opposing team competitors. Give each pair of competitors a different label. Let each competitor place his or her label next to the appropriate poster. If label placement is correct, the team gets two points. If label placement is incorrect, ask the other competitor to place the label by the appropriate poster. If the competitor places it correctly, that team gets one bonus point. After completing the lines, declare one team the winner of the match based on point accumulation. Play the best two out of three matches to see who wins the game.

"Personal Health Concentration"

1. Divide the class into 3 or 4 groups depending on the number of students.
2. Explain that each group will work as a team in scoring points. Have them choose one person to speak for the team.
3. Assemble a board with 20 or more pockets on it. Number the pockets. Explain that half of the cards have a word pertaining to personal health on it. The other half have the definition.
4. Give a demonstration on how the game works.
   Example: Choose 4 and 7 and take the cards out of the pockets. Explain why it is a match or why it is not. If they match, take the cards out; if not, return them back to the pockets.

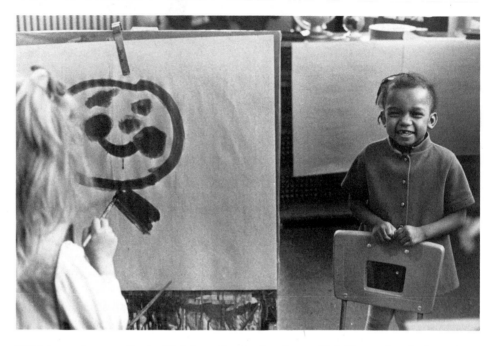

Children must personalize health information by drawing and labeling various body parts.

5. A point is scored for every match that is made.
6. The game proceeds with each team taking its turn in order until all matches have been made. The team with the most points is the winner.

Take Time for Personal Health

Divide students into groups and assign each group a different component of personal health, such as care of the hair, skin, teeth, eyes, or ears, and the need for exercise, sleep, and relaxation. Allow the groups two minutes to list as many roles, functions, or health practices associated with that component as they can. Read each list for accuracy and determine which group won the round. Play several more rounds, explaining that each time listings have to be different. See not only which group can list the most per round, but also which group is able to list the most at the end of the game.

Immunization Game

Fill a bucket or box with names of illnesses written on paper folded so that they cannot be seen. Each student draws one and indicates whether there is an immunization for that illness. Students who are correct draw another illness label and the same procedure is followed until all labels are used. Simultaneously, record the illnesses on the board under "yes" or "no" headings to indicate whether immunization is possible. When the game is over, discuss each illness and immunization technique.

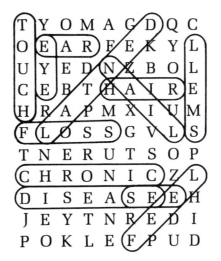

Figure 10.2
Hidden words puzzle format.

Soap

Towel

Comb

Water

Brush

Shampoo

Washcloth

Hidden Words Puzzle

Pass out prepared sheets as shown in figure 10.2. In the figures, the solutions are shown. Find the hidden words that refer to personal health. The words may run from left to right, top to bottom, diagonally, or backwards. Circle each word.

Who Is Knocking?

In playing this game, the students will realize how vitally important their sense of hearing is. You need a chair and a blindfold. A blindfolded child, the doorkeeper, sits on a chair. Another child, the rapper, tiptoes behind her and raps on the floor. The doorkeeper asks, "Who is knocking?" Rapper says, "Guess who," trying to disguise his voice. If doorkeeper guesses correctly, the rapper becomes the doorkeeper. If not, the doorkeeper must remain until she guesses a voice, or has had chances with three different voices. In that case, the last child who spoke becomes the new doorkeeper.

Happy Health Tour—Marching

In playing this game, the students will review daily health habits. You need to make stepping stones from posterboard or construction paper. They bear inscriptions of good health practices. Stones are placed close enough together so that the children can step from one to the other on the classroom floor.

Play this variation of musical chairs. Children line up to walk along the stepping stones. Marching begins with piano or recorded music. When the music is stopped, a teacher asks someone to tell what the inscription she is standing on means. If the answer given explains the inscription correctly, the stone is picked up and the player remains in the game. If she is wrong, she leaves the game. Continue until all the stones have been picked up, or until all players have been eliminated.

Brush Bingo

Make up cards and smile markers as shown below. Remember to rearrange the order and position of words on the card. The first child to cover a row down, across, or diagonally wins.

B	R	U	S	H	😁
DENTIN	ENAMEL	CROWN	INCISORS	CALCULUS	😁
CAVITIES	FLOSS	PLAQUE	FLOSSING	BICUSPIDS	😁
CUSP	PULP	CLEAN TEETH FREE SPACE	DENTIST	CEMENTUM	😁
GINGIVITIS	ROOT	CUSPIDS	PERIODONTAL DISEASE	DENTAL HYGIENIST	😁
FLUORIDE	MOLARS	PERIODONTAL MEMBRANE	TOOTH BRUSHING	FILLING	😁

Dental Crossword Puzzle

Read a definition in the Across group. Decide what health word is being defined. Then find the matching number in the crossword puzzle. Start with this numbered square and write across, filling in the letters of the defined word. Complete the Down letters in the same way, except start with a numbered square and write down.

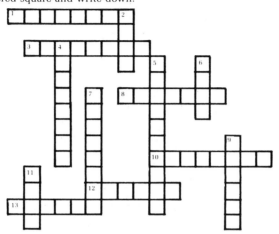

Across

1. Combines with the sugar in plaque to form acid.
3. Tooth that has two cusps
8. Can repair or fix a cavity in a tooth.
10. Teeth in the front of the mouth
12. Hard tissue that forms the body of a tooth
13. Sticky substance that forms on the teeth.

Down

2. Makes holes in the enamel
4. Bonelike tissue that covers the root
5. Sore gums that bleed easily
6. Pointed part on the crown of a tooth
7. Chemical that helps to prevent tooth decay
9. Teeth that grind food
11. The center of a tooth

Source: Meeks, Linda and Heit, Philip. *Health Focus on You.* Columbus, Ohio: Charles E. Merrill Publishing Company, 1984.

Care of the Senses

In each of the corners of the chalkboard and in the middle make a large drawing of an eye, ear, hand, tongue, and nose to indicate each of the senses. Under each drawing, using large stencil letters in bright colors, have students list three rules for the care or safeguarding of that sense.

Healthy Bodies

Create a bulletin board that will remind children of daily health routines for healthy bodies, lots of energy, and a long life. Discuss in class these daily health routines listed and illustrated on the bulletin board: Wash Your Ears Daily; Floss and Brush Your Teeth; Protect Your Eyes; Keep Your Skin Clean; Brush Your Hair; Trim Your Nails, and others.

Food Puzzle

The number and kinds of bulletin boards that can be used to depict personal health topics are limitless. Use your imagination and rely on the creativity of your students.

All of the food words listed below fit into the puzzle. The first word has been done for you. Can you make them all fit into the basket?

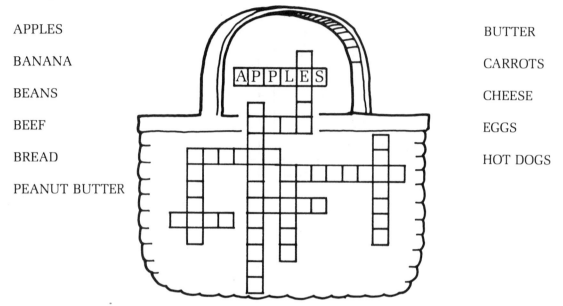

APPLES

BANANA

BEANS

BEEF

BREAD

PEANUT BUTTER

BUTTER

CARROTS

CHEESE

EGGS

HOT DOGS

Smile Awhile

Devise a bulletin board from a display of school photos of students in such a way that each photo is a "tooth" in an enlarged "smile." Figure 10.3 shows an example of this

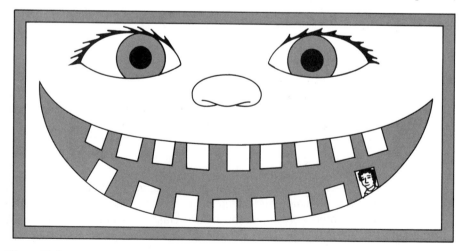

Figure 10.3
Smile Awhile photo collage bulletin board.

bulletin board technique. Underneath the smile, have each student complete the statement: "Happiness is _____" by filling in a personal health preference, such as "Happiness is having good teeth," "Happiness is looking healthy," "Happiness is a clean face," and so forth.

Feel Fit

Create a bulletin board to stimulate the children's interest in feeling fit through exercise. You might ask the children for suggestions about what activities to depict on the bulletin board; volunteers can discuss their favorite activities.

OTHER IDEAS

Storytelling and the Senses

The tale "Little Red Riding Hood" emphasizes the senses. For younger children, read this story and discuss each of the senses as they are brought up in the story. Other stories are also appropriate for this activity, such as "Goldilocks and the Three Bears."

Sense Mobiles

Preface this activity by pointing out that the senses combine to perform many tasks. Then have the students draw or collect pictures that illustrate any or all of the five senses. Have them make mobiles with the pictures and hang the finished products around the classroom.

Dressing for the Weather

Students should understand that dressing appropriately for the weather can help prevent illness. Make an extra large boy paper doll and an extra large girl paper doll along with an accompanying and varied wardrobe for all kinds of weather. Let the students take turns each day dressing the dolls appropriately for the day's weather, or for different seasons.

Immunization Record

Have each student make a chart listing his or her immunization record. Suggest that students should be proud to know that they have contributed to their own health by undergoing these immunizations.

Caution is the Key

Many early warning signs allow an illness to be treated before it becomes severe. Emphasize this point and allow the class to illustrate as a group, by means of a mural or posters in the school cafeteria, signs and symptoms of disease as well as suggestions to follow if these signals occur.

Nice to Nap

Taking a nap is important for younger elementary school students. However, getting the students to take a nap is sometimes difficult. After discussing the importance of sleep with the class, have the students decorate pillow cases. These personal pillow cases should be used by the students during their nap time.

We All Need Rest

Have students draw or cut out pictures of people and animals sleeping. Ask them to write a short paragraph to go with their pictures that discusses the importance of rest for all living things.

Recharging

Explain to students that sleep is the body's way of recharging its energy sources. Put new batteries in a flashlight. Leave it on during class so that it becomes noticeably weak and dimmed. Then, replace the batteries and note the difference. Compare this process to sleep.

Bedtime Records

Have students record bedtime hours for a week. After the assignment has been turned in, determine average sleep time for the boys, the girls, and the class as a whole. Determine whether the students think they are getting enough sleep.

Sleep Machine

Divide the class into groups. Have each group be responsible for designing a "sleep machine." Imagination combined with information provided in class discussion should yield creative results.

Relaxing Can Be Fun

After discussing relaxation with the class, have the students write on a slip of paper a favorite pastime. Each day pick from their list a relaxing activity for the class to do and talk about.

Physical Activity Survey

Before class discussion on the benefits of exercise, have each student keep a record of physical activity for a week. Have the student include exercises and routine physical activities such as walking to school, walking up the stairs, and so on. Have them record time involved. After the reports have been collected, compare the class average to expected norms. Give suggestions for improving physical activity, if needed.

Benefits of Exercise

Explain that exercise provides three benefits—release of stress, improved body posture, and improved fitness. Discuss the significance of each with the class.

Three-Ring Circus

Exercise improves strength, flexiblity, and endurance. Each area is developed through different exercises. Have the students take part in the "three-ring circus of exercises." Decorate the room to give it a circus atmosphere. Divide the class into three groups. Each day have the groups do a different type of exercise. Each type of exercise should be performed in a specific area or station of the room.

> Circle 1—Jump Rope (endurance)
> Circle 2—Stretching Exercises to Music (flexibility)
> Circle 3—Weight Lifting Exercises (strength)

SONGS AND FINGERPLAYS

The following songs and fingerplays can be used to stimulate the learners, enhance personal health practices, or may be used as a warmup in teaching health.

If You're Great and You Know It
(Tune: If You're Happy and You Know It)

If you're great and you know it
clap your hands
If you're great and you know it
clap your hands.
If you're great and you know it
Then your health will surely show it.
If you're great and you know it
clap your hands.

repeat: stomp your feet
nod your head
do all three
shout hooray

Touch Exercise

I'll touch my hair, my lips, my eyes,
I'll sit up straight and then I'll rise;
I'll touch my ears, my nose, my chin,
Then quietly sit down again.

I Wash My Face

I wash my face
I wash my hands
In soap and water cool.   (suit actions to words)
I brush my teeth
I comb my hair
I'm ready to go to school.

Tune: "Yankee Doodle"

I had a little tooth decay
I thought it was temporary;
But it developed everyday
Until it grew quite scary.

Chorus:
    Dentist, dentist, get your drill
    And keep your X ray handy.
    I've got some teeth you've got to fill,
    I've eaten too much candy.

Oh me, oh my! It's something fierce
The way my tooth is aching.
Because I have the toothache so,
A rumpus I am making.

Chorus:
    Dentist, dentist, get your drill,
    Have the filling ready.
    I have this hole you have to fill,
    Be sure your hand is steady.

Tune: "Twinkle, Twinkle, Little Star"

Twinkle, twinkle, little tooth,
Here's a maxim full of truth:
We will keep you from decay,
If we brush you everyday.

Tune: "On Top of Old Smokey"

On top of my molars, are braces so light,
To strengthen my teeth and
    to correct my bite.

When braces come off me,
My teeth will be straight.

So, I'll go to the dentist
And keep every date.

I'll chew hard on apples,
Eat foods that I should.
Brush my teeth daily
So they will look good.

I'm glad to wear braces,
They're setting me right.
My teeth will be stronger,
Straighter and white.

Wake Up Little Fingers

Wake up, little fingers, the morning
   has come.
Now hold them up, every finger and thumb.
Come jump out of bed, see how tall you
   can stand
My, my, but you are a wide awake band
You have all washed your faces
And now you look so neat.
Now come to the table and let us all eat.
Now all of you fingers run out to play.
And have a good time on this beautiful
   day.

(open fingers from
doubled fists)
(raise hands)
(raise hands higher)

(clap hands)
(rub palms together)
(fold hands)
(eating motions)
(wiggle fingers)

Tune: "Row, Row, Row Your Boat"

Brush, brush, brush your teeth
   Brush them up and down.
Cleaner, whiter, stronger teeth,
You don't have to frown.

Brush, brush, brush your teeth
   Gently up and down.
Smile, smile, smile, smile --
Smile and do not frown.

Tune: "Clementine"

She likes candy, she likes ice cream
She likes anything that's sweet
When her mother isn't looking
That is all she ever eats
Not potatoes, not tomatoes,
Not fresh fruit or ever meat

She don't like them, she won't eat them
All she wants is something sweet.

Tune: "London Bridge"

All your teeth are falling out,
　falling out, falling out.
All your teeth are falling out
　if you do not brush them.

So, brush them daily up and down,
　up and down, up and down.
So, brush them daily up and down,
They'll be white instead of brown.

Keep The Germs Away

Here's a rule
Can't be beat
Keep yourself
Clean and neat.
That's the best way to keep the germs away.

Brush your teeth
Take good care
of your fingernails and hair.
That's the best way to keep the germs away.

Why not look your best and stay healthy and well?
When you keep yourself clean and neat, mmmm. . . you sure
　look swell.

You don't need
Brand new clothes
When they're clean everybody knows.
That's the best way to keep the germs away.

Dirty hands
Spread disease
Dirty hair is a home for fleas.
That's not the way to keep germs away.

So why not look your best and stay healthy and well?
When you keep yourself clean and neat, mmm. . . you sure
　look swell.

_____

(Hap Palmer, Learning Basic Skills Through Music: Music, Health, and Safety, #AR526 or AC526)

11. Mental Health

If a child lives with criticism, he learns to condemn.
If a child lives with hostility, he learns to fight.
If a child lives with ridicule, he learns to be shy.
If a child lives with shame, he learns to feel guilty.
If a child lives with tolerance, he learns to be patient.
If a child lives with encouragement, he learns confidence.
If a child lives with praise, he learns to appreciate.
If a child lives with fairness, he learns justice.
If a child lives with security, he learns to have faith.
If a child lives with approval, he learns to like himself.
If a child lives with acceptance and friendship, he learns
  to find love in the world.
—Dorothy Law Nolte

THE IMPORTANCE OF MENTAL HEALTH

Without the sense of inner peace and balance that comes with good mental health, no individual can be considered completely healthy. The links between mental and physical health are clear. Yet the goal of good mental health is in many ways more elusive than that of good physical health. If an individual receives proper nutrition, exercises on a regular basis, gets plenty of relaxation and sleep, and follows good personal health practices, he or she should remain physically fit. Unfortunately, there is no such easy prescription for good mental health. It must be molded on an individual basis. It is also rather intangible—not at all like pounds lost or increases in muscular strength. Mental health is not easily differentiated from mental illness on the surface. Many individuals are functional within society, yet suffer from personality disorders. Lately, there has been a physical fitness boom in this country. But there has been no accompanying mental health boom. On the contrary, we hear reports about increasing alcohol and drug addiction among our teenagers. Suicide is now the second leading cause of death for adolescents. Over one million school-age students run away from home. Depression is prevalent among school-age children (see Health Highlight for this chapter). And, finally, more people in this country are hospitalized because of mental disorders than for all other illnesses combined.

How can teachers, parents, and children make a difference? Becoming familiar with the principles of good mental health and applying these principles can help. We must also assist children to learn how to make successful, positive life adjustments in times of stress or crisis. These life adjustments are learned behavior. No one is born with good mental health. Thus its establishment must begin early in life. We should also teach about becoming more tolerant of others who are mentally ill. This chapter provides information about mental health principles that will assist your students to develop sound mental health. Topics discussed include human needs and the development of self-esteem, behavior and the expression of emotions, stress and its relationship to mental health, values and patterns of decision-making, the role of the family in the development of mental health, the role of the teacher, and rules for developing and maintaining mental health.

HUMAN NEEDS AND THE DEVELOPMENT OF SELF-ESTEEM

Development of positive mental health requires that an individual be immersed in an open and nonthreatening environment that nurtures and supports feelings of self-worth and security. All human beings, young or old, have the same basic needs. Apart from the physical needs of water, food, clothing, shelter, and personal safety, all people need to receive love and affection. Everyone needs to feel a sense of acceptance and importance from others. As a teacher, you should interact with your students in a way that strongly and consistently conveys this message. You should make your classroom into a positive, nonthreatening environment from which students will emerge feeling good about themselves.

The earliest and strongest ties to feelings about one's self and identity develop in the home through interaction with parents and siblings. That is, an individual's perceptions about himself or herself begin to form solidly before the child enters school. Nevertheless, as the teacher you can continue to build upon the positive attitudes and attributes that students bring with them and to help students discover and cultivate additional personal strengths. By recognizing the individuality and special skills of each student, as well as providing support, security, and acceptance, you can enhance self-esteem.

Self-esteem is necessary for developing self-expression and independence. A person with a feeling of self-worth is also better equipped emotionally to show concern for others. As the individual begins to develop meaningful relationships with others that recognize and reward his or her unique qualities of expression, independent thinking flourishes. A strong sense of self-worth permits open and honest communication with others because fears of rejection or disapproval are not seen as great risks as they are to someone with less ego strength.

Thus, with the fulfillment of basic emotional needs like love, affection, acceptance, and a feeling of importance, a person's self-identity and self-esteem become firmly established. This increases the person's potential for successfully interacting with others, meeting individual needs for independence and self-expression, and resolving personal and social conflicts. Improved self-esteem promotes a much more emotionally healthy resolution of such conflicts because of self-confidence to make life adjustments. The person is thus freer to pursue higher human goals, culminating with what Maslow (cited in Hamrick et al., 1986) calls *self-actualization needs*. Maslow's hierarchy of human needs is shown in figure 11.1.

The fulfillment of basic human needs and the establishment of self-esteem are lifelong processes. Their consistent reinforcement is essential to maintaining good mental health. This lifelong quest is more easily attainable if the nurturing of emotional and social well-being has been heavily emphasized in infancy and childhood, thus promoting a sense of security, identity, autonomy, and intimacy early in life.

Other Models of Personality Development

Freud. Freud explained that many of the observable behaviors that are indicative of mental health or illness are the result of motives that are below the conscious level. Freud theorized that a person progresses, either successfully or unsuccessfully, through a series of psychosexual stages. If people successfully navigate their way through these stages, they become emotionally mature persons. However, if any trauma is experienced, the person may become "fixated" on that stage of emotional development and thus have behavioral problems.

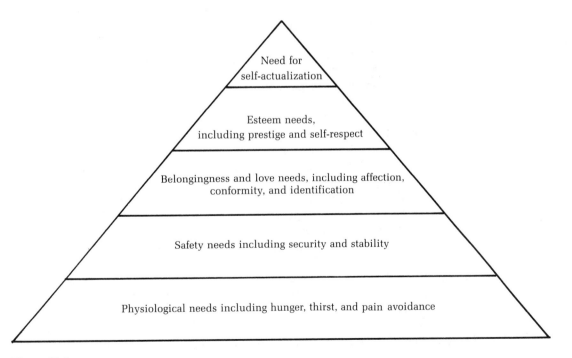

Figure 11.1
Maslow's hierarchy of human needs.

Erikson. Erikson, a student of Freud's, also theorized that individuals progressed through a series of stages toward emotional development. However, where Freud emphasized mastery of sex-related tasks, Erikson stressed a mastery of social behaviors.

BEHAVIOR AND THE EXPRESSION OF EMOTIONS

The most obvious indicator of a person's mental health status is behavior. Psychologists state that there is always a reason for behavior. Admittedly, the reasons may not be immediately apparent either to the individual or to others, but nevertheless there are underlying motives for all behavior. Much of an individual's behavior, both conscious and subconscious, is centered around fulfilling basic emotional needs. Such behavior patterns are often shaped by the ways in which these needs were satisfied or reinforced early in life. Thus, if a change in behavior is desired, new and perhaps more healthy ways of fulfilling basic needs must be learned by the individual. Therefore, in promoting good mental health in the classroom, it is important for you to appropriately reinforce desirable actions so that they will be repeated. Students should also be taught to appropriately express negative emotions, such as anger. By coupling positive reinforcement of desirable behavior with consistent messages of acceptance, affection, and support, your students' emotional well-being and healthy social adjustment will be heightened.

It would be misleading, however, to attribute the complex process of human behavior simply to the results of positive or negative reinforcement. While reinforcement is certainly a significant factor, behavior also arises from many other complicated factors, not all of which are agreed upon by mental health experts. It is generally agreed, however, that all people share not only the same basic needs, but also many of the same emotions. Everyone experiences feelings of sadness, anger, joy, depression, apprehension, pleasure, and the like, but the manner in which these emotions are expressed varies from individual to individual. It is usually the emotional expression of these feelings that becomes labeled as the individual's "behavior." Therefore a better understanding of emotions may lead to greater understanding of human behavior and overall mental health.

The way in which a person expresses his or her feelings is largely determined by the way the person perceives, either consciously or subconsciously, the situation that triggers the feeling. In other words, two people who are exposed to the same situation, say disagreement with a teacher over an answer to a test question, may react quite differently, based on different individual assessments of the situation. Such assessments are based in part on how the situation affects fulfillment of basic needs or efforts aimed at attaining autonomy, identity, or other personal goals. In many cases, the situation is perceived as having little impact and therefore elicits minimal emotional expression. Situations that are perceived as having great influence tend to elicit stronger, more overt expression. Thus emotions are displayed in varying modes of expression as well as varying degrees of intensity. A person is considered more mentally healthy when emotions are exhibited in a positive way to a degree of intensity proportional to the situation's impact. Individuals who *consistently* display

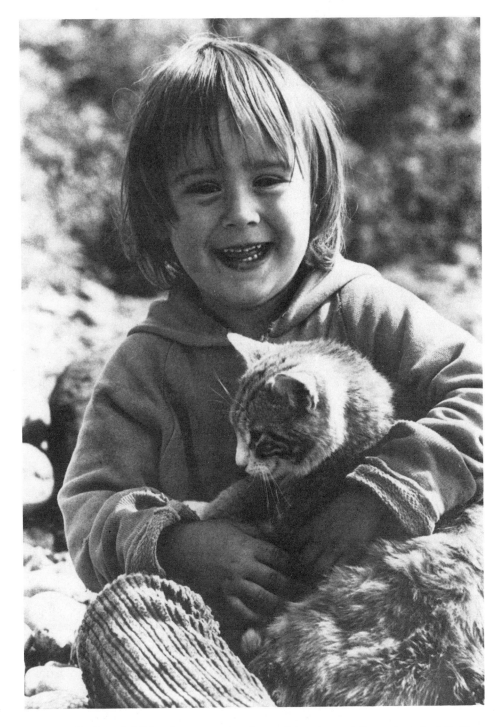

Happy, well adjusted children have a greater chance of growing up to be contented adults than do unhappy, insecure children.

either minimal emotional expression about circumstances generally viewed as having major importance (intimacy with others, successful completion of a difficult task, attainment of career goals, death of a family member) or intense emotional expression about events that are not generally viewed as having major importance (having to redo a homework assignment, misplacing an article of clothing, losing a school football game) are considered less emotionally well-adjusted.

When observing behavior and the expression of emotions, keep in mind that it is not the emotion itself that determines mentally healthy or unhealthy behavior, but rather the degree and frequency of the emotion expressed. All of us have on occasion allowed our emotions to run out of control or be expressed in ways that were not as appropriate, positive, or desirable as they could have been. This type of behavior is a problem only when it becomes a consistent pattern. Often such a pattern of emotional outburst is a result of inner anxiety due to stress originating from conflicts between unconscious drives or needs and conscious values that may not have been self-selected. Stress arising from a temporary crisis can also often trigger inappropriate, unhealthy, uncontrollable, or excessive emotional expression. However, if a crisis is the source of stress rather than anxiety produced from inner conflict, the pattern of undesirable emotional expression will subside as the crisis is resolved.

From an early age children should be provided with learning experiences and reinforcement that teach and foster positive emotional expression, both verbal and nonverbal. Children must understand that all people share the same emotions. They need to know that a feeling or emotion is neither inherently "good" or "bad" but can be expressed in ways that either promote well-being or detract from it. Mentally healthy behavior largely stems from an individual's ability to recognize, analyze, interpret, and communicate feelings in a manner that is consistent, balanced, and positive.

STRESS AND ITS RELATIONSHIP TO MENTAL HEALTH

Because of its influence on behavior and the expression of emotions that may result, stress should be included in any discussion of mental health. Everyone, young and old alike, is exposed to daily stress that must be accommodated to ensure emotional stability. Therefore it is necessary for both children and adults to realize that many situations produce feelings of anxiety or apprehension that cause the same types of fluctuation in levels of mental wellness as those experienced in physical wellness. The key is to learn to reduce anxiety and tension as they arise so that levels of stress are more easily managed. *Stress* is any stimulus that evokes unpleasant or tense feelings of nervousness, agitation, irritation, worry, and the like. In many cases, the stress-producing stimulus is not readily identifiable even though the symptoms exist. Although similar to fear in the psychological and physiological reactions that it evokes, *anxiety* is very different from fear from the standpoint of its *unrealistic* triggers. Fear is triggered by real and concrete threats, such as being physically threatened, whereas anxiety to a great extent is produced by imagined, unfounded, or abstract threats, as in the case of sleep anxiety or anxiety associated with meeting new people.

Causes of Stress

Most children entering school encounter stress from academic pressure and competition with peers (Richardson, Beall, & Jessup, 1983). New demands placed on children to act independently and assume more responsibility are major stressors in a student's life. Fear of not being accepted by peers, coping with various stages of growth and development, and other challenges accompanying maturation are more examples of stressors.

Personality Disorders

In dealing with stress and the resulting anxiety it produces, individuals attempt to cope in a variety of ways, many of which are subconscious and not emotionally healthy. All people to some degree cope with stressful situations by using these subconscious, unhealthy means—neurotic behaviors, also called personality disorders. Like any emotion or action associated with behavior, the degree and frequency of expression of neurotic behaviors generally determines the individual's level of emotional wellness. Thus people who use neurotic behaviors only minimally in facing stressful situations are considered to be functioning at higher levels of mental health than those who rely on neurotic behaviors until they become a constant mode of expression.

By recognizing one's use of neurotic behaviors and making efforts to reduce the degree and frequency to which such behaviors are used to deal with stress, more realistic, positive, and healthy emotional reactions can be fostered. The most common personality disorders associated with stress are anxiety reactions, defense mechanisms, obsessive-compulsive behaviors, phobias, hypochondria, hysterical conversions, and depression.

Anxiety reactions are characterized by physical symptoms that can include a rapid and pounding heartbeat, feelings of faintness or dizziness, shortness of breath, extreme agitation or nervousness, and nausea. The attacks sometimes appear without apparent cause, are sudden, and may last as long as 20 to 30 minutes.

Defense mechanisms are psychological deceptions used to avoid anxiety by hiding an individual's motive from conscious awareness. Examples of commonly displayed defense mechanisms are rationalization, overcompensation, denial, withdrawal, and projection. *Rationalization* is attributing a belief, opinion, attitude, or action to factors more socially acceptable than the real reasons. *Overcompensation* is comprised of attempts to excel or perform in excess in one area of personality development that overshadows another. *Denial* is refusal to recognize or admit to the existence of a stress-causing agent or situation. *Withdrawal* is avoidance of dealing with a stress-causing agent or situation. *Projection* is unjustly attributing one's own faults and negative feelings to another individual or group.

Obsessive-compulsive behaviors arise when an unwanted thought (the obsession) or action (the compulsion) or both continually intrude upon and interrupt conscious functioning. Mild obsessive-compulsive behaviors include constantly looking at one's watch or being preoccupied by the thought of something not particularly important or pleasant. Occasionally, however, there are individuals who demonstrate more pronounced obsessive-compulsive behaviors that can be extremely disruptive to normal daily living.

Like obsessive-compulsive behaviors, *phobias* are neurotic behaviors that can intrude upon normal functioning if they become extreme. Phobias are unrealistic fears of animals, objects, or situations. Common phobias include unrealistic fears of snakes, spiders, heights, elevators, and wide-open spaces. Underlying anxiety is usually at the root of phobias.

Hypochondria is characterized by a constant concern over the possibility of contracting numerous ailments or illnesses. Like other neurotic behavior, hypochondria can be mild or severe.

Hysterical conversions are the manifestations of physical disabilities for which there is no identifiable physiological basis. Examples include hysterical blindness, deafness, and paralysis.

One of the most frequently occurring neurotic behaviors is *depression,* a condition characterized by loss of interest, feelings of extreme or overwhelming sorrow, sadness, and a feeling of debility. Like all neurotic behaviors, depression is a symptom of underlying conflict, tension, or anxiety and may be exhibited in varying degrees for varying lengths of time.

Because neurotic behaviors do not produce a warping of or separation from reality as do psychotic behaviors, they are more treatable or controlled once identified. Neuroses tend to produce feelings of inner conflict in varying degrees and frequencies, some of which may be profound enough to require professional attention from mental health experts.

Effects of Stress

Stress can cause problems in several areas of a student's life. Psychosomatic illness, such as headaches and physical injuries, may result from an abnormal response to stress. A student may withdraw emotionally from others, and experience feelings of worthlessness, apathy, loneliness, anger, hostility, and low self-esteem. Behavior problems like hyperactivity, accident-susceptibility, truancy, substance abuse, and low academic achievement may also result from stress. Stress can affect learning. Low self-esteem and anxiety may lead to a lack of concentration and a disrupted capacity to process information (Jones, 1985).

Dealing with Stress

When trying to limit the use of neurotic behaviors and reduce the amount of stress one is exposed to so that coping with anxiety becomes a more healthy and positive process, several factors must be considered. To begin with, it is essential that individuals try to identify their sources of stress. In identifying sources of stress, it is important to determine which sources arise from intrinsic stimuli, such as being inwardly driven to reach a deadline, and which ones arise from extrinsic stimuli, such as pressure from a teacher to turn in a homework assignment or meet a deadline. Depending on whether the source is intrinsic or extrinsic, ways of remedying stress may vary.

Health Highlight: "Depression in Children"

In the past, the existence of depression as a distinct disorder of children was questionable, but the consensus today is that depression exists among children and adolescents. In fact, the number of cases of depression among this age group may be considerable.

The causes of childhood depression include biological and behavioral explanations. Researchers indicate that depression may stem from biochemical abnormalities and/or genetic factors. Others theorize that depression might be explained by a lack of reinforcement for positive coping behaviors.

School health professionals need to know how depression is manifested among school children. School health professionals also need to become familiar with contemporary approaches to treating childhood depression. A successful program will be a comprehensive plan that focuses on promoting behavior change in each of the child's environments, including home, school, and community.

Source: Epstein, Michael and Cullinan, Douglas, "Depression in Children," *Journal of School Health*, Volume 56, Number 1, January, 1986, pp. 10-12.

It is also beneficial to try to determine whether the source of stress is regular, routine, or consistent, as in the cases of daily conflict, uneasiness, or being self-conscious with peers, respectively, or a more sudden, perhaps isolated or unusual event, such as in the case of the death of a family pet. Sources of stress that are regular, routine, or consistent generally have a greater potential for creating long-term negative effects if not dealt with since they wear on the individual constantly and may therefore demand more time to resolve. Sudden, isolated sources of stress tend to be crisis situations that first require an initial return to some degree of normalcy and may later involve a more lengthy process of conflict resolution.

Thus putting the stress-producing situation in realistic perspective is helpful in objectively evaluating its impact. To do this, mentally classifying events should be done *as they arise.* The individual must decide which situations can be personally handled with relative ease after careful consideration of the possible alternatives. Those events involving either deeper inner conflict or interaction with others may require the assistance of a third party or outside expert. After putting the cause of the stress into perspective and outlining several courses of action, the individual should select the course of action that seems likely to produce the most healthy, positive, or desirable results based on personal values, goals, and conscience. The person should then carry out the course of action and evaluate its effectiveness to determine whether similar courses of action should be repeated for similar circumstances or whether modifications need to be considered.

Apart from identifying and dealing with stressful situations as they arise, an individual should try to become more "stress-resistant." To aid your students in doing this, teach and encourage them to relax, to find joy and pleasure in daily tasks or accomplishments, and to reward or "stroke" themselves just because they are unique and special. These positive personal measures can enhance emotional well-being and promote inner harmony and balance, each of which is a necessary component of good mental health, and each of which can act as a buffer against stress. Stress management and stress reduction skills can help individuals cope with their anxieties, thus increasing the potential for reaching and maintaining high levels of mental wellness throughout life.

VALUES AND PATTERNS OF DECISION-MAKING

Central to the establishment of self-esteem, the expression of emotions and resulting behavior, and the ability to cope effectively with stress are the decision-making patterns that each individual learns in order to make life adjustments in harmony with his or her value system. When decisions about a particular issue reflect actions and attitudes that are in agreement with strongly held values, a person is left intact emotionally since personal behaviors and values remain compatible. If decisions produce behaviors that are contradictory to a person's value system, self-esteem is diminished, emotions are exhibited in an unhealthy fashion resulting from lack of resolution over inner conflicts, and therefore stress increases.

Decision-making patterns can serve as valuable clues to the way individuals perceive themselves, their relationships with others, and the world around them. An individual's actions tell much about that person's underlying value system, which in turn mediates many of the decisions made about life adjustments. Learning to make decisions following clarification and consideration of one's values can help to sustain and enhance the emotional balance crucial to good mental health.

ROLE OF THE FAMILY IN THE DEVELOPMENT OF MENTAL HEALTH

An individual's mental health status can be gauged by assessing the degree to which the basic emotional needs for love, acceptance, and support from others contribute to feelings of self-worth as well as by determining the degree of balance with which behaviors are expressed. In addition, the ways in which individuals face and resolve stressful situations through use of decisions that are compatible with personal values can also serve as a measure of mental health. All these foundations to positive mental health begin to be learned and cultivated within the family from birth. As a result, it is crucial that all teachers have some notion of the influences family structure, interaction, and values have on the behavior and attitudes of children entering the classroom.

The most important individuals in a young child's life are the parents. These are the people who initially supply both physiological as well as psychological needs. Children develop a sense about whether or not they can rely on others based on the quality and constancy of care and support given by parents. With ever-increasing economic demands forcing parents to surrender a significant amount of time in caring for their children, as a teacher you must recognize that some children may have been socialized in quite a different fashion from those who have grown up in a more traditional family setting. Additionally, the high numbers of one-parent and single-parent families that currently exist may greatly affect a child's view of self as well as the world in general. Some children also face the task of having to be incorporated into two different family structures that produce sets of step-parents and step-siblings. Therefore you must be sensitive to these differences in living arrangements and family structure.

Family interaction also contributes greatly to the development of children's mental health. Communication patterns between parents, between parents and their children, and between siblings are all important factors. Communication should allow for intimacy, that is, a sharing of one's innermost fears and concerns, without reprisal or rejection. Interaction patterns between family members set the tone for all other social interaction. It is within the family that children develop a sense about what they can do or accomplish, what their roles in life should be, and what types of behaviors are appropriate, acceptable, and desirable. Criteria for sharing, completing expected tasks, being praised or punished, and many other things are learned according to family modeling and values. The family sets guidelines for all behavior by means ranging from various types of discipline to different ways of expressing love and affection. As a result, children's attitudes, habits, and emotions are reflections of family attitudes, habits, and emotions.

Discipline should be firm, fair, and consistent. Further, the child should be taught decision making as early in life as possible. Even a young child can make decisions if given parameters. For example, a preschool child would be overwhelmed if asked to make a decision without any guidelines or direction. The same student *can* make a choice between two or three appropriate solutions.

Social Influences

Social influences on the family must not be overlooked when considering the overall impact on a child's mental health. Socioeconomic status and ethnic group affiliation as well as parents' job classifications and educational backgrounds can influence how a family meets its needs. In addition, peer group pressure, messages from the media, and changes in cultural mores regarding everything from sex role expectations and drug use to career and lifestyle choices can affect children's behavior and decision-making as well as their values and sense of self-worth. Such influences may interfere with the family's influence on the development of a child's mental health. When considering the behaviors, attitudes, and beliefs that a child brings into the classroom, you need to be aware of the family's contribution to that child's emotional orientation, while recognizing that social factors also influence even the most closely knit families.

ROLE OF THE TEACHER IN THE PROMOTING OF MENTAL HEALTH

Next to family members, the teacher is one of the most significant other individuals in an elementary school child's life. Within the classroom children spend a majority of their waking hours learning not only intellectual skills but those of social interaction and communication. Thus the general emotional climate that exists in the classroom along with the rapport between a teacher and a given student has certain impact upon children's mental health.

There are many ways in which you can promote the already-existing positive emotional characteristics that children bring with them from their family experiences. You can also encourage the development of other healthy aspects of a child's mental well-being. To begin with, constantly keep in mind that you are a role model for your students. A teacher's own conduct during the school day is noted by children and is likely to be modeled in some way. For example by demonstrating fair, balanced, open, and pleasant attitudes, you indicate, both directly and indirectly, the importance of interacting with others in this fashion.

Each child should be dealt with as a unique individual. Offer personal observations or words of praise that let a child know he or she is performing well on a given task or is progressing nicely. This is especially important for shy, withdrawn, or insecure children. Recognition of a child's efforts whenever feasible can do much to foster self-esteem. In addition, you can encourage students to hone their individual talents by providing opportunities for them to do so during the normal course of classroom activity. The chance to work on a special project of personal interest or contribute ideas and opinions without being ridiculed or rejected may enhance autonomy and initiative.

In dealing with your students, provide clear and realistic guidelines about what they are supposed to do. Learning experiences that both challenge and provide success will reinforce students' feelings of competency and mastery. On the other hand, children must also realize that not all tasks, solutions, or skills can be easily acquired. Help children place their inability to meet a goal in the proper perspective so that feelings of doubt, embarassment, or inadequacy do not result. This might best be done by initially providing students with a great deal of direction and assistance, which can later be diminished as they display more understanding and sophistication for accomplishing the desired outcome.

Be alert to any behaviors that might indicate emotional problems. First, be aware that some children with emotional problems become disruptive, while others react in just the opposite way by withdrawing and being very quiet. Some other behaviors that might indicate emotional problems (Jones, 1985, pp. 7–8) are:

- nail biting
- thumb sucking
- problems mixing socially with other students
- destructiveness
- temper tantrums
- inhibition of play
- obsession/compulsion
- hypochondria
- extremely introverted or extroverted
- excessive daydreaming
- very demanding
- excessive crying
- problems controlling emotions

It is especially important for you to realize your limitations in helping an emotionally disturbed student. An interdisciplinary team approach is extremely helpful in assisting these students. Any time these characteristics or obvious bizarre, unusual behaviors are displayed, you should contact the school nurse, psychologist, a social worker, or other appropriate personnel for assistance. These professionals are skilled in many types of counseling and therapy programs that can help the student.

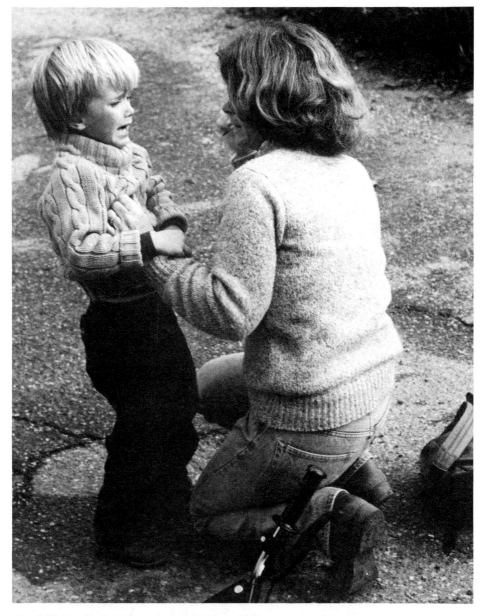

The child develops a sense of whether he or she can rely on others from the quality and constancy of parental care and support.

Finally, it is essential for you to become an effective listener and a skilled observer. Children regularly need opportunities that let them express their feelings and thoughts openly.

Let the students talk and write about their attitudes and opinions concerning the issues that are discussed in class. To foster creativity, allow them to write or talk, but without rigid guidelines. If the students are too young to write, let them express themselves through drawing pictures. This type of expression helps build communication skills as well as building a child's self-confidence.

If this is done, a better understanding of their present emotional status can be determined. All too often, teachers, who by the nature of their professional roles are used to doing all the talking, may not be attuned to listening well. Nonverbal communication can also provide many keys to a child's mental health. Thus allow time during each school day to observe children in various settings, whether it be working alone at their desks, engaged in a group problem-solving activity, playing with other children during recess, or interacting in the school cafeteria during lunch. Teachers who see an individual child in comparison with many other children of the same age are often in a better position than parents to objectively assess the child's adjustment.

The role of the teacher in promoting children's mental health is crucial. The attitudes that teachers demonstrate during their daily interaction with students affect the emotional climate of the classroom. One of the best things a teacher can do to promote mental health in students is to help them learn to accept responsibility for their own behavior. A common mistake made by all of us is to try to shift the blame for something we did on someone else. Students must be taught that a crucial element of emotional development is the ability to accept responsibility and live with mistakes. Children should be given firm, fair guidelines in class, and should be given appropriate guidance and discipline when these rules are disobeyed.

You can help the students learn coping skills that are helpful in alleviating stress or reducing the effects of stress. Such measures as exercise, biofeedback, meditation, imagery, and other relaxation techniques are very effective in helping people deal with stress-related problems (Heide, 1985).

Further, the type of rapport that is established between teacher and child conveys many messages that influence student perceptions about acceptance, trust, support, esteem, competency, and independence. Thus, by relating to each child so that you reinforce special talents and allow the expression of feelings without fear of rejection, you can do much to enhance children's emotional well-being.

RULES FOR DEVELOPING AND MAINTAINING MENTAL HEALTH

Children should be encouraged to practice positive mental health habits in the same way they are taught to practice sound personal health habits. Just as people can take responsibility for their own physical well-being by following health "rules," they can also foster high levels of emotional well-being by following similar mental health "rules." By internalizing certain guidelines and incorporating them into daily living, each individual can promote good mental health and effective life adjustment. Here are ten "rules" that can help achieve this goal:

1. Like yourself. Discover your unique qualities, skills, and talents and be proud of who you are.
2. Be good to yourself. Reward yourself with "strokes"—emotional or material favors—periodically.
3. Learn to be introspective, to examine motives for behavior, and to be insightful about your own conduct.

4. Accept your own limitations. Think in terms of competency levels rather than in terms of "success" or "failure."
5. Deal with a problem or crisis as it arises rather than allowing pressures to mount by worrying about "what ifs."
6. Establish realistic goals, both short-term and long-term, and work toward accomplishing them.
7. Express your emotions in terms of how the emotion makes you feel rather than in terms of how the person makes you feel. "I feel angry for having to do a homework assignment over the weekend," is healthier than, "Mr. Barnes, you make me angry. You shouldn't assign a homework assignment over the weekend."
8. Involve yourself in diversified activities and cultivate many interests. Do not center your life around one person, place, or activity.
9. Develop a sense of humor. Learn to laugh and enjoy life.
10. Be optimistic.

SUMMARY

Fulfillment of the basic human needs for love, security, affection, and a feeling of worthiness is the basis for good mental health. This does much to allow an individual to internalize the belief that he or she is indeed special and important. As an individual's identity and esteem become more firmly established, the person is more likely to feel satisfied with life and to demonstrate these positive feelings through honest and open interaction with others.

All people face many of the same stressful situations in life but learn to adjust to them in different ways. Emotional reactions also vary from person to person depending on how the individual perceives the situation. When emotions are expressed in positive, appropriate ways that arise *after* consideration of the feeling and how best to express it, behavior is much less likely to be impulsive. Unexpressed emotions and feelings, on the other hand, can lead to frustration, hostility, or resentment. Occasionally, all individuals let their emotions and behaviors get out of control. This is understandable and expected. The result may be an emotional outburst or a temporary neurotic response. However, in coping with stressful circumstances, putting the situation into perspective and dealing with it immediately is much healthier. Even if the problem cannot be totally resolved immediately, addressing the issue as it arises should provide a sense of relief and being back in control.

We are all subject to stress, which can result in tension, anxiety, nervousness, agitation, or irritability. Mental health can be improved if individuals consciously attempt to identify factors that contribute to stress. Then measures can often be taken to reduce, or eliminate these stressful sources. Learning to relax effectively can also help individuals cope with stress.

Good mental health can also be fostered by learning to examine individual value systems, which are the basis for decisions made about life issues. People whose behavior is in conflict with their values are in conflict with themselves. The struggle to balance individual drives, wishes, desires, and needs with family, community, or social expectations can be a difficult one. By clearly identifying and clarifying personal values, it becomes easier to make decisions that are compatible with values rather than selecting choices that are put forward by outside forces or social pressure.

Family structure, interaction patterns, and values shape mental health, by serving as the first and often strongest force in the development of a child's emotional well-being. Teachers must recognize the impact of familial socialization on the child entering the classroom and attempt to relate equally objectively to students who come from diverse living arrangements. By recognizing each child as an individual who demonstrates unique qualities and talents, teachers can do much to promote mental health. Words of praise and encouragement as well as appropriate guidance coupled with realistic, clear-cut expectations will help to provide children with a classroom atmosphere that enhances emotional well-being. It is also vital for teachers to listen and show their acceptance, support, and concern.

DISCUSSION QUESTIONS

1. List and discuss the major stressors that school-aged children encounter.
2. Describe the consequences of inadequately dealing with stress.
3. Discuss the problem of depression in school-aged children.
4. Briefly explain Maslow's theory of emotional development.
5. Compare and contrast Freud's and Erikson's theories of emotional development.
6. What are personality disorders? List and describe typical examples of these disorders.
7. What can you do to establish a healthy emotional environment in your classroom? List specific measures that you can take.
8. How can you help children recognize and affirm that they are unique and worthy individuals?
9. Discuss the importance of helping children learn to accept responsibility for their own behavior.
10. Briefly discuss each of the ten rules listed in the chapter for fostering good mental health.

REFERENCES

Epstein, M., & Cullinan, D. "Depression in children," *Journal of School Health, 56,* 1, January, 1986.

Hamrick, M., Anspaugh, D., & Ezell, G. *Health.* Columbus: Merrill, 1986.

Heide, F. "Relaxation: The storm before the calm," *Psychology Today, 19,* 4, April, 1985.

Jones, J. "Promoting mental health of children and youth through the schools," Presentation at the American School Health Association Convention, Little Rock, Arkansas, October, 1985.

Nolte, D. "Children learn what they live," In Olsen, L., Redican, K., & Baffi, C. *Health today, second edition.* New York: Macmillan Publishing Company, 1986.

Richardson, G., Beall, S., & Jessup, G. "The efficacy of a three-week stress management unit for high school students." *Health Education, 14,* 1, January/February, 1983.

12. Techniques for Teaching Mental Health

It's wiser being good than bad; It's safer being meek than fierce; It's fitter being sane than mad.—Robert Browning

MENTAL HEALTH AND LIFE

Mental health is an extremely important part of total health. It is imperative to be able to cope with the daily stresses that individuals of every age face. Individuals who feel loved, secure, and successful as human beings can best cope with stressors. You as a teacher can do much to foster such feelings. In other words, *how* you teach is as important, if not more important, than *what* you teach about mental and emotional health. The classroom environment must be open and accepting; each student must feel welcome and significant. Children should be allowed to express their emotions and they should not feel confined when interacting with you or other students.

Building good mental health must begin in infancy and early childhood. By the time children enter school, their mental health has already been strongly influenced by family and peers. But school experiences are also a powerful shaping influence. By doing all you can to help children build feelings of self-worth and develop effective decision-making skills in harmony with their values, you can ensure that they will be guided toward greater emotional balance.

This goal can be met in part by providing diverse yet related activities that allow children to learn to cope with stress, deal with self-doubt, and develop control over their lives. Your efforts can do much to aid children in building good mental health that can be maintained throughout the challenges of a lifetime.

Concepts to be Taught

- All people share basic human needs for physical safety, love, security, emotional support, and acceptance from others.

- All people experience the same emotions but may express them differently, depending upon individual perceptions, values, and personality traits.

- There are healthy and unhealthy ways to express any given emotion. Mentally healthy expressions of emotion are consistent in frequency and intensity to the impact, influence, or importance of the event that triggers the emotion.

- Each individual has special talents, skills, and attributes that comprise his or her unique personality.

- The attitudes, beliefs, and opinions that an individual has toward himself or herself determine self-concept, self-esteem, and feelings of self-worth. Strong feelings of self-worth are a necessary part of good mental health.

- Feelings of self-worth and self-esteem arise from a variety of influences, especially those involving messages about oneself from family, friends, community, and society as a whole.

- The development of a strong sense of self-worth helps to foster intimate, meaningful relationships with family and friends and vice versa.

- Open and honest communication with others is a necessary part of good mental health.

- All people face stressful situations in day-to-day living. Stressful situations can best be minimized by identifying the situation as it arises, putting the event into perspective, and altering or eliminating the situation if possible.

- Learning to relax and find pleasure in life activities on a day-to-day basis can help to reduce stress.

- Decisions about personal behavior and conduct are an integral part of an individual's mental health and are based on a learned set of values arising from social interaction and from expectations of the culture as a whole.

- Decisions about personal conduct that are compatible with a person's value system can help to balance individual drives, desires, and needs with family, community, and social expectations and therefore lead to a greater potential for emotional balance, unity, and inner peace.

Cycle Plan for Teaching Concepts

Topic	\multicolumn{7}{c}{Grade Level}

Topic	K	1	2	3	4	5	6
Human Needs	***	**	**	***	*	**	***
Self-Esteem	***	***	***	**	*	*	**
Emotion	***	***	***	***	*	***	***
Relationships	***	***	**	***	*	**	***
Communication	***	***	***	***	*	***	**
Stress	***	***	**	**	***	***	*
Decision-Making	**	**	*	***	***	**	*
Values	**	**	*	**	***	**	***

Key: *** = major emphasis, ** = emphasis, * = review.

VALUE-BASED ACTIVITIES

Nametag Descriptors

Ask students to make a large nametag by writing the letters of their first names vertically. Each letter begins a word that the student uses to describe a personality trait or characteristic that the student values. After nametags have been completed, divide the students into small groups to discuss why they value these traits. An example of a nametag might be as follows:

K ind
A thletic
R eliable
E asy-going
N utty

Sentence Completion

On a master ditto, prepare several open-ended statements about mental health. Allow in-class time for each student to complete the statements. Ask volunteers to discuss each sentence. Use open-ended statements such as the following:

1. When I feel happy, I _____ .
2. When I feel sad, I _____ .
3. When I get angry, I _____ .
4. A healthy way to show anger is to _____ .
5. A good friend is one who _____ .
6. The thing I do best is _____ .
7. The thing I wish I could do better is _____ .

Rank Ordering Personality Traits

Tell each student to think of someone he or she admires a great deal and allow a few minutes for the students to write down all the likeable personal qualities that person has. Then ask the students to rank-order those characteristics in terms of the one that is most important, desirable, or likeable, second most important, desirable, or likeable, and so on.

Friends Should Be . . .

Write the following groupings on the board:

A	B	C
_____SMART	_____HONEST	_____LOYAL
_____POPULAR	_____DEPENDABLE	_____CONSCIENTIOUS
_____FUNNY	_____DEDICATED	_____TRUSTWORTHY

D	E	F
_____OPEN	_____QUIET	_____HEALTHY
_____DISCREET	_____BUBBLY	_____HAPPY
_____CLOSED	_____TALKATIVE	_____SUCCESSFUL

Ask each student to rank-order within each grouping the characteristic most important to look for in a friend. Then group the students and ask them to decide upon consensus rankings, which are shared with all other groups. Summarize similarities and differences between group rankings.

"Say" It the Positive Way

Ask each student to list three nonverbal negative behaviors or messages that make others feel bad, such as frowning at someone, making a face at someone, or walking away from someone, and three nonverbal positive behaviors or messages. Divide the students into small groups and have each group record and report results to other groups based on responses in each category.

Mental Health Continuum

Prepare a ditto that contains a blank continuum line and several statements underneath the line relating to mental health. Ask each student to place the letter of the statement on the line wherever it fits with his or her thinking. Draw a large master continuum line on the chalkboard and allow several volunteers to record their ratings for each statement. Follow with general class discussion. An example of a continuum line and statements is shown below.

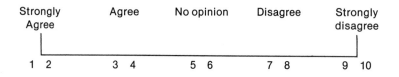

A. Boys shouldn't cry.
B. Some people are better than others.
C. People need to be alone.
D. It's OK to let others know that you are angry.
E. Honesty is the best policy.

The Time of My Life

Have each student draw a circle divided into four sections on a piece of paper. The circle represents a 24-hour time span, with each quadrant equalling approximately 6 hours. From the following categories, ask each student to divide the circle according to the amount of time that he or she thinks *should* be spent on these activities.

    time with friends
    time with family
    time learning at school
    time for homework
    time for sleeping

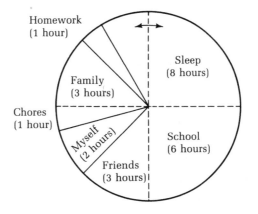

Figure 12.1
Time circle.

time for myself
time for chores

An example of how such a time circle might look is shown in figure 12.1.

Cartoons

There is a saying, "While you laugh, you cannot develop an ulcer." Have students find or draw and label a cartoon that depicts healthy and unhealthy practices. Have students find a cartoon that helps them laugh at themselves. Have them share and describe these cartoons with others.

Source: Linda Brower Meeks and Philip Heit. *Health: Focus on You, Teacher's Annotated Edition.* Columbus, Ohio: Charles E. Merrill Publishing Company, 1982, p. 35T.

Decision Stories

Follow the procedure discussed in Chapter 5 for presenting mental health decision stories such as the following:

Where Did I Put It?

Sally is getting ready for school. She cannot remember where she put her shoes. She looked under the bed, under the chair, and behind the door. Sally begins to cry because she thinks she will be late.

Focus Questions: What could have been done to keep Sally from getting upset? What should Sally do now?

A Nasty Note

Sam was going to the lunchroom when he saw Fred sticking something in Peggy's locker. Later, Sam saw Peggy crying because she found a note in her locker that made fun of her family.

Focus Question: What should Sam do?

A Stolen Gift

John and Bob are in the fourth grade. Bob is new in school and does not have any friends except John. One Saturday, they are in a department store. John picks up a model car and leaves the store. He then gives it to Bob as a present.

Focus Question: What should Bob do?

Into the Bushes

Johnny was playing with a group of friends while walking down the sidewalk to school one morning. The play became a little rough, and Johnny and a friend fell into a neighbor's fence, resulting in a substantial amount of damage to the neighbor's property.

Focus Question: What should Johnny do?

DRAMATIZATION

The Me I Want to Be

Following introductory activities that explain personality and self-concept, divide students into small groups. Have each group write and present a short skit depicting ways to help a main character develop a strong sense of self-worth and thus become "The Me I Want to Be." After presentation of all skits, have a class discussion and emphasize common notions and suggestions.

Role Playing Mental Health

Have students role play the following situations related to various aspects of mental health:

1. A student being praised for receiving a good grade on a test.
2. A student receiving a paper showing that he has failed an important test.
3. A person who has been refused participation in a group activity.
4. A person who has lost a very important object.
5. A person who has unintentionally hurt someone else's feelings.

Another role-playing situation helps the students experience nonverbal communication. Ask volunteers in the class to role play the following emotions without talking:

1. anger
2. happiness
3. sadness
4. humiliation
5. embarrassment

Hidden Messages

Divide students into small groups. Ask half the groups to present a play with a hidden message or moral of their own making using dialogue and ask the remaining groups to give their presentations nonverbally. After all groups have finished, ask for identification and interpretation of the messages and discuss the advantages and disadvantages of verbal and nonverbal communication.

Words Can Hurt

Ask the class as a whole to devise a hypothetical, open-ended situation in which communication could take the form of being either rude or tactful. Then, divide the class into two groups. Ask one group to describe several tactful ways the situation could be handled. Ask the other group to describe several rude ways the situation could be handled. Follow by leading a discussion about students' views concerning each handling of the situation.

The Decision

Provide an open-ended hypothetical situation appropriate for the grade level that involves either rejection by peer group or a family crisis. Then divide the students into three groups. Supply two of the groups with the ending they will enact. Ask the third group to devise their own scenario. Let each group dramatize their ideas and compare differences. If time and attention allow, provide additional situations and rotate tasks.

Pairing

Pair students. Have one member of each pair draw a situation from a box full of hypothetical interactions between two people, such as making a new friend, little brother breaking your toy, or sharing ice cream with a playmate. Use imagination, creativity, and diversity in developing these situations and focus on many areas of mental health. Allow each pair to act out their situation and encourage class discussion after each enactment.

Giving and Gaining

Have several students role play a situation where an individual's personal values must be compromised for the good of the group. Examples might include the mayor allowing an individual to make an unpopular speech, or a police officer enforcing a law he or she does not agree with. Follow with a discussion of why the person made the compromise.

DISCUSSION AND REPORT TECHNIQUES

Getting to Know You

Ask students to print the word PERSONALITY as the heading on a sheet of notebook paper and have them write several phrases that describe their own personalities. Let volunteers share their papers with the class.

Famous Examples

As a library project, have students read a story or book about a famous person. Have them give oral presentations of at least two major life events and how these events affected the famous person. Also ask students to indicate a few of the characteristics they think people should remember about the famous individual.

Provide the class with a chronology of pictures of a famous movie star, singer, politician, or other individual showing how this person appeared as a youngster, adolescent, young adult, and older adult. Discuss the effects of lifecycle stages on this celebrity's personality as well as the perceptions others have about the individual.

Worries Beware

Lead a discussion defining and describing stress. Use probing and illustrative questions that help students understand the meaning of stress, such as: Have you ever moved to a new city or school? Was it hard? What was it like the first day you ever came to school? The first day of school this year? Do you get worried about your report card? Why? What things seem to worry your friends? Your parents? Following the discussion, provide students with several pictures, photos, and drawings that depict people in various stressful situations. Ask them to decide why these people may be uncomfortable or tense. What is the probable source of the stress? Then ask if the students can think of ways to lessen the stress.

Life's Stresses

Divide students into small groups and assign each group a stressful situation to write about, such as the death of a pet, moving, or being accused of something you did not do. Have the groups write how they would handle the situation, using their own ideas, health texts, and encyclopedias. Bind the reports into a booklet entitled "Life's Stresses" and use it as a resource.

Listening Is Important

Read a story that suggests the importance of being a good listener when someone needs to talk about a problem. Ask students what they think of the story and then have them write their own stories about being a good listener. Let volunteers share their ideas.

A Picture of Me

Have students draw several pictures of themselves. The students can draw themselves doing several activities they enjoy, e.g., playing games, listening to music, talking with others. Do not put their names on the pictures. When the pictures are completed, place the pictures around the room, and have the other students guess who drew each picture and what activity each picture represents.

Guest Speakers

Invite a school psychologist, social worker, and other mental health professionals to class to discuss mental health problems among young people and the services available to students with problems.

Different Is OK

To emphasize the fact that all people are different and unique, discuss several categories or groups of plants and animals. Visual aids should be easy to obtain. For example, fruits come in many varieties, sizes, shapes, colors, and tastes, yet all are fruits. People, too, are all different but we are all people.

Ups and Downs

To illustrate that life is not always happy, choose fairy tales such as Red Riding Hood, Snow White, and Cinderella and discuss events in each one. Be sure to note the hard times or sad times as well as "living happily ever after."

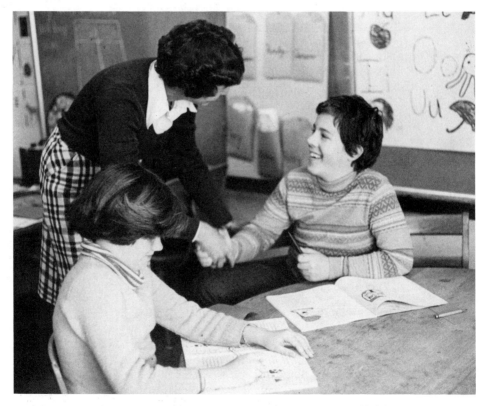

The teacher can do much to foster each student's mental health by reinforcing special talents and allowing expression of feelings.

Caring

Discuss the different needs of a pet dog or cat. When the animal is hungry, we feed it. When it is lonely, we play with it and talk to it. When it is sleeping, we don't disturb it. People have needs that have to be met as well. Discuss how we help meet the needs of others by caring.

Living by the Rules

Sometimes it is hard for young children to understand why it is necessary to follow directions or obey rules. Discuss several rules or laws and the reasons for each. For example, a traffic speed limit helps to prevent accidents, injuries, and deaths. It also helps to conserve fuel. Rules for a game help make the activity fair and fun. Discuss what happens when someone doesn't follow the rules of a game.

EXPERIMENTS AND DEMONSTRATIONS

Likes and Dislikes

Ask five students to step into the hall. Arrange a variety of objects on the table. Allow the students to come in one at a time. Tell each to choose the object he or she would like to have. Do not remove any of the objects until all five students have made their selections. Let the remainder of the class note the different choices and determine why each person made that selection. Then summarize by indicating that differences in choices are an individual matter.

When I Explode

Constant nagging or chiding can cause a person to get angry or upset. Demonstrate this point by blowing up a balloon. After each puff, have the students repeat, "The balloon is getting mad!" Tell students that each puff represents more frustration or feelings of being pushed. Continue to blow until the balloon bursts. This demonstrates a build-up of anger and the resulting "explosion." After this demonstration, ask the students how they handle their anger when they are nagged or constantly chided. Is there a way to keep from "exploding"?

Compliment Circle

Divide students into three groups and have each group sit in a circle. Starting with one person, the group members then anonymously write complimentary comments on separate pieces of paper about that person. The comments are circulated to everyone in the group and then given to the individual. Repeat until all members have been addressed. Rotate groups on two more occasions so that each student receives three anonymous collections of compliments. Then ask each student to prepare a master list by grouping similar compliments. Have the students write a few comments underneath their master lists concerning their feelings about participating in this activity and what they learned from it.

Mental Health in Music

Have students compose songs that describe healthy living. They can bring in records that describe a human relationship. Discuss the feelings depicted in the music. Pay attention to the tone of the music as well as to the words of the song.

Source: Linda Brower Meeks and Philip Heit. *Health: Focus on You, Teacher's Annotated Edition.* Columbus, Ohio: Charles E. Merrill Publishing Company, 1982, p. 38T.

Grab Bag

Give each student a paper bag. Tell students that for three days they are to write their feelings on separate slips of paper as they happen and stick them into the bag. Emphasize that descriptions should not use specific names of people. Instead, have the students refer to "my friend," "my brother," and so on. Also, no names should be placed on the bags. After the time period elapses, divide students into groups of five to seven and have them mix up their bags. Let students try to assign bags to their correct owners by reading comments inside. This activity should demonstrate that each group member felt many of the same emotions since it may be difficult to correctly assign bags back to their owners.

Hearing Is Not Always Listening

Set up several "listening" and "observing" demonstrations to emphasize that these are learned skills. Here are some possible examples:

- Prearrange with a student to share a hypothetical problem with several classmates during lunch or recess. They need to believe that they are being told about the problem in confidence. The following day, reveal the setup to the class and ask each student involved about what he or she heard and understood to be the problem.

- Prearrange with several students to get "lost" during recess. (Have them go to the library or other supervised area.) When the rest of the class returns, ask them to help with descriptions of each missing person. Also have them indicate any reasons they might have overheard during recess as to why these students are gone. After the missing students return, discuss implications of the activity.

- Tell students that you are going to read a story and that you want them to listen carefully. Read aloud a short story with several specific details about a main character's problem or situation and the succeeding events. Immediately following the story, ask each student to write a brief summary of the story, being as specific and accurate as possible. Let volunteers share their versions. Then read the original again. Compare listening skills.

Decisions, Decisions, Decisions!

Divide students into three groups. For a few days, present as many alternatives to the groups as possible concerning decisions about classroom activities. For example, for your recess period today your group can either go for a nature walk with me, go to the gymnasium for supervised games with the P.E. specialists, stay in the room with the teacher's aide to watch a special movie, or have free-play on the playground. Let each group decide what they as a group want to do. You should act as a moderator when needed. Since it is possible that each group may decide to do something different, make sure that all alternatives are feasible and can be implemented with relative ease. Following this experiment in decision making, discuss the process.

PUZZLES AND GAMES

Cooperation Is the Key

Emphasize that cooperation is necessary for most games and group activities. Let the students identify and participate in several activities that require cooperation, such as jumping rope and playing catch. Follow these activities by asking, "Would it be fun to do any of these things alone? Can you do any of these things alone?"

Gossip Go Away

Gossip can hurt, especially when the story gets twisted. Demonstrate how this happens by playing the "whisper" game. Group students in a circle. Think of a sentence and whisper it to one child, who passes it on until the last person says out loud what he or she heard. Note the difference. Rotate the positions of first and last persons and repeat the game.

The Mirror Game

Duplicate a list of 20 to 30 personality traits suitable to the students' age group. Set them up in columns with room for graduated ratings of self and partner (see example below). Have each student pick a partner with whom they are familiar. After passing out the list of traits, stress that they are not to talk while they are evaluating themselves or their partner. They then compare what they marked about themselves

Traits		Self					Partner			
		Never	Seldom	Sometimes	Always		Never	Seldom	Sometimes	Always
Sensitive	+									
Arrogant	−									
Silly	−									
Trusting	+									
Tender	+									
Two-faced	−									

Source: Rosa Sullivan, "The Mirror Game," in Osness, Donna and Thompson, Karen (Editors). *Health Education Teaching Ideas: Elementary.* Reston, Virginia: AAHPERD, 1983, p. 110.

Emotions:
Under each face, write the name of the emotion shown. The emotions are happiness, sadness, anger, excitement, kindness, and fear.

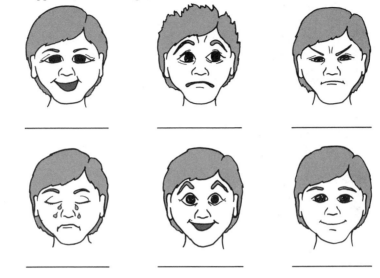

Figure 12.2
Worksheet for identifying emotions.

and each other. This should reveal a number of differences between their self-impressions and how they are perceived by others.

Feelings and Faces

Hand out duplicated sheets to the students showing stylized emotions, as illustrated in figure 12.2. Have each student identify and label the emotion depicted by each face. Follow this activity with a class discussion.

Costume Party

Ask each student to come to class in a costume that depicts as many of his or her personality traits as possible. The class as a whole lists what traits they think are revealed and a secret ballot vote is cast for costumes that are the most accurate, inaccurate, humorous, puzzling, and eye-catching.

Unknown Classmate

Secretly assign each student to observe another student for a few days. Then ask each student to role-play his or her subject, demonstrating personality traits and behavior. The first student to guess the "unknown classmate" gets three points. For wrong guesses, subtract one point from a student's total. Keep score and also time each presentation to see which presenter is the most gifted actor in portraying characteristics.

Silent Steps

Divide students into groups of five to seven. Provide each group with a sealed manila envelope that contains a sheet of colored construction paper cut into five to seven shuffled jigsaw pieces. Each group should receive a different colored puzzle with differently shaped pieces of equal difficulty. Instruct each group member to randomly select a puzzle piece from the envelope upon your signal to start. The students must reconstruct the pieces nonverbally without telling each other where specific pieces should go or fit together. The first group to reconstruct the sheet of construction paper wins and should raise their hands, not talk. Wait until all groups have solved their puzzles. Then discuss the students' feelings about this nonverbal game. Did they feel frustrated? Helpless? Confused? Sharp?

BULLETIN BOARDS

Our Class—We're Special!

Make silhouettes of each student by placing the students between a filmstrip projector and a sheet of black construction paper. Trace the silhouette with white chalk. Let each student write a short personal profile sheet to go with his or her silhouette. Tack the completed silhouettes and profile sheets on a classroom wall.

Relationships

Have students make a collage of their relationships. A picture of the student will be in the center. Around the center, have students put pictures to represent those they are involved with (e.g., teacher, other students, family members).

Source: *Health: A Guide for Grade K Through 12: Level One.* Nashville: Tennessee Department of Education, 1983, p. 25.

Lend a Helping Hand

Let students trace and label their hands on construction paper. Tack the hand outlines to a bulletin board and let students write a caption describing how they help at home, such as by taking out trash, feeding the dog, or sweeping the floor.

Service With a Smile

Obtain photographs of several school personnel, including the custodians, bus drivers, cafeteria workers, librarian, nurse, and principal. Label appropriately. Underneath the pictures, have students design and construct creative awards or citations for the special contributions to a healthy and happy school made by each person.

Steps to the Top

Have students trace their feet on construction paper. Inside the foot outline, ask each student to write a measure, quality, or rule for building mental health, such as self-love, self-respect, consideration for others, open communication, practicing what you preach, and sound decision-making. Tack the footprints on a bulletin board in ascending steps to GOOD MENTAL HEALTH!

Coping with Stress

Divide students into four groups. Ask each group to create a bulletin board that focuses on positive ways to reduce stress. Bulletin boards should be redone each week for a month so that each group's message can be seen and discussed.

OTHER IDEAS

Facial Forecasts

Assign each student an emotion. Provide the students with paper plates and crayons and ask them to draw their own faces indicating that emotion. Have the students use mirrors if necessary. The plates may be used for a colorful wall display.

Communicating with Others

For one day, students observe and record (on paper) accounts of people communicating with others. Note the presence or lack of honesty in what they reveal about their own feelings. Discuss examples of people who did and did not express their true feelings to others.

1. What were the results?
2. Which person would you be most apt to believe?
3. Which person would you most prefer to talk to?
4. What does this tell you about yourself?

Source: Betty Kay Stein, "The Neglected 'R'—Responsibility," in Osness, Donna and Thompson, Karen (Editors). *Health Education Teaching Ideas: Elementary.* Reston, Virginia: AAHPERD, 1983, p. 113.

Two Peas in a Pod

Have students pair off with another student whom they like and know well. Ask each pair to identify on notebook paper a few of the positive characteristics or traits that they share as well as a few that are different. Have the pairs pin their lists on the front of their clothing. Then have each pair spend the rest of the day with one another at lunch, recess, and other free time so that everyone can note the similarities and differences in the partners.

Competencies and Contracts

Divide students into small groups and assign a special task to each group. Let each group member decide how he or she can best contribute to the completion of the task by writing a brief "contract" with the group. When the task is completed, privately assess the outcome of the contribution and contract with each student, being sure to emphasize positive qualities and competencies.

I Remember When . . .

Divide students into pairs and ask each pair to share a personal experience that was stressful. Allow two to three minutes for each person to do this. Rotate pairs until everyone has shared an experience with the others. Ask volunteers to relate the one experience that someone told them that they thought was the most stressful. Compare different perceptions about levels of stress.

Stress Tips

Provide students with an example of a stressful situation, such as playing baseball with friends and accidentally breaking a neighbor's window, bringing home a report card with a bad grade, misplacing library books, or having to perform in a play. Ask students to draw pictures of what they would do in that situation. Compare pictures and ask students to separate the pictures that are "positive" from those that are not.

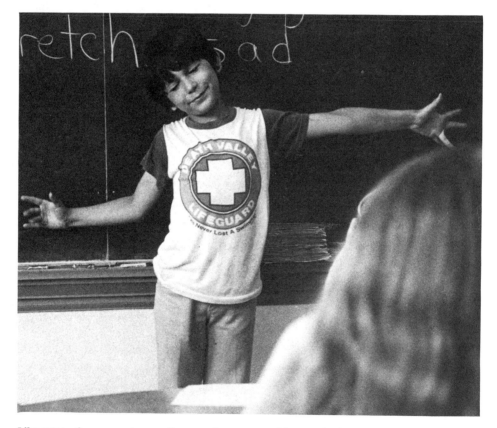

Like most other concepts, emotions can be expressed in a variety of ways. The teacher must explain to the students that in the real world, these ways can be healthy and unhealthy.

Everyone Should Accept Responsibility for His Own Behavior

On a sheet of paper, each student lists new freedoms he has acquired within the past year. Opposite each one, he lists the added responsibilities he has acquired along with the freedom. Then, ask the following questions:

1. Who gave you these freedoms?
2. To whom do you have new responsibilities?
3. What will result if you do not accept the responsibility?
4. How will you feel about yourself if you do or do not fulfill the responsibility?

Source: Betty Kay Stein, "The Neglected 'R'—Responsibility," in Osness, Donna and Thompson, Karen (Editors). *Health Education Teaching Ideas: Elementary.* Reston, Virginia: AAHPERD, 1983, p. 113.

Mental Health Stumpers

Ask each student to write at least two questions about one or more teacher-selected mental health topics. Then give each student a few minutes to ask the questions to the class. Keep a record on the board of those questions that stumped the class and assign additional projects based on this discovery.

Collages

Assist the student in creating collages depicting the following:

> general personality information
> interests
> relationship patterns
> future goals, dreams, and desires for self
> verbal and nonverbal communication

Question Box

Supply a large, colorful question box and encourage students to submit questions that they want to discuss regarding personal fears, worries, or dilemmas. Questions are anonymous. Set aside a particular time for about 30 minutes each week to discuss as many of these as possible.

13. Nutrition

Nutrition is a major determinant of the health and vigor of the school child and sets the pattern for later stages of the life span.—Virginia Beal

KNOWLEDGE AND NUTRITION

Human beings must eat to survive. The well nourished child is more apt to reach her full potential physically, mentally and intellectually. For example, there is now little argument that children perform better in school when they have had a good breakfast (Rapoport & Kruesi, 1983). Yet despite the importance of food, surprisingly few people know very much about ensuring proper nutrition. Although the United States leads the world in food production, many Americans—not just the poor—are malnourished. Ignorance about basic nutritional requirements accounts for only part of this problem; unwillingness to alter lifestyle to meet sound nutritional standards is often at the heart of it. In our fast-paced society, people opt to skip meals, especially breakfast, or to eat a poorly balanced meal at a fast-food restaurant. Many parents fail to provide good examples for their children concerning nutritional habits.

Generally, the nutritional status of American children is good. Clinical evidence of undernutrition showed rates of 2 percent or less in children under 6 years and 5 percent or less in children over 6 years in three national surveys (Beal, 1982). However, many children prefer junk food to a proper diet. This preference is demonstrated especially by snacking behavior. Morgan (1982) found that, in 6 to 11-year olds, the most frequently consumed snacks were bakery products and soft drinks. Nutritious school lunches are picked at or left unfinished because children have learned to prefer candy, potato chips, and soft drinks.

Nutrition education has been listed as a priority by the U.S. Department of Health and Human Services in the "1990 Health Objectives for the Nation," as listed by the Surgeon General (Kolbe & Gilbert, 1984). The need for nutrition education is crucial. For example, American elementary school children demonstrate elevated cholesterol levels compared to children from other countries. Studies indicate that sound school nutrition programs can produce positive outcomes (Perry, Mullis & Maile, 1985). Assisting children to develop sound nutritional habits should be one of your major goals in elementary health instruction. To accomplish this, you must do more than simply provide information. You must counter the impact of television commercials and other sources. You must help children recognize that although the food they eat is strongly influenced by their culture and their lifestyle, they can learn to control these influences. You must also dispel misconceptions associated with food and nutrition, aid children in becoming informed consumers, and develop in them a sense of the importance of nutrition.

FOOD HABITS AND CUSTOMS

Every culture has its own food habits and customs. Approaches to nutrition are based in part on the food resources available. In Japan, where there is little land available for raising livestock, red meat is not a usual part of the daily diet. Animal protein is supplied instead by fish and other seafood, which abound in the waters around the island nation. In southern China, as in Japan, rice is a staple eaten at every meal. However, in the north of China, where rice cannot be grown, wheat and millet are substituted for rice. In Mexico, beans and corn flour tortillas are eaten daily by the poorer, now as in Aztec times. This combination of two simple foods provides all essential protein needed for good nutrition.

Food customs are also often partly a result of religious ideas. Hindus consume no beef, some Jews eat only kosher foods, and some Buddhists are vegetarians. Many

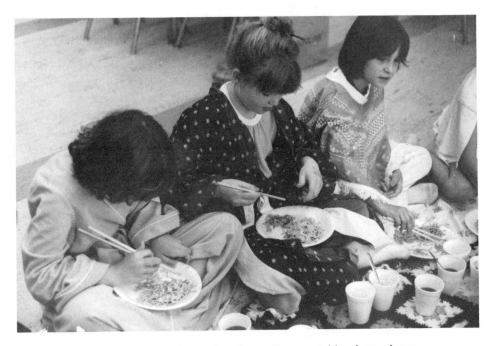

Cooking and eating in class can be a cultural as well as a nutritional experience.

religious dietary rules were originally based on health considerations. For example, the Jewish and Islamic prohibitions against eating pork are probably based on the fact that undercooked pork can harbor parasites that cause such diseases in humans as trichinosis.

Different cultural outlooks also influence food customs. Horsemeat is commonly eaten in France, but is viewed with disdain in England and other English-speaking countries. Milk, which plays such a large role in American diets, is almost never consumed by adult Chinese, who find the taste and idea of drinking it repellent.

Food habits and customs in the United States reflect the multicultural nature of our society. At one time, there were significant regional differences in cooking and food preferences. Seafood was a major part of the diet in the eastern seaboard states. Wild game provided much of the meat eaten in the rural South. Mexican and Indian cultures influenced the cuisine of the Southwest. Today, these regional differences have faded, largely as a result of refrigeration and modern transportation. It is now almost as easy to get fresh fish in Kansas as it is in Massachusetts. Cultural intermixing has also diminished regional differences, while at the same time expanding the range of dishes commonly eaten. Pasta, for instance, is no longer eaten only by Americans of Italian extraction. Chinese, French, German, Mexican, and Middle Eastern dishes have also become popular.

Economic, Personal, and Lifestyle Factors

As an affluent, multiethnic nation, we have a greater variety of foods and dishes to choose from than almost any other people on earth. This does not mean, however, that Americans can afford to eat anything they like. Inflation has influenced the eating habits of all Americans, rich and poor alike—but especially the poor. Those living near or below the poverty level often must subsist on cheap starchy foods, which are filling, if not particularly nutritious.

Although economics influences the American diet, as it does the diet of every nation, most Americans cannot blame lack of money for poor nutritional habits. Instead, we must look for the reasons in personal preferences and lifestyles. Personal preference for a food often is formed by reasons that have little or nothing to do with the nourishment that will be provided by that food. For example, parents typically pass their food preferences on to their children. Persons develop prejudices against foods because of bad experiences, such as when a food causes an allergic response or gastrointestinal upset. The most popular foods eaten by one's subculture and peer group also influence food choices. Finally, a food might be chosen because of the way it looks, smells, and tastes.

The national lifestyle also influences our nutritional habits. When the United States was mostly a rural, agrarian society, breakfast was a major meal. The main meal of the day was served at noon. These two meals provided the necessary energy for performing farm labor and chores. Evening dinner was typically a lighter meal. Today, the reverse is true. Most Americans eat a light breakfast. Some skip breakfast entirely. Lunch is also a light meal, often eaten in haste. The largest meal of the day is consumed in the evening, because there is more time to prepare and eat such a meal. Unfortunately, this meal is then usually followed by general physical inactivity and then by sleep. This is one reason why so many Americans are overweight. Also, many overspice their foods, especially with salt and sugar. Others rush through their meals, which reduces the nourishment received from the foods.

There is not much that you as a teacher can do to change our hectic national lifestyle. However, you can emphasize the importance of starting off the day with a good breakfast that will provide your children with the energy they need for school and studying. You can also point up the value of a balanced, nutritional lunch, and a reasonable evening meal. This is not to suggest that you should criticize the eating patterns of any child's family, and certainly not any religious dietary restrictions a family might heed. But you can be a source of information about sound nutritional practices, and you can encourage your students to consider changes in their diet that could lead to sounder nutrition. For example, you should emphasize that snacking on junk food, such as candy, may spoil a child's appetite for a regular meal as well as contribute to tooth decay. You can also stimulate children's curiosity about trying new dishes that could add needed variety to their diets.

Food is one of the delights of every civilization. Preparation of some dishes in many cultures is an art. Eating a fine meal is an aesthetic experience, not just fulfillment of nutritional requirements, but even the simplest dish can provide great pleasure. Use this positive approach in presenting nutritional concepts. Too often nutrition is taught as a grim and dry subject, divorced from the human perspective. No wonder that children often emerge from health education with scorn for nutritional principles; they associate nutrition with the imagined somber atmosphere of a health food store!

NUTRIENTS

Food's most basic function is to provide nutrients to the body. Nutrients are the substances in food needed to support life functions. One vital way in which this is accomplished is by providing energy that the body needs. This energy, produced as a byproduct of food consumption, is measured in calories. A calorie is defined as the amount of heat energy required to raise the temperature of one kilogram of water one degree Celsius. All foods have specific caloric values, and a given amount of food will produce a certain number of calories when broken down by the body.

The number of calories needed by the body daily depends upon two factors: the individual's basal metabolism, and the amount of energy expended in daily activities. Basal metabolism is the minimum amount of heat produced by the body when at rest. This heat, among other things, is necessary to maintain a normal body temperature. The amount of energy expended by an individual varies, depending upon the activities of the individual. Thus someone who engages in heavy physical labor each day needs more calories than someone who works in an office. Young children need fewer calories per day than active adults, because of the difference in body sizes.

Although caloric requirements differ with age, basal metabolism, and daily activities, the Food and Agricultural Organization of the United Nations recommends a daily minimum intake for adults of 2650 calories. However, more than half the people in the world exist on fewer than 2200 calories per day (Jones, Shainberg, & Byer, 1986). During the periods of rapid growth, children also need more calories. For example, a 10-year-old boy requires an average daily intake of about 2300 calories, with this amount rising to 2900 calories by age 13. A 10-year-old girl requires an average daily intake of 2200 calories, and 2400 calories at age 13. Three categories of nutrients provide caloric energy: carbohydrates, fats, and proteins. Together, they make up most of the elements in the foods we eat.

Carbohydrates

Foods rich in carbohydrates form about half of the typical American diet. Carbohydrates are either simple sugars, derived from such foods as sugar and honey, or more complex compounds, derived from such foods as cereals and potatoes. The sweet taste of corn and peas is due to the presence of carbohydrate compounds.

The metabolism of carbohydrates produces energy. Four calories are produced per gram of carbohydrates. If carbohydrates are not abundant in the diet, protein and fat have to be metabolized to produce needed energy. Carbohydrates must be constantly replenished in the blood, either by eating or by breaking down glycogen stored in the liver and muscles.

Carbohydrates are important in a child's diet. Foods rich in carbohydrates include rice, spaghetti, noodles, bread, breakfast cereals, and potatoes. Many vegetables, fruits, and fruit juices also contain some carbohydrates. Although candy and cookies are good sources of carbohydrates, the refined sugar they contain contributes to tooth decay and does not provide additional nutrients. For this reason fruits and juices make healthier snacks.

Proteins

Protein means "to come first." This suggests that proteins are essential nutrients. No organism can live and almost no biological process can take place without protein.

A protein molecule is composed of smaller structures called amino acids. Some amino acids are termed essential, which means they must be provided by the diet, and some are termed nonessential, which means they are synthesized by the body. These amino acids are building blocks necessary for several body functions. Proteins are present in every cell, in enzymes, and in body secretions. Proteins provide calories but also serve other important and complex functions. They are important components of DNA and RNA molecules, which determine the genetic makeup of our bodies. Also, proteins help build new cells and tissues in growing children, maintain tissues that are already built, and are involved in the manufacture of blood, enzymes, hormones, and human milk. Further, antibodies, which combat infection, are synthesized from proteins in response to infectious agents.

Milk and meat products are excellent sources of protein. Poultry is another good source of this essential nutrient. If a person eats a vegetarian diet, enough protein must be ingested to support normal growth and development, especially in children.

Nonmeat sources of protein include soybeans, dried beans, and nuts. Cereal grains, vegetables, and fruits contain vegetable protein, which must be augmented by other protein sources, as in the tortilla and beans example mentioned earlier.

Fats

Fats, or lipids, are the most concentrated source of calories we ingest. Fats provide nine calories per gram as compared with four for proteins and carbohydrates. Approximately 40 percent of our food energy is provided by fats.

Fats are important parts of our diets. Their vital role is sometimes overlooked because of the association of fats with cardiovascular problems. However, fats serve several vital functions. The energy they provide spares protein for tissue synthesis. Fats also serve as carriers of fat-soluble vitamins A, D, E, and K. As food, they provide satiety because the rate at which a meal is emptied from the stomach is related to the fat content. The higher the fat content, the slower the food empties from the stomach. Fats are an important part of all cells, membrane structures in the body, and tissues.

Additionally, they provide protection in the adipose tissue just under the skin. This layer of adipose tissue also helps in maintaining the body temperature at a constant level despite changes in the environmental temperature. Similarly, fats provide a layer of protective shock-absorbing tissue between the kidneys, reproductive organs, and other organs. They also provide padding for the cheeks, palms of the hands, and balls of the feet. Finally, fats make foods more appetizing and flavorful. The major food sources of fat are animal and vegetable fats, such as butter, cream, lard, and salad dressings. Olives and nuts also have a significant fat content.

In addition to the three major nutrients, water, minerals, and vitamins are vital to human nourishment.

Water

In considering nutrition, water is often overlooked, but it is second only to oxygen in importance to body functioning. A person can survive longer without food than water; there can be no life without water.

Water is an essential component of body structure. It also acts as a solvent for minerals and other physiologically important compounds. In the body, it transports nutrients to and waste products from the cells. Further, water helps to regulate the body temperature (Katch & McArdle, 1983). Water comes from fluids and solids in the diet and is also produced by the metabolizing of energy nutrients within the tissues. The amount of activity and the climate are important factors influencing the amount of water a person needs. Since children usually participate in more physical activities, they perspire more and therefore need more water than many adults. Water is also lost through exhaled air. The recommended daily intake is the equivalent of six to eight glasses of water. Much of this is gained from solid foods.

Minerals

The body needs organic compounds such as carbohydrates, fats, and proteins for proper nutrition, but it also needs inorganic materials, such as minerals. These inorganic elements are present in the body in small amounts, but they play a vital role in nutrition. The major minerals needed by the body are calcium, phosphorus, potassium, sulfur, sodium, chlorine, and magnesium. Other mineral elements, known as trace elements and required in lesser amounts, are iron, zinc, selenium, magnesium, copper, iodine, fluorine, chromium, molybdenum, and cobalt.

Minerals function in the body in several ways. After the organic compounds have been oxidized, minerals remain to form actual body parts. For example, calcium, magnesium, and phosphorus are components of the bones and teeth. Minerals also act as regulators and are necessary to certain body functioning. For example, minerals contribute to the water and electrolyte balance of the body and are important in the functioning of the transmission of nerve impulses.

Minerals serve as catalysts in a number of physiological reactions. They do not actually become part of the end product, but the reaction could not take place without them. For example, the production of insulin in the body depends on the presence of zinc, and the clotting of blood depends on calcium. Minerals contribute to the osmotic pressure of body fluids. They contribute to the maintenance of neutrality—the acid-base balance of the blood and body tissues. Finally, they make possible the normal rhythm in the heart beat.

A lack of essential minerals can cause malnutrition. For example, iron-deficiency anemia is a major health problem in the United States and Canada and even more so in the rest of the world. Children deprived of iron show psychological disturbances, such as hyperactivity, and reduced IQ (Whitney, Hamilton, & Boyle, 1984). This deficiency occurs most frequently in infants, adolescent males, and females during child-bearing years.

Vitamins

No group of nutrients has captured the imagination of the public more than vitamins. Vitamins were discovered fairly recently, when physicians sought the cause of several diseases such as scurvy. They concluded that the chemical compounds called vitamins can make a great deal of difference to health. These vitamin-related discoveries have led people to equate good nutrition with vitamins, and some even thought vitamins contained the essential element for life. Quacks have exploited this belief by promoting the unproven use of megavitamins as disease cures (Jarvis, 1984). The enrichment of food with vitamins and the use of vitamins as diet supplements are commonplace in our country.

Vitamins are organic compounds that must be provided by the diet since the body is not able to synthesize them in the required amounts. Vitamins foster growth, promote the ability to produce healthy offspring, maintain health, aid in the normal function of the appetite and digestive tract, and help the body's resistance to bacterial infections.

The fat-soluble vitamins transported by lipids through the body are A, D, E, and K. Vitamin A is important in promoting growth and health of body tissues. This vitamin also enhances vision by aiding the retina to function properly, permitting us to distinguish between light and shade and see various colors distinctly. Vitamin D is needed to prevent and cure rickets, a deficiency disease in which bones fail to harden. Vitamin E is an activator in certain enzyme reactions, and it protects vitamins A and C from being used up too quickly. Vitamin K is essential for the synthesis of prothrombin, a substance needed for normal blood coagulation.

The water-soluble vitamins include the B vitamins and vitamin C, or ascorbic acid. The B vitamins are essential to daily human nutrition. Known as the B-complex group, they help body systems combat stress and maintain energy reserves. The B-complex group is comprised of vitamin B-1 (thiamine), vitamin B-2 (riboflavin), vitamin B-3 (niacin), vitamin B-5 (pantothenic acid), vitamin B-6 (pyridoxine), vitamin B-12 (cobalamin), folic acid, and biotin.

Thiamin is necessary for carbohydrate metabolism. It aids in the release of energy from food. Riboflavin assists body cells to use oxygen, promotes tissue repair, and helps the nervous system function properly. Niacin is essential to growth; without niacin, thiamine and riboflavin could not function properly in the body. Pantothenic acid helps increase vitality and influences glandular functions. Pyridoxine is necessary for healthy teeth and gums, and helps maintain normal body cholesterol. Further, it aids in the production of antibodies. Cobalamin works in conjunction with folic acid and iron to build normal blood cells and prevent pernicious anemia. Folic acid aids in the proper growth and reproduction of blood cells, and contributes to healthy skin. Biotin is necessary for the proper utilization of fats, carbohydrates, and protein. Biotin also helps produce antibodies.

Ascorbic acid is vital in the prevention of scurvy, in the formation and maintenance of collagen (the cementing material that holds cells together), in the normal metabolism of some amino acids, and in the function of the adrenal glands.

Vitamins are similar to minerals in that they sometimes serve as catalysts for important body functions, are required only in small amounts, and are vital to nourishment. They are unlike minerals, however, in that they do not become part of the body, as calcium does in the teeth and bones.

NUTRITIONAL NEEDS

About 50 different nutrients are needed to maintain health. No food contains all the nutrients needed, not even milk, which is highly regarded in our society. Therefore a variety of foods is required to satisfy nutritional needs. One way to assure this variety and to establish a balanced diet is to select foods each day from each of four established groups identified by the Institute of Home Economics of the United States Department of Agriculture in 1957. The four basic food groups are shown in figure 13.1.

The Four Food Groups

The milk group is comprised chiefly of dairy products such as milk (whole, evaporated, and buttermilk), and cheeses. These are excellent sources of calcium, protein, and riboflavin. Vitamin A and phosphorus are also provided by foods in this group. Elementary school children need three servings per day from this group.

Protein, iron, and other minerals come from the meat group. Foods in this group include lean beef, veal, lamb, pork, liver, heart, and kidneys. Fish and poultry are also part of this group, as are dried beans, peas, nuts, and peanut butter. Children need two servings from this group daily.

A good source of vitamins A and C is the fruit and vegetable group, which includes citrus fruits, cabbage, peppers, salad greens, tomatoes, melons, berries, dark

Nutrients for Health

Nutrients are chemical substances obtained from foods during digestion. They are needed to build and maintain body cells, regulate body processes, and supply energy.

About 50 nutrients, including water, are needed daily for optimum health. If one obtains the proper amount of the 10 "leader" nutrients in the daily diet, the other 40 or so nutrients will likely be consumed in amounts sufficient to meet body needs.

One's diet should include a variety of foods because no single food supplies all the 50 nutrients, and because many nutrients work together.

When a nutrient is added or a nutritional claim is made, nutrition labeling regulations require a listing of the 10 leader nutrients on food packages. These nutrients appear in the chart below with food sources and some major physiological functions.

Nutrient	Important Sources of Nutrient	Some major physiological functions		
		Provide energy	Build and maintain body cells	Regulate body processes
Protein	Meat, Poultry, Fish Dried Beans and Peas Egg Cheese Milk	Supplies 4 Calories per gram.	Constitutes part of the structure of every cell, such as muscle, blood, and bone; supports growth and maintains healthy body cells.	Constitutes part of enzymes, some hormones and body fluids, and antibodies that increase resistance to infection.
Carbohydrate	Cereal Potatoes Dried Beans Corn Bread Sugar	Supplies 4 Calories per gram. Major source of energy for central nervous system.	Supplies energy so protein can be used for growth and maintenance of body cells.	Unrefined products supply fiber—complex carbohydrates in fruits, vegetables, and whole grains—for regular elimination. Assists in fat utilization.
Fat	Shortening, Oil Butter, Margarine Salad Dressing Sausages	Supplies 9 Calories per gram.	Constitutes part of the structure of every cell. Supplies essential fatty acids.	Provides and carries fat-soluble vitamins (A, D, E, and K).
Vitamin A (Retinol)	Liver Carrots Sweet Potatoes Greens Butter, Margarine		Assists formation and maintenance of skin and mucous membranes that line body cavities and tracts, such as nasal passages and intestinal tract, thus increasing resistance to infection.	Functions in visual processes and forms visual purple, thus promoting healthy eye tissues and eye adaptation in dim light.
Vitamin C (Ascorbic Acid)	Broccoli Orange Grapefruit Papaya Mango Strawberries		Forms cementing substances, such as collagen, that hold body cells together, thus strengthening blood vessels, hastening healing of wounds and bones, and increasing resistance to infection.	Aids utilization of iron.
Thiamin (B₁)	Lean Pork Nuts Fortified Cereal Products	Aids in utilization of energy.		Functions as part of a coenzyme to promote the utilization of carbohydrate. Promotes normal appetite. Contributes to normal functioning of nervous system.
Riboflavin (B₂)	Liver Milk Yogurt Cottage Cheese	Aids in utilization of energy.		Functions as part of a coenzyme in the production of energy within body cells. Promotes healthy skin, eyes, and clear vision.
Niacin	Liver Meat, Poultry, Fish Peanuts Fortified Cereal Products	Aids in utilization of energy.		Functions as part of a coenzyme in fat synthesis, tissue respiration, and utilization of carbohydrate. Promotes healthy skin, nerves, and digestive tract. Aids digestion and fosters normal appetite.
Calcium	Milk, Yogurt Cheese Sardines and Salmon with Bones Collard, Kale, Mustard, and Turnip Greens		Combines with other minerals within a protein framework to give structure and strength to bones and teeth.	Assists in blood clotting. Functions in normal muscle contraction and relaxation, and normal nerve transmission.
Iron	Enriched Farina Prune Juice Liver Dried Beans and Peas Red Meat	Aids in utilization of energy.	Combines with protein to form hemoglobin, the red substance in blood that carries oxygen to and carbon dioxide from the cells. Prevents nutritional anemia and its accompanying fatigue. Increases resistance to infection.	Functions as part of enzymes involved in tissue respiration.

Guide to Good Eating...

A Recommended Daily Pattern

The recommended daily pattern provides the foundation for a nutritious, healthful diet.

The recommended servings from the Four Food Groups for adults supply about 1200 Calories. The chart below gives recommendations for the number and size of servings for several categories of people.

Food Group	Recommended Number of Servings				
	Child	Teenager	Adult	Pregnant Woman	Lactating Woman
Milk 1 cup milk, yogurt, OR **Calcium Equivalent:** 1½ slices (1½ oz) cheddar cheese* 1 cup pudding 1¾ cups ice cream 2 cups cottage cheese*	3	4	2	4	4
Meat 2 ounces cooked, lean meat, fish, poultry, OR **Protein Equivalent:** 2 eggs 2 slices (2 oz) cheddar cheese* ½ cup cottage cheese* 1 cup dried beans, peas 4 tbsp peanut butter	2	2	2	3	2
Fruit-Vegetable ½ cup cooked or juice 1 cup raw Portion commonly served such as a medium-size apple or banana	4	4	4	4	4
Grain, whole grain, fortified, enriched 1 slice bread 1 cup ready-to-eat cereal ½ cup cooked cereal, pasta, grits	4	4	4	4	4

*Count cheese as serving of milk OR meat, not both simultaneously.

"Others" complement but do not replace foods from the Four Food Groups. Amounts should be determined by individual caloric needs.

B164 [2] 1977. Copyright © 1977, 4th Ed., National Dairy Council, Rosemont, Il 60018
All rights reserved.

Figure 13.1
The four basic food groups.

Source: Courtesy of the National Dairy Council.

green vegetables, yellow vegetables, and potatoes. Four servings from this group are recommended daily for children. Because overcooking removes much of the vitamin content from vegetables, they should be steamed, cooked briefly, or cooked in a small amount of water. Fresh fruits are best, but when these are unavailable, canned or frozen fruits are acceptable. Fruits canned in heavy syrup should be avoided, however.

The bread and cereal group includes breads, cooked grain, and other foods such as macaroni, spaghetti, and noodles. Grains are the basis for breakfast cereals popular with elementary school children. Whole grain or enriched breads are recommended when selecting foods from this group. These foods provide primarily carbohydrates but are also sources of thiamin, iron, and niacin. They are fairly inexpensive. Also, they are easily digested and they enhance the peristaltic movements in the alimentary tract. Four servings from this group are recommended daily.

Recommended Dietary Allowances

The Food and Nutritional Board of the National Academy of Sciences-National Research Council has established a chart of recommended dietary allowances that suggests the nutritional needs of individuals in the United States. This chart is shown in table 13.1. The recommendations have been set specifically as determined by the climate and general energy needs of the American population. Statistics were obtained from large groups of people living in the United States to establish the criteria for the recommended allowances. These recommended daily allowances are only estimates of the nutritional needs of Americans, but they are useful for dietary planning to ensure proper amounts of various nutrients.

FOOD PROBLEMS

Problems concerned with food have been a part of human life from the earliest times. In past ages, crop failures have led to famine and war. Even today, starvation kills hundreds of thousands of children and adults in very poor nations each year. Although there is also poverty in the United States, few children actually face the threat of starvation. Unfortunately, this does not mean that our nation does not have food problems. Many Americans are undernourished or malnourished. Overweight and obesity are also common.

Undernutrition

Typically, an undernourished person is also underweight, but this is by no means always the case. Undernutrition implies that the individual is not getting enough nutrients. This can occur even if the person is consuming more than enough calories. Thus personal weight is not necessarily an indication of nutritive status. In the United States, malnutrition due to undernutrition is most likely to occur in infants, children, and adolescents, when nutritional requirements for tissue growth and development are high. Undernutrition may inhibit growth, delay maturation, limit physical activity, and interfere with learning (Beal, 1982). The causes of undernutrition are many; poverty and lack of nutrition education are two major factors. Additionally, many

Table 13.1

Food and Nutrition Board, National Academy of Sciences–National Research Council recommended daily dietary allowances[a] (revised 1980). *Designed for the maintenance of good nutrition of practically all healthy people in the United States.*

	Age (years)	Weight (kg)	Weight (lb)	Height (cm)	Height (in)	Protein (g)	Fat-Soluble Vitamins Vita-min A (µg RE)[b]	Vita-min D (µg)[c]	Vita-min E (mg α-TE)[d]	Water-Soluble Vitamins Vita-min C (mg)	Thia-min (mg)	Ribo-flavin (mg)	Niacin (mg NE)[e]	Vita-min B-6 (mg)	Fola-cin[f] (µg)	Vitamin B-12 (µg)	Minerals Cal-cium (mg)	Phos-phorus (mg)	Mag-nesium (mg)	Iron (mg)	Zinc (mg)	Iodine (µg)
Infants	0.0–0.5	6	13	60	24	kg × 2.2	420	10	3	35	0.3	0.4	6	0.3	30	0.5[g]	360	240	50	10	3	40
	0.5–1.0	9	20	71	28	kg × 2.0	400	10	4	35	0.5	0.6	8	0.6	45	1.5	540	360	70	15	5	50
Children	1–3	13	29	90	35	23	400	10	5	45	0.7	0.8	9	0.9	100	2.0	800	800	150	15	10	70
	4–6	20	44	112	44	30	500	10	6	45	0.9	1.0	11	1.3	200	2.5	800	800	200	10	10	90
	7–10	28	62	132	52	34	700	10	7	45	1.2	1.4	16	1.6	300	3.0	800	800	250	10	10	120
Males	11–14	45	99	157	62	45	1000	10	8	50	1.4	1.6	18	1.8	400	3.0	1200	1200	350	18	15	150
	15–18	66	145	176	69	56	1000	10	10	60	1.4	1.7	18	2.0	400	3.0	1200	1200	400	18	15	150
	19–22	70	154	177	70	56	1000	7.5	10	60	1.5	1.7	19	2.2	400	3.0	800	800	350	10	15	150
	23–50	70	154	178	70	56	1000	5	10	60	1.4	1.6	18	2.2	400	3.0	800	800	350	10	15	150
	51+	70	154	178	70	56	1000	5	10	60	1.2	1.4	16	2.2	400	3.0	800	800	350	10	15	150
Females	11–14	46	101	157	62	46	800	10	8	50	1.1	1.3	15	1.8	400	3.0	1200	1200	300	18	15	150
	15–18	55	120	163	64	46	800	10	8	60	1.1	1.3	14	2.0	400	3.0	1200	1200	300	18	15	150
	19–22	55	120	163	64	44	800	7.5	8	60	1.1	1.3	14	2.0	400	3.0	800	800	300	18	15	150
	23–50	55	120	163	64	44	800	5	8	60	1.0	1.2	13	2.0	400	3.0	800	800	300	18	15	150
	51+	55	120	163	64	44	800	5	8	60	1.0	1.2	13	2.0	400	3.0	800	800	300	10	15	150
Pregnant						+30	+200	+5	+2	+20	+0.4	+0.3	+2	+0.6	+400	+1.0	+400	+400	+150	h	+5	+25
Lactating						+20	+400	+5	+3	+40	+0.5	+0.5	+5	+0.5	+100	+1.0	+400	+400	+150	h	+10	+50

[a]The allowances are intended to provide for individual variations among most normal persons as they live in the United States under usual environmental stresses. Diets should be based on a variety of common foods in order to provide other nutrients for which human requirements have been less well defined.

[b]Retinol equivalents. 1 retinol equivalent = 1 µg retinol or 6 µg β carotene. See text for calculation of vitamin A activity of diets as retinol equivalents.

[c]As cholecalciferol. 10 µg cholecalciferol = 400 IU of vitamin D.

[d]α-tocopherol equivalents. 1 mg d-α tocopherol = 1 α-TE.

[e]1 NE (niacin equivalent) is equal to 1 mg of niacin or 60 mg of dietary tryptophan.

[f]The folacin allowances refer to dietary sources as determined by *Lactobacillus casei* assay after treatment with enzymes (conjugases) to make polyglutamyl forms of the vitamin available to the test organism.

[g]The recommended dietary allowance for vitamin B-12 in infants is based on average concentration of the vitamin in human milk. The allowances after weaning are based on energy intake (as recommended by the American Academy of Pediatrics) and consideration of other factors, such as intestinal absorption, see text.

[h]The increased requirement during pregnancy cannot be met by the iron content of habitual American diets nor by the existing iron stores of many women, therefore the use of 30–60 mg of supplemental iron is recommended. Iron needs during lactation are not substantially different from those of nonpregnant women but continued supplementation of the mother for 2–3 months after parturition is advisable in order to replenish stores depleted by pregnancy.

Americans are undernourished because they resist changing nutritionally deficient eating habits and patterns. Other practices dictated by cultural taboos, religious beliefs, and cultural patterns also sometimes lead to nutritional health problems. Occasionally, the cause is physiological. A poorly functioning body might fail to use nutrients supplied to it. For example, a disease such as hyperthyroidism can affect growth regardless of the quality of diet.

Psychological factors can also lead to undernutrition. Hurried meals in haphazard settings may be deleterious because of the type and amount of food as well as how the food is eaten. The noise and confusion that often accompany rushed meals can affect proper digestion. An improper concept of one's nutritional state can bring on health problems such as anorexia nervosa. This is a condition, typically seen in adolescent girls, in which the person perceives herself as overweight even when body weight is extremely low. The anorexic person controls weight by severely restricting food intake and exercising to extremes. A related condition is bulimia, in which a person eats large quantities of food during short periods of time and attempts to control weight by self-induced vomiting or laxative use (Mallick, 1984). This condition can have serious health consequences, and medical help and counseling are essential.

The symptoms of undernutrition include lusterless hair, poor teeth, pale skin, dermatitis, inflamed eyes, sore tongue, fissures at corners of the lips, muscular weakness, apathy, increased susceptibility to infections, shortness of breath, extreme nervousness, irritability, and sometimes weight loss. A seeming contradiction occurring in undernourished children is that though they might be lacking physical endurance they are often hyperactive. Some researchers believe this could be due to dyes or refined sugars in the foods the child is eating (Mailman and Lewis, 1983). A simple solution to the problem of undernutrition is to eat more of the proper nutrients, assuming these foods are available. If lack of knowledge is the only cause of the problem, then suggestions for proper food selection might remedy the situation. A balanced diet that includes a variety of foods, sufficient complex carbohydrates, a

Health Highlight: 1990 Health Objectives for Nutrition

The following are the U.S. Department of Health and Human Services' 1990 nutrition objectives for the nation that can be directly attained or influenced in important ways by schools.

1. By 1990, over 75 percent of the population should be able to identify the principal dietary factors known or strongly suspected to be related to the following: heart disease, high blood pressure, dental caries, and cancer.
2. By 1990, 70 percent of adults should be able to identify the major foods which are low in fat content, low in sodium content, high in calories, and good sources of fiber.

3. By 1990, 90 percent of adults should understand that to lose weight, people must either consume foods that contain fewer calories or increase physical activity, or both.
4. *By 1990, all states should include nutrition education as part of required comprehensive school health education at elementary and secondary levels.*
5. By 1990, 50 percent of school cafeteria managers should be aware of and actively promoting USDA dietary guidelines.

Source: Kolbe and Gilbert, 1984.

minimal level of fat, sodium, and cholesterol can be extremely beneficial to an under-nourished student (Hamrick, Anspaugh, & Ezell, 1986).

HUNGER AND LEARNING

Hunger is a physiological and psychological state that occurs when food needs are not met satisfactorily. Research has shown that hunger definitely has an effect on learning behavior. Hunger increases nervousness, irritability, and disinterest in a learning situation. As Williams (1973) notes, "A lack of interest in what is being taught and an inability to concentrate tend to isolate a hungry child and the negative responses to the child's behavior heighten feelings of isolation to create a vicious circle. The child fails to learn for social and psychological rather than biological reasons" (p. 210).

The Role of the Teacher

As a teacher, you should provide accurate information concerning nutrition to help prevent undernourishment among students. Emphasize the importance of eating a good breakfast and lunch. Also, encourage sociability among students when they are eating. Help the students enjoy the taste, smell, color, and texture of food to increase interest in it. In addition, you have an excellent chance to be an exemplary role model by eating the right foods in the right way while at school.

OVERWEIGHT AND OBESITY

Approximately one out of four of school-aged children is obese, and fat children tend to become fat adults (DeWolfe & Jack, 1984). The health risks of obesity, such as degenerative diseases and shorter life span, may not be of immediate concern to elementary school students, but there are many other reasons for maintaining a correct weight.

Obesity can be considered a physical handicap at any age because it affects physical activity. Also, overweight students face many emotional problems. In a society where "thinness" is emphasized, overweight children may be isolated and shunned, ridiculed, stared at, and rejected socially. As a result, overweight students may lose their sense of self-worth and withdraw from others. A complicating problem occurs when overweight children find satisfaction in nothing else except eating, which causes them to gain even more weight, further alienating them from peers.

Being overweight becomes a health problem when the person is 15 to 20 percent above normal. Of course, body build and an individual's lean-to-fat ratio also have to be taken into consideration. A person might have a stocky build and be over the desired weight for the person's height and age, but the percent body fat might be within the normal range. More often than not, however, obesity is self-evident.

Obesity is a problem influenced by the individual's physical, social, and emotional environment. Usually the condition is due to overeating, improper food habits, or emotional problems. Some people simply enjoy food too much. Others overeat to reduce anxiety, using food as a tranquilizer. Still others eat out of anger or to relieve boredom. Family habits sometimes play a role in contributing to obesity. A family's pattern of overeating and oversnacking is easily incorporated into a child's lifestyle through imitation, perpetuating obesity in the family.

Weight Control

Weight reduction demands self-discipline and commitment. An overweight individual must accept personal responsibility for the condition. If an emotional problem is the cause, that problem must be treated first to ensure long-lasting success at weight control because the overweight condition is only a symptom of a deeper problem. Before any reducing plan is implemented, a physician should be consulted.

Obese persons must consume fewer calories than they expend daily, but this is easier said than done. Dieters should use a diet that is similar to the one to which they are accustomed so they do not feel as restricted and tempted to quit dieting. Weight reduction programs that incorporate behavior modification techniques, daily exercise, and a reducing diet have been successful in helping obese school children lose weight (DeWolfe & Jack, 1984).

Other techniques that have helped people lose weight are to

- Arrange to eat in one place only
- Remove all unnecessary fat when cooking and eating meat
- Avoid gravies, using herbs and spices for seasoning instead
- Start meals with filling, low calories dishes like soup or celery sticks
- Eat fresh fruit instead of canned
- Eat regular meals—a missed meal may make you even more hungry during the day
- Use raw vegetables for snacks
- Eat baked, broiled, or boiled foods without adding fat
- Use a salad-sized plate rather than a dinner plate so the portions look larger
- Cut food into small bites and eat *slowly*
- Brush the teeth after each meal; sometimes the aftertaste of food can stimulate the appetite
- Exercise moderately and regularly
- Develop hobbies; sometimes people substitute food for friends and outside activities

Therapy and Counseling

Weight reduction is usually more successful when using a "buddy system" or peer support groups. Teachers can help by getting together several students who have a similar goal of weight reduction. Have them eat together and share their concerns and problems. You can also educate obese and overweight students about proper nutrition and encourage physical activity. To nurture the emotional health of the obese student, offer security and acceptance without pitying or overprotecting the child. Try to reduce the child's anxiety while helping build self-esteem and independence.

OTHER FOOD-RELATED ISSUES

Food Quackery

Obese individuals may understand the need to diet but may want to do so as painlessly as possible. Such individuals are vulnerable to fad diets advertised to help a person lose weight quickly. Some of these fad diets are restricted in variety, expensive, useless, and sometimes even detrimental to health. Most fad diets are directed at adults, rather than children, of course, but children are impressionable. It is important to put these diets into proper perspective. The fact is that most people who are overweight do not need to read a book on what to eat to lose weight. Simply eating somewhat less of everything will usually produce results, if the diet is followed conscientiously.

Food quackery is by no means confined to diet books or dieting clinics that employ dubious methods. The whole "natural and health foods" industry is considered quackery by many nutritional experts. Both of these areas prey upon natural fears and uncertainties about foods and nutritional requirements. There is no accepted legal definition of what "natural foods" actually are, and no way to keep entrepreneurs from selling granola, dried fruits, and so on at inflated prices, all the while hinting that these products are somehow healthier for a person to eat. "Health foods," such as bee pollen and algae extracts, fall into the same category. Such foods are not harmful to health, but they are no better than foods obtained from ordinary sources. Advocates of "natural," "organic," and "health" foods claim that additives or pesticide residues in regular foods can cause disease or even lower the nutritional value of the food, but these claims are highly exaggerated. By and large, the Food and Drug Administration and other supervisory agencies do a good job in preventing possibly harmful or unsafe foods from reaching the market. Help children become informed consumers of food products and develop a good knowledge of nutritional principles. But nutrition should not become an obsession, as it is with many food faddists. Children should also be taught to recognize the difference between nutrition and food nostrums.

Food Myths

In spite of the level of education and communication in our country, nutritional myths and misconceptions are still commonplace. There are many false beliefs about food that people cling to without regard to research findings or physicians' advice. The sad thing about these fallacies is that many people become malnourished by believing these myths and by implementing them in their diets. Some of the more common myths according to the Center for Science in the Public Interest (1982, p. 4) are:

- Watermelon is rich in Vitamins A and C
- Corn syrup contains no nutritional values other than calories
- Salt is not used in excessive quantities in processed foods
- Megadoses of Vitamin C can cure the common cold
- Skipping meals helps to lose weight
- Middle-aged spread is inevitable

The most effective means of destroying these myths is through nutrition education. Develop lessons designed to enlighten your students about these food misconceptions.

Food Labeling

There is a tremendous amount of nutritional information available today, but many Americans are still misinformed and confused about the foods they buy and eat. The U.S. Food and Drug Administration has attempted to ameliorate this problem by establishing regulations for advertising and labeling of food products (Hamrick, Anspaugh, & Ezell, 1986). These regulations have resulted in improved labeling designed to give a listing of nutrients in the product, and to make the information on food labels more meaningful to consumers. Manufacturers must use nutritional labeling when they add any nutrient to packaged food or when they make some nutritional claim for their products. Labeling is also meant to stop unsupported generalizations and fraudulent statements. Nutritional labeling of food products is being sought for nearly all foods. This would be difficult for some foods, such as fresh fruits, but labeling of all food products would be beneficial to the consumer.

Nutrition Education

In emphasizing sound nutrition to your students, make sure that the learning opportunities you provide are interesting and personalized. Students should be taught to help themselves make responsible food choices. Of course, the home and school have to work together to make the nutrition education of the child a success.

The School Lunch Program

A well planned school lunch program provides excellent learning opportunities in nutrition. The federal school lunch program was established to provide nutritionally sound meals at low cost to students. These lunches can help students make good food choices while at school. This lunch consists of one-half pint of whole milk; two ounces of lean meat, poultry, fish, or cheese; a three-fourths cup serving of two or more vegetables or fruits or both; one slice of whole-grain or enriched bread or its equivalent; and one teaspoon of butter or fortified margarine. Some schools now offer alternative lunches of salads and/or sandwiches.

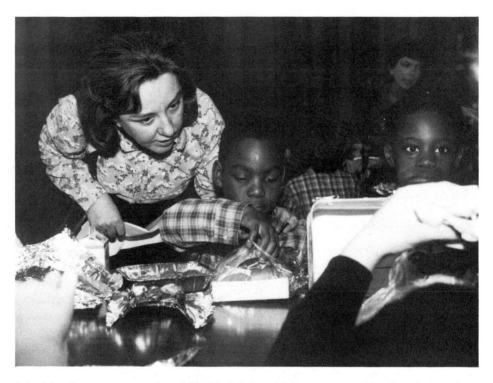

School lunch programs are often critical in helping children meet nutritional goals.

The educational impact of a lunch program can be important if used correctly. For students who bring their lunches from home, you should provide several examples of nutritious sack lunches. The cafeteria can be used as a place in which to help children learn table manners, sitting posture, and appropriate social behavior. The planning, preparation, and serving of meals by the cafeteria staff can also provide excellent learning opportunities for students.

SUMMARY

Although food is basic to human existence, food choices often have little to do with good nutrition. Socioeconomic factors, personal preferences and habits, cultural customs, and religious beliefs are all determining factors in the foods we select.

The eating habits of American children are often poor. This is due primarily to the habits of their parents, hurried lifestyles, lack of nutrition education, and improper attitudes about eating.

The food we eat can be measured by the caloric energy it provides. The major categories of energy nutrients in foods are carbohydrates, proteins, and fats. Other important nutrients are water, minerals, and vitamins.

Foods can be classified in four basic groups as an aid to selecting a balanced diet. The four are the milk group, the meat group, the fruit and vegetable group, and the bread and cereal group. Recommended dietary allowances have also been established in the United States to help promote and maintain health through proper nutrition.

The major health problems related to nutrition are undernutrition and overeating. These problems are caused by lack of nutrition education, poverty, improper dietary habits, and emotional problems.

All the nutrition information that is available to Americans can lead to confusion and misinformation. Some food quacks attempt to capitalize on this confusion by making misleading claims concerning their food products or weight-reducing programs. A contributing problem is that of food fallacies, which many people still adhere to. The Food and Drug Administration is attempting to eliminate some of this confusion and aid the consumer in making wise food choices through labeling regulations of all packaged food products.

Nutrition education is the key to solving many of the health problems associated with foods. Classroom teachers should promote sound nutrition by helping students make responsible food choices and by providing good role models.

DISCUSSION QUESTIONS

1. Why is nutrition education needed early in a child's life?
2. Discuss the relationship between some religious beliefs and nutrition.
3. Discuss the factors that determine personal food preferences.
4. Define basal metabolism.
5. List the food sources of complex carbohydrates.
6. Enumerate the vital functions that fats serve in our bodies.
7. Name the good food sources in the meat food group.
8. Differentiate between anorexia and bulimia.
9. Discuss the techniques that will help a person lose weight.
10. Discuss the importance of a well planned school lunch program.

REFERENCES

Beal, V. "Nutrition and growth patterns of young children." *Contemporary Nutrition, 7,* 10, October, 1982.

The Center for Science in the Public Interest, *Nutrition Action.* Washington, D.C.: 1982.

DeWolfe, J. & Jack, E. "Weight control in adolescent girls," *Journal of School Health, 54,* 9, October, 1984.

Hamrick, M., Anspaugh, D., & Ezell, G. *Health.* Columbus: Merrill, 1986.

Jarvis, W. "Vitamin use and abuse," *Contemporary Nutrition, 9,* 10, October, 1984.

Jones, K., Shainberg, L., & Byer, C. Dimensions VI. New York: Harper & Row, Publishers, 1986.

Katch, F., & McArdle, W. *Nutrition, weight control, and exercise,* second edition. Philadelphia: Lea & Febiger, 1983.

Kolbe, L., & Gilbert, G. "Involving the schools in the national strategy to improve the health of Americans." *Prospects for a healthier America.* Washington, D.C.: U.S. Department of Health and Human Services, 1984.

Mailman, R., & Lewis, M. "Food additives and childhood hyperactivity." *Contemporary Nutrition, 8,* 6, June, 1983.

Mallick, M. "Anorexia nervosa and bulimia." *Journal of School Health. 54,* 8, September, 1984.

Morgan, K. "The role of snacking in the american diet." *Contemporary Nutrition, 7,* 9, September, 1982.

Perry, C., Mullis, R., & Maile, M. "Modifying the eating behavior of young children." *Journal of School Health, 55,* 10, December, 1985.

Rapoport, J., & Kruesi, M. "Behavior and nutrition." *Contemporary Nutrition, 8,* 10, October, 1983.

Whitney, E., Hamilton, E., & Boyle, M. *Understanding nutrition, third edition.* St. Paul, Minn.: West Publishing, 1984.

Williams, R. *Nutrition against disease.* New York: Bantam Books, 1973.

14. Techniques for Teaching Nutrition

The ultimate reality of nutrition rests with the chemistry of the food we eat and its effects on the processes of life.—R. M. Deutsch, *Realities of Nutrition*

A FLEXIBLE APPROACH TO NUTRITION

The concept of nutrition is quite abstract to younger elementary school children, often seen as somehow connected with but divorced from eating. Your job in teaching nutrition is to make that concept more concrete and real to your students by presenting learning opportunities that relate nutritional information to daily life. In other words, you must personalize the information so that students will internalize it and recognize its relevance to health.

Avoid a rigid, by-the-rules approach, and do not reduce nutrition education to a set of rules. Not only will this approach make nutrition seem grim, it will also cause children to reject sound principles as unrealistic. Help students to understand the motivations for choosing and eating certain foods, and that some of these motivations have little to do with the amount of nutrients to be attained from a certain food. For example, a person might be choosing a certain mid-afternoon snack because that snack was the one always offered by his parents, but that snack might not be as nutritious as another readily available snack.

Children—and adults—will change their habits only when they personally recognize the importance of doing so. Do not expect changes overnight. Encourage introspection and foster positive decision-making skills. Act as a role model for changes you wish to bring about. Respect differences in tastes, likes, and dislikes. Slowly, you will begin to see that your message is getting through.

Concepts to be Taught

- There are many reasons why people eat the food they eat.
- A good breakfast is important for growing and learning.

- Food is an important part of our lives.

- Food provides the body with energy and nutrients for growth and body maintenance.

- Food nutrients can be classified as carbohydrates, fats, proteins, water, minerals, and vitamins.

- Nutrients perform a wide variety of specific functions in the body.

- Eating a variety of carefully selected foods is the best way to ensure that the body receives the proper amounts of the nutrients it needs.

- The four basic food groups can serve as an aid in planning balanced, nutritious meals.

- Lack of certain nutrients can lead to certain diseases.

- Being underweight or overweight can lead to physical and emotional problems.

- Maintaining a proper weight is an individual responsibility, but others can help if there is a weight problem.

- Even if an individual does not have a weight problem, the person can be malnourished.

- Simple foods can be nutritious and provide a well balanced diet, if properly selected.

- Trying new and different foods can be fun.

- Junk foods, such as candy and soft drinks, can cause health problems if consumed too regularly.

- Many people in the world do not have enough to eat.

- Many people wrongly believe in food myths and food nostrums.

- Food labels can provide useful nutritional information.

- Money spent for food should be spent wisely.

Cycle Plan for Teaching Topics

Topic	Grade Level						
	K	**1**	**2**	**3**	**4**	**5**	**6**
Food Habits and Customs	**	***	**	**	**	*	*
Nutrients	**	**	**	**	**	*	*
Nutritional Needs	**	**	**	***	**	*	**
The Four Food Groups	*	**	**	**	***		
Snacks and Junk Foods	**	**	**	***	***	***	**
Overweight and Underweight	*	**	**	**	*	*	**
Meal and Diet Planning	*	*	*	**	**	***	***
Food Myths and Quackery	*	*	**	**	**	**	***
Food Sanitation	*	*	*	**	**	**	**
Consumer Product Knowledge	*	**	**	**	***	***	***
World Food Problems	*	**	*	**	**	**	***

Key: *** = major emphasis, ** = emphasis, * = review.

VALUE-BASED ACTIVITIES

Nutrition Sentence Completion

Have students complete the following statements with phrases that come to mind immediately upon hearing the key phrase beginning the statement:

The most important meal of the day for me is _____ .
Eating a good breakfast is _____ .
My favorite foods are _____ .
Eating right means _____ .
I think that my present diet is _____ .
Between-meal snacks should be _____ .
One problem about nutrition for me is _____ .

Rank Ordering Favorite Foods

Have each student prepare a list of three or four favorite foods or dishes from each of the four food groups. Then tell the students to rank order each food or dish, with most favorite being labeled "1." Now, have the students compare their lists. What class preferences seem to emerge? What are some individual preferences? Follow with a discussion of personal likes and dislikes.

Would You Like It?

Ask the students to bring in photographs from magazines of different food dishes or recipes. These should be dishes that the students are unfamiliar with or have not tried themselves. Discuss each dish. What do the students think it might taste like? Would they like to try it? If possible, bring in small portions of some foods that are unfamiliar to students and have them taste each one. Stimulate curiosity.

Values Continuum

Pass out continuum sheets. One end of the continuum represents a lifestyle where every meal is eaten at home under relaxed conditions. The other end of the continuum represents a lifestyle where every meal is eaten outside the home under hurried or hectic conditions. Have each student place an X on the continuum representing his or her assessment of eating lifestyle. Follow with a general discussion of how eating lifestyle may affect growth and development as well as emotional state.

Decision Stories

Follow the procedure outlined in Chapter 5 for presenting nutrition decision stories such as these:

Snacktime

John came home from school hungry. His mother told him that dinner would be late, so he could have a snack. She told him to go to the kitchen and get a piece of fruit to eat.

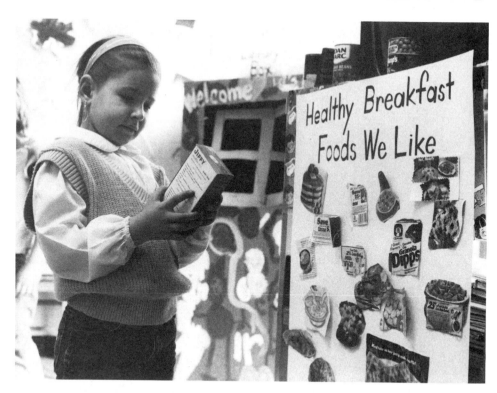

Bulletin boards may be used to teach values.

But John remembered a candy bar that he had in his lunch box and thought of having that instead, even though he knew that the fruit would be better for him.

Focus Question: What should John do?

Just a Few

Andrea was taken to the doctor for a routine checkup. The doctor said that Andrea was overweight. He advised that she not eat between meals and not eat junk food, such as candy bars and potato chips. A few days later, Andrea is visiting her friend Mary. Two other of her friends are also there. Mary opens up a large bag of chips and passes them around. Andrea is sensitive about her weight problem, but she doesn't want her friends to know that she must watch her diet. Mary offers the chips to Andrea.

Focus Question: What should Andrea do?

Fast Food

Tim doesn't like the food they serve in the school cafeteria. Some of his friends go to a fast-food restaurant near the school instead. He would like to go with them, but he knows that his parents want him to eat in the cafeteria.

Focus Question: What should Tim do?

The Big Test

Tomorrow you have a big test at school. You want to get enough sleep and you need to study for the test. You also plan to get a good breakfast. It is 9 PM and you are tired. Should you study another hour right now or should you skip breakfast to study?

Focus Questions: What are some good reasons for staying up another hour? What are some reasons for studying in the morning? Which choice will help you think more clearly on your test? Give reasons for your choice.

From Linda Brower Meeks and Philip Heit. *Health: Focus on You.* Columbus, Ohio: Charles E. Merrill Publishing Company, 1982.

DRAMATIZATION

Food Puppets

After discussing the four basic food groups and the nutrients they provide, have the class make puppets representing the various food groups or foods within each group. Prepare a skit that explains how the foods work together to provide a balanced diet containing all essential nutrients, including water.

Marco Polo

To tie in with a discussion of food customs of different lands, have the students write a short play about the adventures of Marco Polo in China. The play should emphasize the many kinds of new dishes that Marco Polo was exposed to in his travels. Supposedly, for example, Marco Polo brought back the recipe for noodles (pasta) when he returned to Italy.

Stranger in a Strange Land

Divide the class into small groups. Have each research the foods and dishes eaten in a different nation, such as Mexico, India, Malaysia, Germany, Japan, and Greece. Then have the students in each group prepare models or drawings of different typical dishes served in their assigned nation. You act the part of a traveler, just arrived in the country and very hungry. Ask about each dish the children have to offer. What is it made of? How does it taste? How does one actually eat it? Follow with a general discussion of different ethnic foods.

Junk Food on Trial

Have the students stimulate a courtroom trial. The defendant, played by a volunteer student, is Junk Food. Other students act the parts of judge, prosecuting attorney, defense lawyers, witnesses, and jury. Junk Food is accused of misleading people into thinking that they are getting proper nutrition by eating candy, chips, and so on. The defendant claims only to be giving people what they want. Have evidence presented by both sides in the case. Then have the jury agree on a verdict.

Dramatization/Role Play

1. Have students role play about good health practices when they are on a picnic and cannot wash their hands.
2. Have students role play good health practices when they are preparing for lunch after playing outside.
3. Plan a skit showing different ways people can eat, such as with chopsticks or sitting on the floor. Discuss the reasons why people eat differently in other cultures. Ask why it is important to learn about and respect different ways of eating.

From *Health: A Guide for Grade K through 12, Level One.* Nashville, Tennessee: Tennessee Department of Education, 1983.

DISCUSSION AND REPORT TECHNIQUES

Presentation by Health Professionals

Invite a nutritionist or institutional menu planner to class to discuss the elements of a balanced diet. Have the person explain not only the nutritional requirements that must be met, but also how foods are prepared to provide visual and taste appeal. The person in charge of planning your school cafeteria meals could also be invited to speak to the class and answer questions.

Pie in the Sky

If possible, invite a representative from a commercial airline to discuss how nutritious meals are prepared for a jumbo jetful of passengers. Also have the person discuss special meals that can be prepared for passengers with dietary restrictions.

World Hunger

Present a lecture on the problems of hunger in the world today. Focus on the problems of poor, third-world nations but also note that there is hunger in our own nation. Discuss what is being done to alleviate the situation in various places. Mention the work of such agencies as Oxfam and Care.

Candy Machines in the Schools Debate

Should candy machines be placed in the school cafeteria? Have two debate teams argue the issue. Act as moderator and keep the debate on track. Then follow with a general class discussion.

Food Label Report

Have students research the regulations concerning labeling of packaged foods and present their reports either orally or in writing. Individualize the activity by having each student prepare a report on a specific food product. Then have the student discuss his or her findings in class, explaining what information is contained on the label of the package. Later, put all the packages on display so that students may examine them.

Activity Masters

Have students complete the activity masters on pp. 282–84: What Makes You Go?; I'm Full of High Protein Foods; and I'm Full of Energy Foods.*

Deficiency Diseases

Divide the class into small groups and have each group research a deficiency disease such as scurvy, rickets, beriberi, and kwashiorkor. Have the students find answers to the following questions: What is the cause of the condition? What are its consequences? Can the condition be cured? If so, how? Is the condition prevalent in this country? Why or why not? In what parts of the world is the condition a problem? What can be done to lessen the problem? Have the students present the results of their research in a panel setting. Each student should be prepared to answer questions from the rest of the class.

Case History

A case history is a short description of an event that can be used to illustrate a health concept such as nutritional lifestyle. Develop a case history about a person who has poor eating habits, e.g., skips breakfast, salts food heavily, eats several meals a week from fast-food restaurants. Ask students to read the case history and to identify the poor eating habits.

From Linda Brower Meeks and Philip Heit. *Health: Focus on You.* Columbus, Ohio: Charles E. Merrill Publishing Company, 1982.

EXPERIMENTS AND DEMONSTRATIONS

Animals in the Classroom

Obtain some white rats or guinea pigs and keep them in separate cages. Feed one group of animals a healthy, balanced diet. Provide an insufficient diet for the others. Observe the differences in behavior and appearance for a while. Then restore a proper diet to the experimental animals and note any changes for the better. Be careful not to cause undue suffering to any of the animals and discontinue the experiment if you have any doubts.

---

*All from Joanne Sockut and Lowell F. Bernard, *Nutrition Action Pack.* Cleveland, Ohio: Cleveland Health Museum (in cooperation with the McDonald's Corporation), 1985.

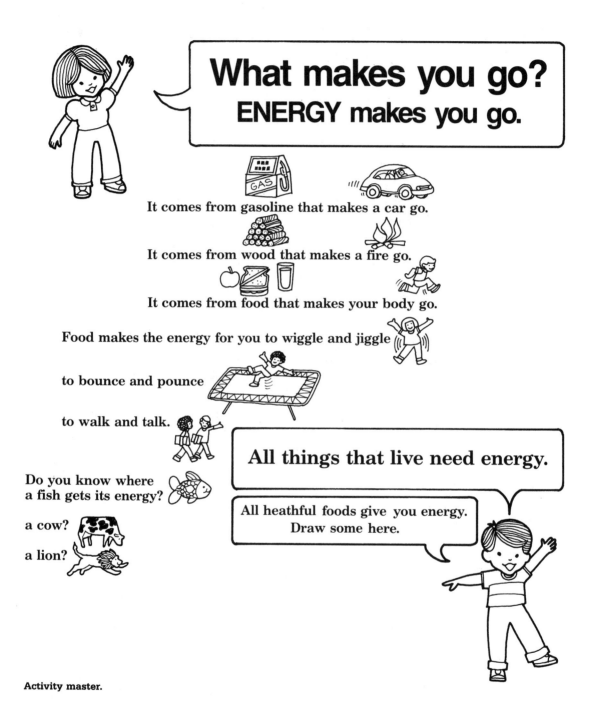

What makes you go?
ENERGY makes you go.

It comes from gasoline that makes a car go.

It comes from wood that makes a fire go.

It comes from food that makes your body go.

Food makes the energy for you to wiggle and jiggle

to bounce and pounce

to walk and talk.

All things that live need energy.

All heathful foods give you energy.
Draw some here.

Do you know where
a fish gets its energy?

a cow?

a lion?

Activity master.

*All from Joanne Sockut and Lowell F. Bernard, *Nutrition Action Pack.* Cleveland, Ohio: Cleveland Health Museum (in cooperation with the McDonald's Corporation), 1985.

I'm full of high protein foods.

1 Do you see foods from the fruit and vegetable group?

_____

2 Do you see foods from the bread and cereal group?

_____

3 Do you see foods from the meat and protein group?

Name them. _____

_____

4 Do you see foods from the dairy group?

Name them. _____

5 Circle the food groups that are high in protein.

DAIRY GROUP   FRUIT AND VEGETABLE GROUP

BREAD AND CEREAL GROUP   MEAT AND PROTEIN GROUP

Activity master.

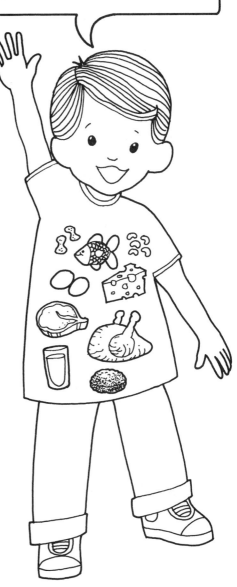

*All from Joanne Sockut and Lowell F. Bernard, *Nutrition Action Pack*. Cleveland, Ohio: Cleveland Health Museum (in cooperation with the McDonald's Corporation), 1985.

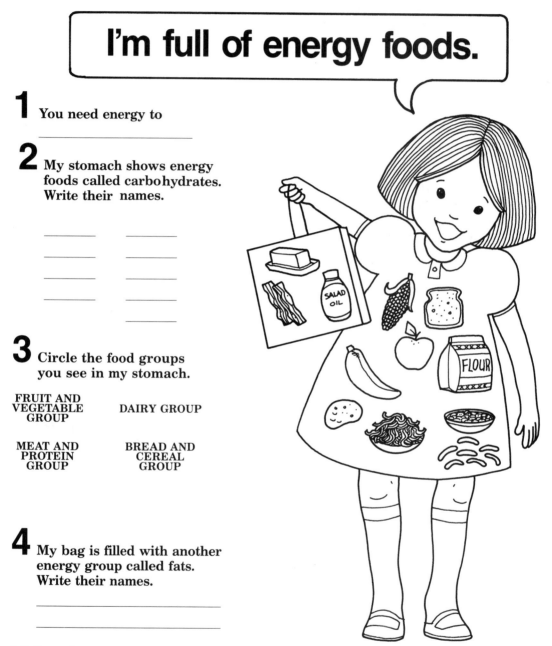

I'm full of energy foods.

1 You need energy to
_____

2 My stomach shows energy
foods called carbohydrates.
Write their names.

_____ _____

_____ _____

_____ _____

_____

3 Circle the food groups
you see in my stomach.

**FRUIT AND
VEGETABLE
GROUP**

DAIRY GROUP

**MEAT AND
PROTEIN
GROUP**

**BREAD AND
CEREAL
GROUP**

4 My bag is filled with another
energy group called fats.
Write their names.

_____

_____

Activity master.

_____

*All from Joanne Sockut and Lowell F. Bernard, *Nutrition Action Pack*. Cleveland, Ohio: Cleveland Health
Museum (in cooperation with the McDonald's Corporation), 1985.

Make Sure It's Fresh

Discuss the importance of keeping some foods refrigerated, not eating foods that have gone bad, and so on. Note the risk of food poisoning that can occur as a result of eating contaminated foods. To demonstrate how microbes and mold can grow on food that is left out, place a piece of bread and a piece of cheese in a dish. Expose the food for an hour, then cover the dish and put it in a warm, dark place. Examine the food with the class each day for the next few days. Note the mold that soon grows. If you have a microscope or strong hand lens, have students examine the growing mold.

Tasting Party

Set up four tables, each containing dishes from the four basic food groups. Label each collection of dishes. Then have the students sample some of the foods from each group. For the milk group, you might supply small cubes of a few different kinds of cheeses—some mild, some stronger, some hard, and some soft. For the meat group, include bits of salami or other sandwich meat. Slices of fresh fruit and vegetables that can be eaten raw should be included in the fruit and vegetable group. Crackers, breakfast cereals, and bread can represent the bread and cereal group. Try to include some foods that children might not be familiar with.

Experiments

1. Testing for Carbohydrates Test a food for carbohydrates by putting a drop of iodine on the food. If carbohydrate is present the food will change color to deep blue-black.

2. Testing for Fat Test a food for fat by rubbing the food on a paper towel. After allowing time for drying, fat is present if the spot remains.

3. Water in Fresh Foods Compare dried and dehydrated foods to fresh foods to show the amount of water in them. For example, place a beet on a plate and leave overnight. Compare the dehydrated beet with a fresh one brought in the next day.

All from *Health: A Guide for Grade K through 12, Level Two*. Nashville, Tennessee: Tennessee Department of Education, 1983.

Comparison Shopping in Class

Provide the students with copies of supermarket ads from a local paper. Using only the items advertised, have them prepare a list of foods they would buy for a complete day's meals. Then have the students add up the total they estimate they would have spent on the items.

Plants Need Nutrition, Too

Grow two seedling plants under controlled conditions. Provide one plant with good soil and give it the proper amount of water and light. Place the other plant in sandy soil and limit the amount of water and light it gets. Compare the two plants after a few weeks. Relate the results to human nutritional needs.

Table Manners

Prepare your students for this activity by noting that the atmosphere in which people eat has an effect on nutrition. Point out that eating is not enjoyable if the atmosphere is unpleasant. Then lead into a discussion of proper table manners. Set up a table, chairs, and place settings for a few students and have them demonstrate good table manners.

Cooking in the Classroom

Prepare a simple dish that does not require heating and serve samples to your students. Have the students help you in preparing the dish, but supervise them closely and do all cutting and other potentially hazardous tasks yourself. One dish that you might prepare is a Middle Eastern salad called tabouli. The recipe is as follows:

1 cup cracked wheat (bulgur)
3 cups chopped Italian parsley
2 tablespoons chopped fresh mint leaves
5 green onions, bulbs, and green tops chopped together
3 tomatoes
juice of 2 lemons, or to taste
½ cup olive oil
salt
sliced mushrooms (if desired)

Soak the bulgur in warm water to cover for 1 hour. Drain and squeeze out as much water as possible. Combine with parsley, mint, green onions, tomatoes, lemon juice, olive oil, salt, mushrooms. Chill and serve cold.

PUZZLES AND GAMES

Have students complete the following activities (from *Our Vegetable Parade—A Teacher's Guide* by the Potato Board):

Scrambled Vegetables

Unscramble these vegetables
cetutel   hspcian
eakrothic   rdshia
toopat   ebrmccuu

Vegetable Riddle

Provide students with the following riddles:

1. What is good but makes you cry? (onion)
2. What has eyes but cannot see? (potato)
3. What has a bulb but isn't used in a lamp? (garlic, onion, or shallot)
4. What has an ear but cannot hear? (corn)

Find as many vegetables as you can.
You may go horizontal, vertical, or
diagonal. There are eighteen in all!

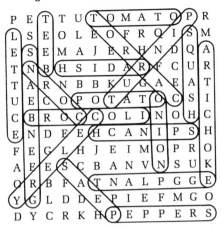

Figure 14.1
Puzzle sheet.

Mixed Vegetables

Pass out prepared sheets as shown in figure 14.1.

Food Group Tic-Tac-Toe

Prepare visually appealing game sheets such as the one shown in figure 14.2 and pass them out to the class. Develop game sheets for each of the four basic food groups. Note that there should be only one way to "win" the game.

Play tic-tac-toe.
Mark an X on the foods in the **Bread-Cereal Group.**

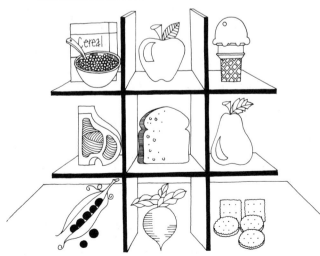

Figure 14.2
Tic-Tac-Toe sheet.

Source: *Fun with Good Food*, U.S. Department of Agriculture, Food and Nutrition Service Program Aid, Washington, D.C., 1981.

Puzzling Over Good Nutrition

The words in this puzzle run across, up and down, and diagonally. Circle each word neatly as you find it in the puzzle from the list of words below:

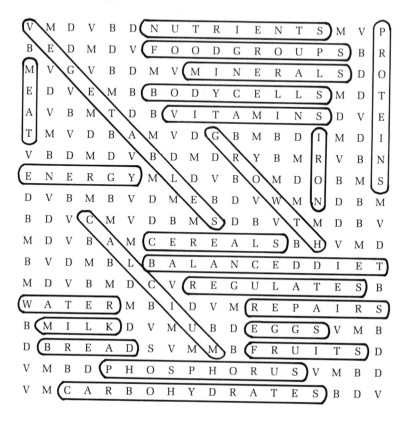

Balanced Diet	Vitamins	Fruits
Vegetables	Cereals	Repairs
Nutrients	Phosphorus	Milk
Regulates	Food Groups	Eggs
Carbohydrates	Body Cells	Iron
Breads	Proteins	Growth
Water	Minerals	Energy
Calcium		Meat

Figure 14.3
Nutrition puzzle.

Food Alphabet Game

Divide the students into teams and assign each team a number of letters of the alphabet. For example, one team can be assigned letters A through E, the next team letters F through J, and so on. Challenge each team to write down at least one food for each letter assigned to their team.

Matching Game

Prepare visually appealing game sheets such as the one shown in figure 14.4 and have the class complete the activity. Also allow students to make their own game sheets and try them on one another.

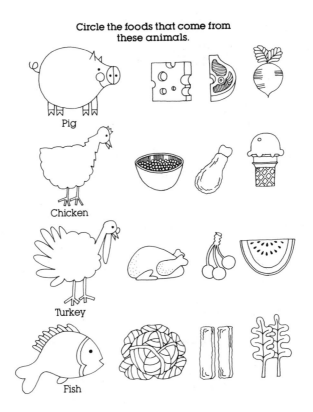

Circle the foods that come from these animals.

Pig

Chicken

Turkey

Fish

Figure 14.4
Matching game sheet.

Source: *Fun with good food*, U.S. Department of Agriculture, Food and Nutrition Service Program Aid, Washington, D.C., 1981.

Got It

Object:

The object of the game is to get five cards each representing a different culture of food.

Equipment Needed:

1. 1 package index cards 3 × 5 inches.
2. Pictures of foods from countries studied. These pictures can either be cut out of magazines, from food boxes, or drawn. Foods from Mexico, France, China, Germany, Italy, and Hawaii are especially interesting to study.

Instructions:

To make cards, paste or draw pictures of food in the center of the card. Write name of food at the top of the card. The player must recognize the country when he sees name of food. Suggested number of cards is 30 for 2 to 4 players, more for larger groups.

How to Play:

1. Shuffle the deck well.
2. Deal five cards to each player face down.
3. The player on the dealer's left draws one card from the deck. He may either keep the card, or discard it right side up next to the pile. If he keeps the card, he must discard another (at all times the player must have five cards in his hand).
4. The opponent (s) may either take the card that is right side up or draw from the pile. He discards.
5. The game continues until a player has five different cultures of food represented by his cards.
6. The player lays down his hand for his opponent (s) to see and check. If correct, he is then declared the winner.

Variation:

Players can decide to play for one culture of food. In which case 6 cards should be made for each of 5 cultures. When a player sees the first five cards he is dealt, he can decide which country he has more food representing. This will determine which country he plays for and he will try to get a "set" of cards for that country. The first player to get a set is the winner.

Food for Thought*

Teaching Objectives: To teach the students practical knowledge of various foods important for a well balanced diet, and to increase their appreciation of these foods by discussing and discovering unique aspects of the food item.

Number of Players: The class is divided into two teams, each with a team captain.

Game Materials: Pencils and paper, basic cookbook or food text, and an encyclopedia, if available.

How to Play: Each team chooses two basic food items. The teacher should check the choices to make sure there are no duplicates, and that the choices are basic and familiar to all. Each team confers privately and establishes eight clues for each item. The students can use the following clues as guidelines.

1. Food group to which the food item belongs
2. Caloric content of an average serving of the food
3. Major vitamin or mineral content
4. Historical origin of food
5. Classic recipe which uses food
6. Major geographical location where food is cultivated or processed

*by Cece Krumrine

7. Color of food
8. Texture or consistency of food
9. Market price of food

Some examples of foods and their clues are listed below:

CORN

1. This food is considered America's great contribution to the cereal group, although the food is a vegetable.
2. Starch, syrup, oil, and flour can all be processed from this food.
3. The food is available fresh, frozen, and canned.
4. The food was so important to the American Indians that they often referred to it in their mythology and religious practices.

EGG

1. The food is used in cooking to thicken, leaven or bind, or to color or garnish.
2. The food is a breakfast staple.
3. The food is a good source of protein, Vitamin A, and iron.
4. One serving of the food contains about 80 calories.

APPLE

1. Newton is said to have discovered gravity with the use of this food.
2. The food is a good supplement to the diet since it is high in carbohydrate, cellulose, Vitamins A and C.
3. One serving contains 75 calories.
4. The food is in peak season in late summer, early fall.

PEANUTS

1. A polyunsaturated oil is processed from this food.
2. The food is high in fat and contributes a substantial amount of protein.
3. The food must be shelled before it is eaten.
4. A spread processed from the food is a favorite with children.

After the team develops their clues, the competition begins. Team #1 presents the first clue of the first food item to team #2. The captain of team #2 confers briefly with the team and submits a guess as to the food item's identity. If the guess is incorrect, team #1 is awarded 10 points. When the identity of the food is guessed by team #2 and/or all the clues are given, whichever comes first, team #1 will proceed to the second food.

If all the clues are given and the food item is not correctly guessed, the captain should then reveal the answer. When both food items are guessed and/or all food clues are given, the game ends. The score for team #1 is then tabulated. At this point, team #2 presents their first food clue and the game is repeated until both food items are guessed and/or all the clues are given. The team which scores the highest number of points wins. The maximum number of points each team can score is 160.

Food Squares*

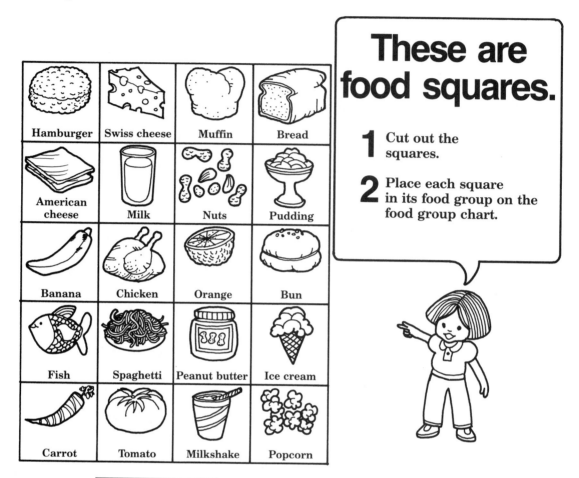

These are food squares.

1 Cut out the squares.

2 Place each square in its food group on the food group chart.

---

*From Joanne Sockut and Lowell F. Bernard, *Nutrition Action Pack.* Cleveland, Ohio: Cleveland Health Museum (in cooperation with the McDonald's Corporation), 1985.

I'm Hungry*

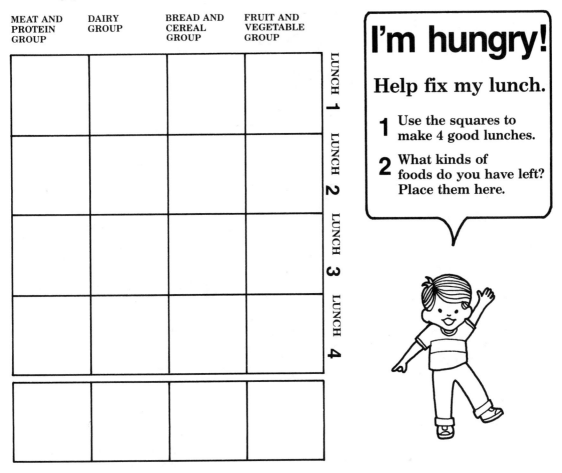

MEAT AND PROTEIN GROUP	DAIRY GROUP	BREAD AND CEREAL GROUP	FRUIT AND VEGETABLE GROUP	
				LUNCH **1**
				LUNCH **2**
				LUNCH **3**
				LUNCH **4**

I'm hungry!

Help fix my lunch.

1 Use the squares to make 4 good lunches.

2 What kinds of foods do you have left? Place them here.

*From Joanne Sockut and Lowell F. Bernard, *Nutrition Action Pack*. Cleveland, Ohio: Cleveland Health Museum (in cooperation with the McDonald's Corporation), 1985.

Vitamin Quiz*

Make a vitamin quiz card

Use this page and the next one to make a vitamin quiz card. When you finish you will have something to take home to show to your parents and friends.

This is what to do:

1 Cut out the questions and answers on this page. Can you tell the answer to each question?

2 Cut out the quiz card from the next page. Fold it and paste the two halves together.

3 Paste the questions and answers in the right spaces on each side of the quiz card.

4 The person you quiz will see only the questions. You will be able to turn the card over to show the answers.

5 Color the foods you see. They are some of the foods that give you vitamins.

Eat foods from the four food groups every day.

To live, to grow, and to stay well in every way.

How can you get your vitamins?

A, B, C, D, E and K.

Why does everybody need vitamins?

Can you name some vitamins?

---

*From Joanne Sockut and Lowell F. Bernard, *Nutrition Action Pack*. Cleveland, Ohio: Cleveland Health Museum (in cooperation with the McDonald's Corporation), 1985.

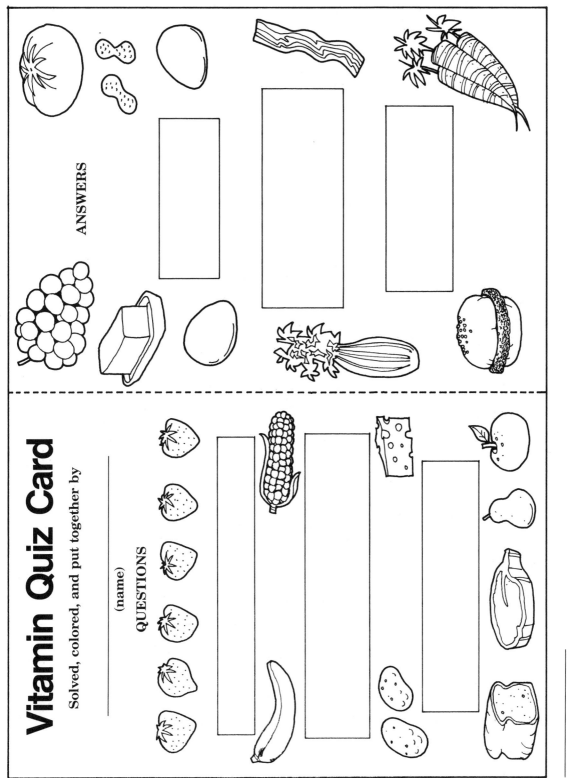

Vitamin Quiz Card

Solved, colored, and put together by

_____
(name)

QUESTIONS

ANSWERS

*From Joanne Sockut and Lowell F. Bernard, _Nutrition Action Pack_. Cleveland, Ohio: Cleveland Health Museum (in cooperation with the McDonald's Corporation), 1985.

Name that Nutrient

Place large pictures of specific foods on the chalkboard. Include such foods as cheese, beef, spinach, spaghetti, fish, oranges, and peanut butter. Write the names of various nutrients on small pieces of paper and place them in a box. Divide the class into teams. Have the first player on each team draw a slip from the box. The challenge is to match the nutrient with the correct source pictured on the board. Score two points if it is a good match, one point if it is a fair match, and no points for an incorrect match. As most foods contain many nutrients, supply duplicate slips.

BULLETIN BOARDS

Food in Other Countries

Each month, emphasize the foods of a different nation or culture in a colorful bulletin board display. If possible, combine the activity by serving food representative of the featured culture.

Climbing the Ladder to Good Nutrition

Construct the outline of a tree from burlap, as shown in Figure 14.5. Make a ladder from cardboard and twine. Place felt apples on the branches of the tree. On the back of each apple, write a nutrition question. Students "pick" one apple apiece and try to answer the question. A correct answer means one rung of the ladder to good nutrition has been climbed. Let students record their progress by writing their names on

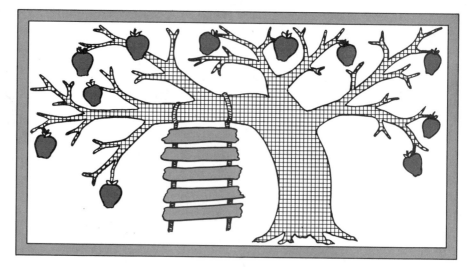

Figure 14.5
The ladder to good nutrition.

the rungs as they progress upward. Place new questions on the apples from week to week until everyone has had a chance to reach the top rung.

The Wisdom Tree

Using the same tree from the last bulletin board suggestion, prepare a fact or fallacy quiz that students can try in their free time. On the front of each of the apples, write a statement about food, either a fact or a fallacy. To check the correct answer, students turn the apples around, where either the word "fact" or the word "fallacy" appears. Statements you can use might include the following:

> Water is a vitamin. (fallacy)
> Liver is a good source of vitamin K. (fact)
> Carbohydrates give the body quick energy. (fact)
> Brown eggs are more nutritious than white ones. (fallacy)
> Most children need to take extra vitamins. (fallacy)
> Lettuce is a good source of calcium. (fact)

Nutrition Tips

Construct bulletin boards giving tips for good nutrition. Two examples are illustrated in figure 14.6.

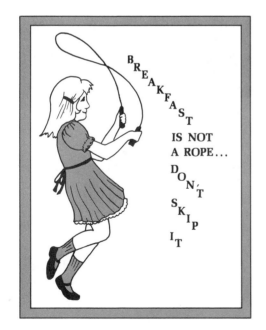 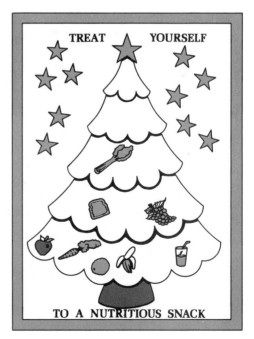

Figure 14.6
Nutrition tips bulletin board examples.

Food Groups Collage

Have the students assist you in constructing a collage of the four food groups. Write the name of each group in large letters. Then have students cut out colored pictures from old magazines showing representative foods from each group.

Good Nutrition for Good Health

Each week, assign a small group of students to illustrate a nutrition rule, such as, "Eat a good breakfast every day." Place the completed group drawing in a prominent place.

OTHER IDEAS

Field Trips

Arrange to take the class on a field trip to a dairy, bakery, food processing plant, or other nutrition-related operation. Be sure to prepare your class thoroughly for the trip before they go. Discuss the nature of the operation that they will see. Explain the processes they will observe, and have the students prepare a list of questions they will want to ask.

Snack Food Charts

Have students keep a personal record of every between-meal snack that they eat for a week. To encourage honest reporting, emphasize that the lists will not be turned in. At the end of the week's work, ask each student to assess the kinds of snacks eaten. Were the snacks mostly junk food, consisting of empty calories (sugar without other nutrients)? Do students feel that there is room for improvement in the snacks they eat? What changes do they suggest?

Self-Portrait

Have students draw pictures of what they think they would look like if they ate nothing but candy and soda pop for a month. Keep the activity light-hearted, but make the point that good nutrition is necessary for good health.

Owl Mobile

Have the students help you construct an owl mobile as shown in figure 14.7. Each leaf hanging from the branch should be brightly lettered with the name of one of the four food groups.

School Cafeteria as an Activity Center

The school cafeteria can serve as an excellent activity center for students to learn about nutrition, food planning, sanitation, food preparation, and food economics.

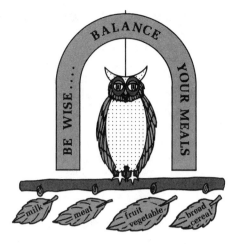

Figure 14.7
Owl mobile illustrating the four food groups.

Here are just a few of the learning opportunities that you can provide in this setting:

Have students observe the kitchen workers to note sanitation procedures followed.
Ask the person in charge to provide a tour of the facilities, pointing out the dozens of things that must be done each day to provide students with nutritious meals.
Have your students weigh the food that is wasted by fellow students at one lunch period and ask them to estimate the amount of money that was also wasted.
Note the sanitation procedures followed by cafeteria workers.

Poster Contest

Each week assign a theme for individual posters, using such topics as the four food groups, table manners, essential nutrients, and so on. Post the completed art in the classroom or in the school cafeteria.

Making It Strange

Point out to your class that food habits can restrict our diets. We think of certain foods as being linked only to certain meals. Toast and jelly, for example, is a breakfast food. But there is nothing nutritionally unsound about having very different foods instead of traditional ones. Why not a bowl of soup for breakfast, for instance? Have the students come up with examples of very nontraditional—but nutritious—ideas for meals.

More Ideas

1. Visit the local drugstore and make a list of the over-the-counter reducing aids available.
2. Visit a library or bookstore and note the number and titles of books on dieting.

3. Compile magazine and newspaper advertisements on diets, diet aids, and slimming devices. Evaluate the reliability of these advertisements analyzing the use of objective facts.

4. Write to adolescent summer weight camps and adult "fat farms" for brochures. Figuring length of stay and desired weight to be lost, determine how much each pound of weight loss would cost.

5. Make a survey of family and friends to determine if they ever dieted; types of diets; aids, products and/or facilities used; success rate, and cost.

From Marilyn Mudgett and Dorothy Culjat, "Sensible Dieting," in *Health Education Teaching Ideas: Elementary.* Editors: Osness, Donna, and Thompson, Karen. Reston, Virginia: American Alliance for Health, Physical Education, Recreation and Dance, 1983.

15. Safety and First Aid

"As long as accidents continue to increase, there will be a need for. . . safety education. If students will acknowledge the importance of safety and practice it, we will have made an important step forward in the quality of their lives."—Warren E. Schaller, Ball State University

CHILDREN AND ACCIDENTS

It is a sad fact that accidents are the leading cause of death among elementary school children (Payne and Hahn, 1986). The reasons for this are not hard to discover. Children are extremely active. They are constantly exploring and testing their environment. They are often ignorant or unmindful of the risks they take. And, finally, they have simply not yet learned to be as cautious as they should be.

Fortunately, most accidents that happen to children are not serious or fatal. Unfortunately, enough are to make safety an extremely important part of elementary health instruction. As a teacher, your involvement in safety education is imperative because fully half of all accidents involving children occur at school (Willgoose, 1979). Your efforts, combined with those of the school administration, *can* make a difference. Indeed, for the most part, the schools have been doing a good job, as evidenced by statistics that show that, over the past 50 years, the accidental death rate for children in the 5-to-14 age range has dropped more than that of any other age group (Cornacchia & Staton, 1979).

The number of accidents that occur among children is still unnecessarily high, however. Although accidents will always occur given the characteristics of children, accidents don't just "happen." In most instances, they are caused by human error or carelessness, and these factors can be positively influenced by safety education. Children do not have to learn safe behavior through trial and error; they do not have to have continued accidents to recognize the importance of safety. They can be taught the elements of safety in a positive way that will result in fewer accidents of all types, both at school and away from school. As a teacher of health education, this should be one of your major goals.

This chapter presents an overview of the elements of safety education. Topics include risk taking and safety procedures, positive characteristics of safety, accident prevention, types of accidents, and the school safety program. Emergency first aid procedures will also be discussed. Partly because of liability considerations, you should not attempt to provide medical help to students unless you have no choice. However, if a life-threatening situation arises, you must know what to do.

SAFETY AND RISK TAKING

We do not live in a "safety-first" world, despite slogans that proclaim the contrary. There is some physical risk in almost everything we do, from going to school or work in the morning, to cooking or eating a meal, to engaging in daily tasks and recreational activities. If safety were paramount, logically many of these efforts would have to be curtailed: one could be hit by a truck while crossing the street, choke on a piece of food, or suffer a fatal injury while at work or at play. What is an "acceptable" degree of risk depends upon the individual and the activity. Some adults, for instance, make their living by engaging in highly risky activities—race drivers, deep sea divers, law enforcement officers, and so forth. Such individuals are often held in high esteem by the rest of the population, demonstrating that risk taking is viewed positively in our society.

Children pick up these cues early in life. They develop an unrealistic view of risk taking that may tempt them to enter into situations that are potentially very hazardous. This, combined with their natural inquisitiveness and energy, can greatly increase the chance of serious accidents. Part of your job in teaching safety education is to make children aware that unnecessary risk taking is not socially endorsed behavior. This cannot be accomplished, however, by simply providing your students with a list of safety "don'ts." Children, especially younger children, should be emphatically warned of dangers in the environment. However, the "don't" approach to safety education is a negative one, and one that is not likely to influence behavior.

A Positive Approach to Safety

If you are to influence children's behavior toward safer personal practices, you must take a positive approach. Emphasize that safety is largely a matter of individual volition and responsibility. While an acceptance of risk is a part of living, embracing risk without recognizing and accepting the possible consequences is not wise. In considering role models, point out that even adults who make their living in the most hazardous of ways do all they can to minimize the risk involved.

As in all areas of health education, stress the importance of personal decision-making skills. Accidents happen not because of chance or fate, but because of the inherent risk involved in the activity combined with the possibility of human error. When children understand and internalize this concept, they will be in a better position to enhance their own personal safety. By recognizing their own volition and responsibility, they will begin to be better able to assess the risk involved in a given activity and to take steps to minimize the possibility of making errors when engaged in that activity.

ARE YOU SAFE IN YOUR HOME?

YES NO

IN THE KITCHEN:

1. Do you wipe up spilled liquids promptly?

2. Is a sturdy step stool available for use in reaching high cabinets and shelves?

3. Are all household poisons like lye, bleaches, cleaning materials, kerosene, rat and bug killers stored where small children cannot get them?

4. Do you keep matches in metal containers out of reach of small children?

5. Do you keep handles of cooking utensils turned inward on the stove?

6. Do you keep knives in a rack with points protected and out of reach of children?

7. Do you make it a rule never to use gasoline or kerosene for starting fires?

IN THE BATHROOM:

8. Are aspirin and other medicines properly stored out of reach of children?

9. Are old medicines destroyed?

10. Do you have non-skid mats in the tub or shower and non-skid rug on floor?

11. Is there a hand-hold near the bathtub?

12. Are electric pull-chains properly insulated?

13. Are electric appliances kept out of reach from basin and tub?

14. Do you stay in the bathroom with small children to prevent their being drowned or scalded?

IN THE BEDROOM AND LIVING ROOM:

15. Are screens fastened to protect children from falling through open windows?

16. Do you have a metal screen for the fireplace or is your stove jacketed?

17. Do you keep passageways clear of electric cords?

18. Are rugs anchored with non-skid materials?

19. Is the furniture arranged so that low tables and footstools will not be tripped over?

20. Do you make sure all matches, cigars, and cigarettes are out before going out or to bed?

21. Do you make it a rule never to smoke in bed?

22. If you have a gas or oil heater in your bedroom, is the room well-ventilated?

23. Is there a light near the bed so that you need not walk and stumble in the dark?

24. Does the baby have a separate bed?

ON THE STAIRS:

25. Do you keep all toys, brooms, mops, and other articles off the steps to prevent falls?

26. Are all stairways well-lighted and equipped with suitable handrails?

27. Do you have gates at the bottom and top of stairs to keep the baby from falling?

IN THE BASEMENT AND/OR GARAGE:

28. Do you avoid accumulation of old papers, oily rags and other inflammable rubbish?

29. Do you use tightly-covered metal containers for storing paints, oils, gasoline, and other inflammable and/or poisonous liquids?

30. Are insecticides labeled and stored properly out of the reach of children?

31. Are there racks for storing garden tools properly?

GENERAL:

32. Are fuses of no more than 15 amps. used for 110 volt circuits?

33. Are electrical appliances, fixtures, and switches so installed and maintained as to prevent electric shock when handled?

34. Are firearms kept unloaded and out of the reach of children?

35. Are porch floors and outside steps in good repair?

36. Are garden tools and outdoor playthings stored in proper places promptly after use?

37. Are the yard and driveway kept free of trash and clutter to eliminate tripping hazards?

38. Are cisterns and wells adequately covered?

Householder _____

Address _____ County _____

Figure 15.1
Home safety checklist.

Source: Reprinted with the permission of the Tennessee Department of Public Health, Nashville, Tennessee.

To become safety-minded, a person must become analytical. What are the risks involved in the activity contemplated? What can be done to lessen those risks? After determining the probable answers to these questions, the individual can then act accordingly. The process of becoming analytical about decision making begins in childhood. You can do much to assist children to develop analytical decision-making skills by providing a variety of learning opportunities that require them to think before they act.

Of course, you cannot expect a child to have the analytical skills of a competent adult, and therefore you must also supervise children's activities to prevent needless accidents. This supervision should take place in the classroom, gymnasium, cafeteria, hallways, and playground. As much as possible, however, relate your supervision to individual decision-making skills. Always keep the approach to safety a positive one.

THE ACCIDENT-SUSCEPTIBLE INDIVIDUAL

Everyone has heard the terms *accident-prone* or *accident-susceptible* and among your students there will be a few who could be so characterized. It is important to recognize that being accident-susceptible is usually not synonymous with being unlucky.

Children and adults who have more than the typical number of accidents are often psychologically disposed to self-harmful behavior. Some of the emotional factors related to accident susceptibility are subconscious guilt for which the accidents serve as punishment, viewing accidents as a means of escape from anxieties or responsibilities, and perceiving accidents as a means of gaining sympathy or attention (Jones, Shainberg & Byer).

Accident-susceptible individuals are often impulsive, unable to form close relationships, or hostile to authority. For such individuals, simply providing information about safety procedures and encouraging the development of decision-making skills may not be enough. Special attention and counseling are often necessary to help the person understand the root of the real problem. Personality characteristics of children are often good indicators of their proneness to accidents. Special attention should be given to children who are daydreamers, who tend to be absentminded, children who are easily frustrated and tend to lose their tempers quickly, and those who try to gain attention by showing off. All such individuals may have a higher accident rate than average for their age group (Strasser, Aaron, & Bohn, 1981).

ACCIDENTS

Causes of Accidents

Before the solution to a problem or the cure for a disease can be found, the source of the problem or cause for the disease has to be examined. About 85 percent of all accidents are attributable to human error. The implication is that appropriate safety education aimed at changing human behavior could reduce accidents. Many of these accidents are due to inadequate knowledge, improper attitudes and habits, or insufficient skill.

Some physiological factors play a role in the causation of accidents. Some physiological factors that could contribute to accidents are sensory impairments (e.g., faulty vision), fatigue, and medical disorders (e.g., epilepsy). Cultural factors, such as a hurried lifestyle and poor attitudes toward competition, often contribute to accidents as well (Olsen, Redican, & Baffi, 1986).

Types of Accidents

Accidents involving school children can be classified into five categories: school, traffic, recreational, home, or disaster. Disaster situations include floods, hurricanes, tornadoes, and earthquakes. As these are general emergencies involving a large segment of the population, they will not be detailed here.

School Accidents. Most school accidents occur in physical education classes, during playground activities, and in sports contests. These activities expose the students to greater levels of risk. Plan carefully to ensure maximum safety. First of all, the teacher in charge should make sure that sports and playground equipment are in good condition and suitable for the activity. Work closely with school administrators, other faculty members, and the school custodians. Equipment that is not in use should be stored so that it does not interfere with the ongoing activity. Swings and other play equipment should be inspected regularly. The playground should also be routinely inspected for hazards, including broken glass, damaged fencing, and so forth.

Next, be sure that all physical activities are properly supervised by an adequate number of faculty members. Confine all activities to designated areas, and be sure that the activity of one group of children does not interfere with that of another group. Keep any activity that you are supervising well ordered and watch for signs of fatigue. When a child becomes tired, the chances for an accident increase. Finally, when your students have finished the activity, make sure that equipment is properly stored. Lock all equipment cabinets to prevent unauthorized, unsupervised use.

Safety in the hallways, stairways, cafeteria, and other parts of the school outside the actual classroom should be maximized by teacher supervision. Stress the importance of polite, considerate behavior rather than simply demanding that students follow rules. Hall monitors should not be allowed to function as prison guards. Work with school administrators and custodians to keep the school environment free of potential hazards. Stairways should have banisters and adequate lighting. Water fountains should have the appropriate amount of water pressure—not too low to cause children to bump their teeth and not too much to cause water to spill on the floor. Spills of any sort should be wiped up promptly, and litter should be removed. Doors to maintenance areas should be locked.

In the classroom itself, make sure that you also maintain a safe environment. Keep equipment and supplies stored until they are needed. Supervise all activities closely. If you prepare any experiment or classroom demonstration that could be hazardous, do not take unnecessary risks. For example, if a demonstration involves the use of a sharp object or a chemical, do not have students help you. Also, be especially careful with any electrical apparatus.

Traffic Accidents. Going to and from school accounts for few school accidents. This is surprising when one considers the potential dangers that children face as pedestrians, bicyclists, and bus and auto passengers. The low accident rate speaks well of school safety patrols and pedestrian and bicycle safety programs. Nonetheless, traffic accidents do occur, and they are often serious. Help your children recognize the importance of following established safety procedures when they are pedestrians, bicyclists, and vehicle passengers.

As pedestrians, children should understand how they interact with motor vehicles. Traffic laws are designed not only for operators of motor vehicles but also for pedestrians. Each has an obligation to the other, a point that you should stress. Help younger children learn the meaning of traffic signs and signals, and explain the reasons behind traffic regulations. Youngsters usually do not appreciate the physical principles involved in the operation of a motor vehicle and do not understand that a car cannot stop on a dime. Further, children often become so engrossed in their own activities that they simply do not consider the vehicular traffic around them. They may dart into the street after a ball without thinking.

Bicycle safety should also be emphasized. Children often assume that traffic laws and regulations apply only to motor vehicles. They see themselves not as operators of vehicles—which they are—but rather as mounted pedestrians. To some degree, this is a values-related issue and must be approached as such. That is, children do not see themselves as being irresponsible when they fail to heed traffic regulations because they place themselves in another category when they ride their bikes.

Most children are regular passengers on school buses and in family vehicles. Nearly 50 percent of all students in public elementary and secondary schools are transported to and from school on buses (Bever, 1984). The numbers of students riding to and from school on buses in the future will increase (Miller, 1982). Children need to become aware of proper safety practices in buses and cars.

Drivers of school buses are responsible for supervising students during their ride. Cooperate with drivers in establishing firm guidelines for safe student behavior while loading, riding, and unloading the buses. Unruly students can easily distract a driver so that an accident results. Make clear the possible consequences of unruly behavior and point out that the well-being of many individuals can be affected by poor behavior. Also provide instructions for safe behavior. Children should enter the bus in an orderly manner and move to their seats swiftly but with care. They should remain seated during the ride. Books, lunch boxes, and other objects should be kept out of the aisles. Windows should remain closed unless the driver opens them. If windows are opened, children should not stick their arms out or throw trash from them. Finally, students should remain well clear of the bus when it is approaching the bus stop and after they have departed.

As automobile passengers, children should also be aided in developing safety practices. Emphasize that even though it may look easy, driving a car requires the full attention of the operator. Children should not distract the driver and should not lean out of windows. Stress the importance of wearing seat belts, even if the parents of some children do not regularly use them. Some states in America, e.g., New York and Ohio are now requiring the use of seat belts by some passengers. Many other states are considering such legislation. Not wearing a seat belt is *essentially* irrational behavior. Reasons given for not using belts are many. Some drivers find them constricting or uncomfortable. Others say that they are not needed for short trips. A few claim to fear being trapped inside the vehicle in case of an accident. None of these reasons hold up. The truth is that people refuse to wear seat belts either because of simple laziness or because of a belief that somehow preparing for an accident by wearing a belt will actually allow an accident to take place! Not wearing a belt is a psychological device called denial.

Health Highlight: Require Seat Belt Use On School Buses?

One proposal to reduce the number of student traffic fatalities is to require the use of seat belts by all passengers on school buses. The argument in favor of such a proposal is the reduction of fatalities to students who travel to and from school on buses.

However, there are several arguments against such a proposal. The installation of such equipment would be very time-consuming and costly. School systems who operate their own buses would pay directly for the installation of seat belts, while those systems who contract bus transportation would pay indirectly for the overhead costs incurred by private bus companies. Another argument against seat belts regards supervision. The bus driver has many responsibilities while driving the bus. Will the driver also be asked to ensure that every student is buckled in a seat belt during the entire trip?

A required seat belt legislation appears sound on the surface, but many related issues must be resolved before passage.

Recreational Accidents. A large portion of recreational accidents happen to children in and around water. Thus water safety should be an important component of the instruction that you provide. All children should be taught to swim at an early age. This is something that you can encourage by getting parents and children involved in organized recreational programs. Even if children know how to swim, the danger of accidental drowning always exists. Most drownings happen to people who are not dressed for swimming, which implies that they were not planning to be in the water. Victims usually fall into the water, whether in a home pool, from a boat, or by a river or lake. Emphasize to your children that any body of water should be treated with respect and caution, including a flooded drainage ditch. Also include the rules for boating safety, such as always wearing a life preserver, in your discussion of water safety.

Camping and hiking activities contribute to many recreational accidents. Falls from cliffs and other high places result in hundreds of fatalities and injuries each year. Stress the importance of being cautious in unfamiliar terrain. Skateboards also cause many recreational accidents among children. The popularity of skateboards is currently on the wane, but use it still high, as is the number of resulting accidents. Emphasize the need for proper protective equipment. Also note that skateboards should not be used on streets. A collision between a car and a child on a skateboard can be fatal for the child.

Your treatment of recreational safety should also include any forms of recreation popular in your area, such as snowmobiling, iceskating, hunting, and fishing. The following suggestions (Jones, Shainberg, & Byer, 1985) increase safety in winter sports.

1. Always have warm, comfortable clothing and adequate equipment.
2. Ski, sled and skate on *supervised* slopes and rinks if possible.

Home Accidents. "There's no place like home" implies that home is a pleasant place to be. Unfortunately, there's no place like home for accidents, either. More accidents happen in the home than in any other place, partly because most people spend a great deal of time at home. The leading cause of death in the home is fire. Most home fires occur in the kitchen and bedroom. For the latter, smoking in bed is often the cause. Home safety, including fire safety, is primarily a parental responsibility, but you can help by making your students aware of possible hazards. Work with parents and children to ensure that every family has a fire safety and fire evacuation plan.

For younger children, emphasize the danger of playing with matches or with the kitchen stove. Encourage parents to install smoke detectors. Teach children what to do if a fire breaks out in the home, especially at night. Too often, frightened children seek shelter in a closet or other enclosed area rather than fleeing. Follow each fire drill in school with a discussion of home fire drills. Every member of the family should know the evacuation route and an alternative route if the primary one is blocked by smoke or flames.

Poisonings are another common home accident, especially among younger children. Explain the dangers of ingesting any substance, such as medicines, food that may have gone bad, and household chemicals. Make sure that parents understand the dangers of accidental poisonings from such substances as aspirin, and encourage them to keep a list of emergency procedures on hand. Also, inform parents and children of the telephone number of the local poison control center. Electrical appli-

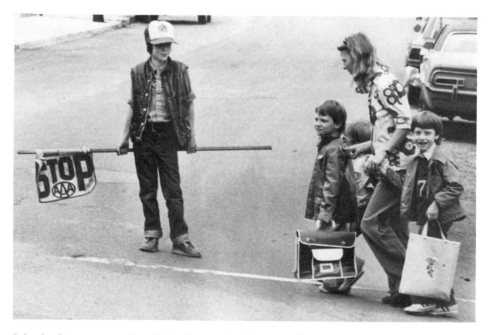

School safety programs have helped to minimize traffic accidents involving students going to and from schools, but these accidents still occur and are often serious.

ances are a common source of home accidents. Make sure that your children understand the danger of playing with any electrical device. Also discuss how electrical overloads can lead to home fires.

Your instruction in home safety techniques should include specific recommendations, such as not leaving toys or other objects on stairs or sidewalks, having adequate ventilation when running internal combustion motors, and wearing protective eye equipment when using power tools or lawn equipment. Encourage parents to do all they can to keep the home a safe environment for themselves and their children. For example, you may wish to prepare a checklist for children to take home to their parents. Discussion of items on the checklist can provide a valuable learning experience for all involved.

Just as a family should have a home evacuation plan in case of fire, it should also have a general disaster plan. Encourage children and their parents to work out a plan for any disaster that might hit their community. Depending on the locale, disasters might include earthquakes, floods, tornadoes, or extreme blizzards. Each family member should know what to do in case a disaster strikes.

THE SCHOOL SAFETY PROGRAM

Instruction in safety education should be only one part of your school safety program. The total program should consist of these components.

1. Providing instruction by and for faculty, staff, and students.
2. Planning and implementing safety procedures.
3. Providing safe transportation, including bus travel, walking, and bicycle safety.
4. Establishing accident reporting and record-keeping procedures.
5. Making sure there is liability insurance protection for staff.
6. Providing emergency health care for all persons attending or employed by the school.
7. Creating a safe environment.

The school should define the responsibilities of each person involved in the safety program, and instruct each person regarding specific duties or responsibilities. Supervision should be provided for all school activities, including travel to and from school, physical education, playground time, and after-school gatherings.

Some schools have established school safety councils to develop rules, policies, and procedures for safe living within the school and for school activities. Safety councils provide excellent learning opportunities and allow for student involvement. For example, a school safety council could do a needs assessment or accident survey for the school. This procedure makes the students and others involved aware of the accident situations in their school environment, helping to prevent future accidents.

Generally, any accident that causes a student to miss school, go home from school, or that involves property damage should be reported. Some schools have specific forms for reporting any type of accident in or around the school. An example of such a form is shown in figure 15.2. Accident reports can provide data for studying accident trends in the school environment. They are also valuable in the event of lawsuits filed against the school.

STANDARD STUDENT ACCIDENT REPORT FORM
Part A. Information on ALL Accidents

1. Name: _____ Home Address: _____

2. School: _____ Sex M☐: F☐ Age:_____Grade or classification:_____

3. Time accident occurred. Hour_____ A.M.;_____P.M. Date: _____

4. Place of Accident: School Building☐ School Grounds☐ To or from School☐ Home☐ Elsewhere☐

5. NATURE OF INJURY				DESCRIPTION OF THE ACCIDENT
Abrasion	_____	Fracture	_____	How did accident happen? What
Amputation	_____	Laceration	_____	was student doing? Where was
Asphyxiation	_____	Poisoning	_____	student? List specifically unsafe
Bite	_____	Puncture	_____	acts and unsafe conditions
Bruise	_____	Scalds	_____	existing. Specify any tool, machine
Burn	_____	Scratches	_____	or equipment involved.
Concussion	_____	Shock (el)	_____	
Cut	_____	Sprain	_____	
Dislocation	_____			
Other (specify)	_____			

5. PART OF BODY INJURED			
Abdomen	_____	Foot	_____
Ankle	_____	Hand	_____
Arm	_____	Head	_____
Back	_____	Knee	_____
Chest	_____	Leg	_____
Ear	_____	Mouth	_____
Elbow	_____	Nose	_____
Eye	_____	Scalp	_____
Face	_____	Tooth	_____
Finger	_____	Wrist	_____
Other (specify)	_____		

6. Degree of Injury Death☐ Permanent Impairment☐ Temporary Disability☐ Nondisabling☐

7. Total number of days lost from school: _____ (To be filled in when student returns to school)

Part B. Additional Information on School Jurisdiction Accidents

8. Teacher in charge when accident occurred (Enter name) _____ Present at scene of accident: No _____ Yes _____

9. IMMEDIATE ACTION TAKEN

First aid treatment _____ By (Name): _____
Sent to school nurse _____ By (Name): _____
Sent home _____ By (Name): _____
Sent to physician _____ By (Name): _____
Physician's Name: _____
Sent to hospital _____ By (Name): _____
Name of hospital: _____

10. Was a parent or other individual notified No _____ Yes _____ When _____ How _____
Name of individual notified: _____ By whom? (Enter name): _____

11. Witnesses: 1. Name: _____ Address: _____
2. Name: _____ Address: _____

12. LOCATION		Specify Activity		Remarks
Athletic field	_____	Locker	_____	What recommendations do you have for preventing other accidents of this type? _____
Auditorium	_____	Pool	_____	
Cafeteria	_____	Sch grounds	_____	
Classroom	_____	shop	_____	
Corridor	_____	Showers	_____	
Dressing room	_____	Stairs	_____	
Gymnasium	_____	Toilets and	_____	
Home Econ.	_____	washrooms	_____	
Laboratories	_____	Other (specify)	_____	

Figure 15.2
Accident report form.

Source: Reprinted with the permission of the National Safety Council, Washington, D.C.

Teacher liability should be an important consideration in the school safety program. Teachers may be held legally liable if an accident occurs because of a variety of contributing factors (Bever, 1984). These include:

1. Teacher absence from the classroom while school is in session
2. Use of faulty equipment
3. Lack of proper instruction
4. Lack of care with regard to the age and maturity of pupils

To avoid liability situations, you must become aware of your legal and moral responsibilities as a teacher. You must also practice foresight and engage in prudent behavior in all school activities, including planning, administering, and supervising, as well as maintaining equipment in the classroom, gymnasium, and playground.

Considerations of liability are especially important in physical education and playground activities because of the greater potential for accidents in these situations. Activities normally considered potentially dangerous, such as tumbling and gymnastics, actually result in relatively few liability suits against teachers and schools because instructors are alert to the risks and take proper precautions to ensure a safe lesson. However, activities that are more common present more of a problem for liability suits. Teachers often assume that students are familiar with the activity and fail to be as careful in supervision as they should be. Liability insurance coverage should be a part of the school safety program to protect teachers from lawsuit damage payments. This type of coverage is usually included as part of membership in professional education organizations such as the National Education Association. Physical education teachers and others who may be particularly vulnerable to lawsuits should consider adding to the basic coverage.

Another aspect of the school safety program should be fire and disaster drills and preparations. These drills are usually mandated under state law. They should be carefully planned and implemented. As a classroom teacher, impress upon your students the importance of fire and disaster drills. As a role model, you should take them seriously so as to encourage your students to do likewise.

FIRST AID SKILLS

First aid means just that—providing aid before more qualified medical help can be obtained. Adults and children alike should have some knowledge of first aid procedures so they can aid an accident victim in an emergency. Often, such knowledge can make the difference between life and death in extreme cases. However, first aid should never be dispensed casually, and not at all if more qualified help can be obtained quickly. Improper first aid can actually cause more damage than good in some instances. As a classroom teacher, you should learn basic first aid procedures and instruct your students in them. Rarely will you or any of your students meet a life-threatening situation. More often, first aid procedures are used in common, everyday incidents involving cuts, nosebleeds, sprains, and so on. Still, you should be prepared for more serious circumstances.

Begin your own preparation by checking with the school administration and medical personnel to determine established procedures for handling medical prob-

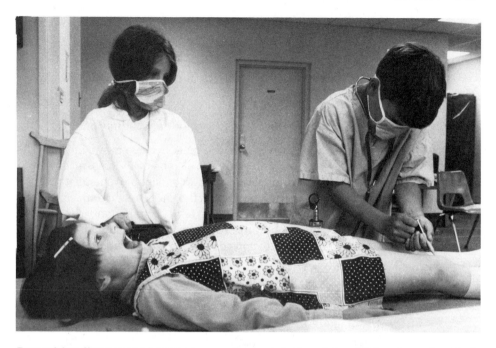

Dramatizing disasters and how the community reacts to them helps children learn about both safety and first aid.

lems and emergencies. This is extremely important as far as liability is concerned and cannot be stressed too strongly. In most instances, you will probably be told not to offer any medical assistance except under clearly life-threatening circumstances or when there is no possibility of obtaining more qualified assistance. In some instances, however, administering first aid may be acceptable and provided for in the school safety program.

Keep in mind that first aid is not treatment; instead it is protection of the victim until treatment can be given. The purpose of first aid is to offer emergency care, prevent further injury, lessen the victim's pain, and ward off unnecessary complications, such as shock. While this is being done, help should also be sought.

When administering first aid, your first task is to determine where help is needed most if there is more than one victim. Often you must rely on your own judgment on the basis of visible injury. Never assume that anyone who has been involved in an accident is without injury or trauma, even if there is no apparent evidence of such. There could be internal bleeding or brain injury. Shock is also a common complication that may not be readily visible in the victim at first. Remain calm and communicate your calmness to the victim. Reassure the person that help is on the way—and make sure that it is. Do all you can to prevent panic. Staying in control yourself will be easier if you are thoroughly familiar with basic first aid procedures. Providing emotional support is an important part of the aid you give.

If the victim is conscious, ask what happened. This information can be vital to the assistance you give both to the victim and to those qualified medical personnel who arrive on the scene later. If the victim is not conscious, immediately check for vital signs. Mouth-to-mouth resuscitation at this point may save a life. You should be qualified to administer this technique in an emergency. Generally it is best to keep the victim lying down to prevent further injury, fainting, or shock. Do not move the victim unless there is no choice, as in a traffic accident where a fire has broken out. Then, get help so that the person can be moved without likely injury to the spinal cord or neck region.

In many school accident situations, crowd control is necessary. Keep other children away from the victim and restore order. Do not let anyone else attempt to give aid. Do what you can for the victim until help arrives. Then provide follow-up care as required, if you are asked to do so.

Emergency Situations

The best way to prepare yourself to handle an emergency medical or accident situation is to take a course sponsored by the American Red Cross or other health agency. You will gain hands-on experience in dealing with a variety of situations and will have a chance to practice basic first aid skills before you actually have to use them. In this section of the chapter, information is provided about handling some of the serious emergency situations you may encounter. Simply reading about these emergency procedures, however, is a poor substitute for actual first-aid coursework.

Breathing Problems. The major causes of breathing difficulties involve chest injuries, cardiovascular problems, head injuries, obstruction (choking or swallowing), carbon monoxide poisoning, drug intoxication, electrical shock, lack of oxygen in the air, and drowning. Symptoms include dizziness or unconsciousness, shortness of breath or difficulty in breathing, chest pain, bluish tint to the skin, and dilated pupils. A victim might not have all these signs but will likely manifest a combination of most of them.

The general procedures to follow when caring for a person with a breathing difficulty are:

1. Clear the mouth of any objects that might be blocking the airway.
2. Send someone to get medical assistance.
3. Position the victim in a supine position with jaw and head extended to keep the air passages clear.
4. Loosen any tight clothing around the neck or stomach.
5. Maintain body temperature.
6. Begin resuscitation if needed.

Mouth-to-mouth resuscitation is the best method of assisting a person who is not breathing and is unconscious. The procedure is :

1. Keep the jaw extended with your hand or a blanket under the neck.
2. Pinch the nostrils shut with thumb and forefinger of the other hand.
3. Cover the victim's mouth with your mouth. If the victim is a very small child, you may cover the mouth and nose with your mouth.
4. Breathe four times quickly, then once every five seconds.

Throughout the administration of resuscitation, the pulse should be monitored periodically. If no pulse is evident, then external heart massage (or cardiopulmonary resuscitation) should be given. Locate a proper position on the sternum so as not to break off the bottom portion of the sternum or to fracture any ribs. Then compress the sternum one to two inches 15 times at an 80 per minute rate, breathe twice into the victim's mouth, and repeat the procedure. Continue these resuscitation efforts until more qualified medical help arrives.

One of the best methods for treating choking victims is the Heimlich maneuver. This is a method for forcing objects out of the mouth and throat of a choking victim by externally compressing the air in the lungs, thereby causing a sudden flow of air up through the trachea that will expel the object. Stand behind the person and wrap your arms around the torso. Place your fist, thumb side, against the victim's stomach slightly above the navel and below the rib cage and press upward with a quick thrust. This action can be repeated several times if needed.

Bleeding. Loss of blood can be life-threatening and may require immediate attention. If an artery has been severed, the blood will be bright red and will spurt from the wound. If a vein is affected, the blood will be darker red and will ooze from the wound. There may be little visible blood loss from a puncture wound or bad contusion (bruise) but internal bleeding may be taking place.

The general procedure for treating a bleeding wound involves stopping the bleeding, protecting the wound from infection, treating for shock, and getting medical attention in cases of severe bleeding. In most instances, try to stop the blood loss by applying direct pressure with a sterile cloth right over the wound. It is also helpful to elevate the bleeding part, if possible. This will reduce the amount of blood going to the affected part due to the force of gravity. If the blood loss is too heavy for these methods, to curtail the bleeding, various pressure points can be used. The four major pressure points are the brachial arteries in each arm and the femoral arteries in each leg. Press these arteries against the corresponding bone to close off most of the blood supply to the affected part. A tourniquet should only be used as a last resort. A tourniquet may be fashioned from a cloth, a tie, or a belt. Place it above the wound and tighten until the blood supply is squeezed off. *Remember that a tourniquet should only be used as a last resort to save a life.*

When the bleeding has been stopped, bandage the wound. Place a sterile cloth directly over the wound to reduce the chances of infection. The bandage should be tied tightly enough to help control the bleeding, but not too tightly. As you administer aid, watch the fingers of the victim if the wound is on an arm. If the fingers turn pale or bluish, loosen the bandage. Keep the victim lying down with the affected part elevated.

Nosebleeds are common among elementary school children. There are many misconceptions concerning the proper handling of a nosebleed. Many people still think that the victim's head should be tilted back. This action will prevent the blood from coming out of the nose, but it does not stop the bleeding. Rather, have the victim be seated and lean forward. Provide support to keep the person from falling forward if he or she faints. Then pinch the nostrils together to stop blood loss. If this method does not work, apply ice to the nose. If bleeding persists, place cotton gauze in the nostrils and pinch them together.

Shock. Every first aid treatment should include treatment for shock. Regardless of the nature or severity of the injury, the victim could go into shock either from physical or mental stress. If you treat an injury successfully but fail to prevent the victim from going into shock, then you could be considered negligent. When a victim goes into shock, blood pressure drops. The heart beats faster in order to circulate more blood, but the vessels constrict so the extremities (arms, legs, head) do not get enough blood or oxygen.

You must be able to recognize the early signs of shock in order to prevent the victim from going deeper into a severe shock state. The signs of shock are pale skin, dilated pupils, shallow and irregular breathing, weak and rapid pulse, cool and moist skin, vomiting, nausea, and lapsing into unconsciousness. The victim's eyes will look dark and hollow and the person will appear to be staring into space. When these signs are evident, immediately try to maintain the victim's body temperature, and monitor vital signs closely.

Placing the victim in a proper position can prevent or minimize shock. If there is a severe wound to the lower face or jaw, place the victim on his or her side to allow for fluid drainage. If there is a breathing problem, place the victim in a supine position, with the head and shoulders raised. If there is a head injury, keep the victim flat or propped up slightly. If no major injuries are evident, raise the feet about 12 inches in order to improve the blood flow to the brain. When you have any doubt as to the proper shock position, keep the victim in a horizontal position so as not to damage any body part.

Poisoning. The vast majority of poisonings involve young children. Young children are especially vulnerable to poisoning because of their tendency to explore new things by putting them into their mouths. You should be aware of the signs of poisoning. Have the phone number of the local poison control center in a handy place. Also keep a poison control chart in the classroom. These precautions are very important since speed is vital when treating a poison victim.

The major causes of poisonings in children are swallowing poisonous substances, bites, stings, contact with poisonous plants, and inhalation of toxic fumes. The primary objective in first aid for a poison victim is to get medical assistance quickly. Keep the victim from moving around and keep the person lying down.

If a person suffers a bite from a poisonous snake, there is usually extremely rapid swelling within 30 minutes, and the skin will be discolored. With snake bite, there is a possibility of breathing difficulty, vomiting, and shock. Monitor the vital signs of the victim closely in case mouth-to-mouth resuscitation is needed. If a noncorrosive poison, such as floor wax or furniture polish, has been swallowed, get the victim to a treatment center immediately. Do not induce vomiting unless recommended by a physician or the poison control center. If the ingested poison is a corrosive, such as petroleum product, have the victim drink water or milk to dilute the substance if the person is conscious and not convulsing. Do not force a person who has swallowed a corrosive poison to vomit because the substance could damage the esophageal lining on the way back up the esophagus.

If the victim has been poisoned from an inhaled gas, such as carbon monoxide, remove the person from the source as quickly as possible. Do not just ventilate the building and leave the victim inside. Disconnect the source of the poison if possible (for example, a car engine). Monitor the vital signs closely in case there is a need for mouth-to-mouth resuscitation.

Contact with poisonous plants will produce the following signs: itching, redness, rash, headache, and fever. If you are with the person immediately following the contact with such a plant, remove contaminated clothing, flush the affected skin with water, and wash with soap and water for several minutes. Calamine lotion can be applied to the affected skin. If the contact poison is a corrosive substance or pesticide, get medical assistance immediately.

For minor insect stings, use cold applications and soothing lotions. In the case of bee sting, try to remove and discard the stinger and venom sac. Because of the possibility of violent allergic response, always obtain medical help for afflicted students.

Burns. The primary objectives for treatment of burns are relieving pain, preventing or treating shock, dressing the wound, and maintaining body fluids. Burns are usually categorized as first, second, or third degree. *First degree burns* are superficial. Usually the top layer of skin is reddened. Treat this type of burn with cold, wet compresses or with ice packs. This lessens the pain and the degree of tissue destruction. You can also coat a first degree burn with an antiseptic ointment. Be sure not to use butter as an ointment and do not apply the ointment with cotton, which will adhere to the wound. *A second degree burn* is characterized by blisters on the skin. This type of wound should be immersed in cold water. Gently blot with sterile gauze or a clean towel, taking care not to open the blisters, and keep the affected parts elevated. Obtain medical assistance as soon as possible. *Third degree burns* are typically distinguished by charred skin. A third degree burn is a medical emergency. The victim may not be in as much pain as with a second degree burn only because the nerves in the affected area might have been destroyed. Do not remove any clothing that adheres to the burn. Cover loosely with a sterile dressing, keep the burned part elevated, give psychological assurance, treat for shock, and get medical assistance.

If the burn is a chemical burn, the affected part should be copiously flushed with water. Remove any contaminated clothing. If the burn is on the body, have the victim take a shower if possible. If an eye is burned, flush it out with plenty of water. Make sure the burned eye is below the other eye so as not to affect both eyes.

Exposure to Extreme Temperatures. Young children like to play in ice and snow, and many times they do this for too long at a time. This makes them susceptible to hypothermia—the lowering of the body temperature through prolonged exposure to cold and wet weather that can result in frostbite, which occurs when the tissue in the extremities becomes frozen. The signs of frostbite are gray skin, discomfort, and loss of pain in the frozen part due to the nerves becoming dysfunctional. To give first aid for frostbite, cover the frozen part and wrap the body in a blanket. If possible, move the victim indoors and give warm fluids to drink if the person is conscious and not convulsing. Gradually rewarm the frozen part in water that is approximately 100 to 110 degrees Fahrenheit (Hafen, 1985).

Do not rub the frozen part, and never use a heat lamp or hot water bottle for heat. Also, do not allow the person to get too close to a fire or hot stove to warm up. Because of loss of feeling in affected nerves, the victim cannot gauge the degree of heat.

The body can also be affected detrimentally by exposure to too much heat. When a person is exercising vigorously on a hot day and water is not adequately replaced, blood circulation diminishes and organs are affected. This condition, known as heat exhaustion, produces such symptoms as headache, dizziness, nausea, weakness, profuse sweating, weak and rapid pulse, pale, cool, and sweaty skin, and rapid, shallow breathing. To treat for heat exhaustion, move the victim to a cool place and remove as much clothing as possible. Sponge with cold water, have the person lie down, and raise the feet approximately 12 inches. Then loosen the remaining clothing. If the victim is not lapsing into unconsciousness, provide sips of salted drinking water.

A serious complication of exposure to extreme heat is heat stroke or sun stroke. Overweight individuals and the elderly are especially susceptible to heat stroke, but it can happen to anyone. The signs of heat stroke are red, dry, hot skin, cessation of perspiration, headache, rapid and strong pulse, nausea, and dizziness. Essentially, the sweating mechanism in the body has quit functioning; there is no sweat on the body to cool it off, and the body temperature goes up dramatically and dangerously. Treat heat stroke by moving the victim to shade or a cool place. Loosen clothing, cool the person with wet towels or by immersing in cold water, give sips of water if conscious, and seek medical assistance.

Bone and Joint Injuries. The signs of a fracture vary greatly in different situations. Many people make the mistake of asking the injured person to move the body part, assuming that a broken bone cannot be moved, but this is a misconception. Do not ask the victim to move the affected part, as this might further aggravate the injury. If the person is conscious, ask how the injury occurred. Sometimes there will be an obvious deviation in the bone alignment, pain and swelling, and discoloration due to contusions surrounding the fractured bone. If there is any doubt as to whether the injury is a fracture or not, treat it as if it were a fracture to be safe.

The proper way to care for a fracture is to immobilize the injury with a splint. With an open fracture, where the skin has broken as well as the bone, dress and bandage the skin wound before splinting the limb. Wide, flat materials, such as boards, should be used for splinting. They should be padded if placed next to the victim's skin. The injured extremity should be splinted beyond the joints above and below the fracture to lessen the amount of movement. If the victim is allowed to move the fractured limb, the possibility of further injury, more pain, and shock are increased. If the skull is fractured, do not apply pressure as this might force bone fragments into the brain. Any fracture that might involve the skull or vertebrae should be splinted with a long board that covers the entire body. A person who has suffered a fracture should not be moved unless in a dangerous situation, such as a burning building or a busy street.

Sprains are often associated with fractures. They occur when ligaments and other tissues around a joint are stretched beyond their normal range of motion. Sprains can be caused by severely twisting a joint, a direct blow to the joint, or a fall. The signs are similar to fractures: pain, swelling, and discoloration. If you are unsure as to whether the injury is a sprain or a fracture, treat it as a fracture to be safe. To treat a sprain, elevate the affected body part to reduce swelling. Do not allow the victim to walk; do not encourage the person to "walk it out." Pack the injured part in ice to control internal bleeding, pain, and swelling. Then bandage firmly. As with all bandages, check the toes and fingers to make sure the splint and bandage are not so tight as to cut off circulation to the extremity.

Dislocations also occur from moving the joint beyond the normal range of motion in twisting injuries and falls. Specifically, a dislocation happens when one bone is separated from another bone at a joint. There is typically marked deformity, pain, swelling, loss of use, discoloration due to damage to blood vessels and nerves, and possible shock. A dislocation should be treated just as a fracture. Immobilize the victim, treat for shock, and get medical assistance. Cold applications can be used on dislocated bones to reduce pain, swelling, and internal hemorrhaging.

Eye and Ear Injuries. If something is in the eye, wash your hands and then take the lower lid down and check. If you can find nothing, pull the upper lid out, roll it up on a swab and check the eye. Use a clean handkerchief to dab at the foreign particle in the eye. Do not let the person rub the eye and do not attempt to remove anything that is penetrating the eyeball. If you have to bandage the eye, bandage both eyes loosely so the object will not be forced deeper into the eye. When both eyes are bandaged, the victim is less likely to move the eyes as much and further damage the injured eye.

Earaches and ear drainage are the two most common problems of the ear experienced by young children. Both of these conditions can be treated with either ice packs or hot-water bottles applied to the ear. If allowed, pain medication can be given. If either of these conditions persist, they should be reported to a physician.

Fainting. Fainting is usually a physiological manifestation resulting from an emotional response. Fainting is similar to shock in that it is caused by a lack of oxygen to the brain. There are a variety of causes ranging from the sight of blood to a reaction to an injury. You can often prevent fainting by having the person lie down, with the head lower than the legs.

Convulsions. As a teacher, you first need to understand the emotional aspects of a child who has frequent convulsions. These are symptoms of a behavior pattern, not a disease. Affected children are often ostracized by the peer group because of misconceptions about convulsions. Students should be instructed as to the causes of convulsions, emotional aspects related to convulsions, and what procedures to follow if a convulsion occurs in the classroom or anywhere at school.

To treat a child who is having a convulsion, call the school nurse immediately. While waiting for help, remove all objects from around the person. Soften the impact of head, arms, and legs by padding the floor. Remove other children from the scene if possible. Loosen the convulsing child's clothing. If the victim vomits, turn the head to one side to allow for drainage of fluid from the mouth and nose.

Emergencies Related to Diabetes Mellitus. Diabetic coma results from insufficient insulin in the body. The signs of diabetic coma are flushed face, cherry red lips, dry skin, breathing difficulty, and acetone breath (very sweet smelling). If a child lapses into diabetic coma, summon medical assistance immediately and treat for shock.

Insulin shock occurs when there is too little sugar or too much insulin in the blood. The signs of insulin shock are ashen appearance, moist and clammy skin, rapid pulse, and slow and shallow breathing. Give the victim sugar under the tongue or fruit juice if conscious. Summon medical aid immediately.

Unconsciousness. Any time that a person is found unconscious, a true emergency exists. Always monitor the vital signs of an unconscious victim, treat for shock, and obtain medical help immediately. Be sure to check for other injuries and give treatment as necessary. Determining the cause of unconsciousness is often difficult. The condition can result from a blow to the head, a fall, a lack of oxygen, reaction to extreme temperature, or a secondary reaction to illness or shock. If the skin is bluish, there is usually a lack of oxygen. If the skin is pale, there might be severe blood loss or shock. If the skin is red, the condition might be caused by heat stroke, concussion, or a convulsion.

Asthma. Asthma is a chronic allergic reaction caused by extreme sensitivity to some allergen. During an asthmatic reaction, the muscles in the victim's respiratory system constrict spasmodically, preventing air from moving freely to and from the lungs. Such an asthmatic attack can last up to four hours. The condition is complicated when the victim becomes anxious during the coughing spells and wheezing. To provide first aid, support the person in a sitting position during the reaction, provide reassurance, humidify the air, keep the victim warm, and obtain medical assistance.

Acute Appendicitis. A person suffering acute appendicitis will experience a sudden, intense pain in the lower right abdominal area, rigid stomach muscles, nausea, vomiting, fever, and fatigue. Summon medical help immediately. In the meanwhile, keep the victim quiet and immobile, and apply cold applications to the lower right abdominal area. No water or fluids should be given, as these might complicate the problem.

KEEPING A FIRST AID KIT

Check with your school administration, and if endorsed by school district policy, keep a first aid kit ready for use. This kit should be available for classroom, playground, and other situations in which accidents frequently occur. An accessible first aid kit can be of tremendous assistance in preventing further injury. Suggested contents for such a kit are as follows (Brennan & Crowe, 1981, p. 178):

1. Sterile gauze dressings, 4 by 4 inches individually wrapped, for cleaning and covering wounds.
2. Roll of gauze bandage, 2 inches wide, to hold dressings in place.
3. Adhesive tape to hold dressings in place.
4. Assorted adhesive dressings (Band-Aids, Curads, etc.) to cover small cuts and abrasions.
5. Small bottle of mineral oil to be used for small burns.
6. Absorbent cotton may be used to wash skin or apply mineral oil.
7. Petroleum jelly, such as Vaseline—may also be used for small burns.
8. Box of baking soda. This may be moistened and used to soothe insect bites.
9. Scissors to cut bandages and tape.
10. Medicine dropper for rinsing eyes.
11. Tweezers to remove stingers from insect bites.
12. Thermometer for recording body temperature.
13. Ice bag to help prevent swelling of sprains.
14. Hot water bottle to be used to reduce swelling of sprains.
15. Flashlight.

SUMMARY

Elementary school children are subject to many hazards. This age group is the most significantly affected by accidental deaths. Thus safety education should be a vital part of health instruction.

Safety education will help students to increase their awareness of the accident problems and causes, provide them with factual knowledge about safety, help them adjust to new, unfamiliar environments, and heighten their potential for living full, productive lives. Safety should be seen by the students as a vital part of living.

The emphasis in safety education should be on positive attitudes and values. Learning opportunities in safety should be designed to help students recognize potentially hazardous situations and develop a sense of responsibility for their own safety and others. Do not provide safety instruction that is limited to accident statistics, safety rules, or scare tactics. Instead, stress that living is much more enjoyable when a person is safe.

As the teacher, you should set a good safety model for your students. The classroom and other parts of the school environment should be examples of safe, efficient places to work and live.

Because so many accidents happen to children while they are attending school, teachers should learn basic first aid skills to treat injuries resulting from accidents, when other help is not immediately available. Students should also learn how they can be of help in emergency situations. If school policy permits, a first aid kit should be available for use in the various sections of the school in which accidents most frequently occur.

DISCUSSION QUESTIONS

1. Discuss the major human and environmental causes of accidents.
2. Describe the characteristics of an accident-susceptible person.
3. List the main contributing factors for liability situations in the schools.
4. Compare the advantages and disadvantages of requiring all students to wear seat belts in school buses.
5. Discuss the first aid measure to take for an earache.
6. Why should risk taking be considered a necessary evil?
7. Contrast a positive approach to safety education with a negative approach.
8. Describe the major parts of a school safety program.
9. What factors should a teacher consider when administering first aid to a student?
10. List the major items that should be included in a first aid kit for the classroom.

REFERENCES

Bever, D. *Safety: A personal focus.* St. Louis: Times Mirror/Mosby College Publishing, 1984.

Brennan, W., & Crowe, J. *Guide to problems and practices in first aid and emergency care,* fourth edition. Dubuque, Iowa: William C. Brown, 1981.

Cornacchia, H., & Staton, W. *Health in the elementary schools,* fifth edition. St. Louis: C. V. Mosby, 1979.

Hafen, B. *First aid for health emergencies,* third edition. St. Paul, Minnesota: West Publishing Company, 1985.

Jones, K., Shainberg, L., & Byer, C. *Health science,* fifth edition. New York: Harper and Row, Publishers, Inc., 1985.

Miller, D. *Safety: An introduction.* Englewood Cliffs, New Jersey: Prentice-Hall, Inc., 1982.

Olsen, L., Redican, K., & Baffi, C. *Health today,* second edition. New York: Macmillan, 1986.

Payne, W., & Hahn, D. *Understanding your health.* St. Louis: Times Mirror/Mosby College Publishing, 1986.

Strasser, M., Aaron, J., & Bohn, R. *Fundamentals of safety education,* third edition. New York: Macmillan, 1981.

Willgoose, C. *Health education in the elementary school,* fifth edition. Philadelphia: W. B. Saunders, 1979.

16. Techniques for Teaching Safety and First Aid

As long as accidents continue to be the leading cause of death among children and youth there will be a continuing need for improved and expanded safety education in our schools. . . . Unfortunately there is no Salk vaccine for accidents. No, there is no panacea; no magic amulet to ward off the accident demon. But there is a cure, and the schools can—indeed, must—play a major role in that cure, by teaching their students from kindergarten through college that accidents can be prevented, that the consequences of accidents can be lessened.—Vincent L. Tofany, President, National Safety Council

FOSTERING SAFETY BEHAVIOR

Progress has been made in virtually every area of health education in this century, including disease prevention, environmental sanitation, and nutritional habits. If there is one area of health education that has lagged behind, it is safety and accident prevention. Many laws have been passed, especially in the area of traffic safety. Some states are passing mandatory seat belt and stiffer drunk-driving laws. These laws should help save more lives on the road; however, in spite of these and other legislative safety efforts, thousands of Americans die or are injured each year because of needless accidents. The situation will not change significantly until Americans reject an attitude of apathy toward safety, and adopt a lifestyle of safe behavior.

Concepts to be Taught

- Each person is to a large degree responsible for his or her own personal safety.
- Risk taking is a part of living, but unnecessary risk taking greatly increases the risk of harm to oneself and to others.
- The degree of risk in any particular activity can often be determined by analytical thinking.
- Most accidents can be prevented by taking proper precautions.
- Elementary school children have more fatal accidents than any other age group.

- More than half of all accidents involving children happen at school.
- Acting without thinking often results in an accident.
- Individuals who are accident prone often have ulterior motives for such behavior.
- Basic first aid skills are important for everyone.
- Improper first aid can do more harm than good.
- Safety is not just a matter of "luck." Safe behavior must be learned.

Cycle Plan for Teaching Topics

Topic	Grade level						
	K	1	2	3	4	5	6
Causes of Accidents	**	**	**	**	***	**	**
Safety at School	***	***	***	***	**	**	**
Traffic Safety	**	**	**	***	***	***	***
Recreational Safety	*	*	*	**	**	**	***
Home Safety	**	**	**	**	**	**	**
Coping with Disasters	*	**	**	**	*	*	*
Accidents and Emergencies	*	**	**	**	*	***	**
Providing First Aid	*	*	*	*	**	**	**
Preventing Accidents	**	**	***	***	**	**	**
Safe Behavior	***	***	***	***	**	**	**

Key *** = major emphasis, ** = emphasis, * = review.

VALUE-BASED ACTIVITIES

Safety Sentence Completion

Have your students complete the following statements. Then, on a volunteer basis, discuss the values implicit in each statement.

All students should be required to participate in fire drills because _____ .
Safety education to me means _____ .
Accidents are the result of _____ .
As a pedestrian I should know _____ .
People who drive should be aware of _____ .
The costs of accidents are _____ .
I would become personally involved if someone was hurt in an accident if _____ .
Accidents could be reduced by _____ .
The greatest number of accidents are _____ .
Educating others about preventing accidents can be organized by _____ .

Decision Stories

The Hill

George and Frank like to ride their bikes to school. There is a hill on the way to school. Near the top of the hill there is a stop sign. If they stop, getting over the hill is difficult.

George usually stops, but Frank never does. George has to get off his bike and start again. Frank kids him about this and calls him a chicken. George does not want to seem a coward to his friend but he knows that he should stop for traffic signs.

Focus Question: What should George do?

The Model

Chieko is working on a model car made from wood. This is the first one that she has ever tried to make. Usually her older sister helps her, but today her sister is away. Chieko wants to cut some parts for the model. She sees a very sharp knife that her older sister usually uses. Maybe she should wait for her sister to come home. Maybe she should go ahead by herself, even if she doesn't know how to use the knife properly.

Focus Question: What should Chieko do?

The Raft

Jason and his friends are playing by a river near their home. Some of the boys decide to build a raft. They are going to use it to cross the river on. They find some wood on the riverbank and start making the raft. But it doesn't look too sturdy to Jason. When the time comes to put the raft in the water, Jason has his doubts. What if the raft falls apart while the boys are on it? Jason knows how to swim, but swimming might be difficult with his clothes on. And he is not sure the others can swim.

Focus Question: What should Jason do?

The Stranger

Beth and her sister Harriet are walking home from school. Just then a car pulls up by the curb. The driver is a man Beth and her sister have never seen. He asks them their names, and they tell him. Then the man says that he is a good friend of their father. He says that their father has asked him to pick them up and take them for a ride. The stranger offers to buy the girls some ice cream, too.

Focus Question: What should Beth and her sister do?

The Swimming Pool

Candy and her friends were at a party one evening. The party was outside and everyone was having a good time. Someone suggests climbing over the fence to swim in the neighbor's pool. Everyone agreed. Candy was hesitant. Candy has a heart problem and she can't swim for long periods of time. She has never told her friends about her heart problem.

Focus Question: Should Candy swim in the neighbor's pool?

The First Real Party

Tammy was a shy girl. She rarely got invited to parties. Sam, a friend at school asked Tammy if she would like to come with him to a big bash this Friday night. Tammy accepted, thinking this would be her chance to get to know some more people. At the party some of the kids are smoking and drinking. Sam wanted Tammy to smoke and drink too. This would help her come out of her shell.

Focus Question: Should Tammy smoke and drink at the party?

The Fire

Susan is having a slumber party. Her parents have gone away for the weekend and they have trusted her with the house. Susan is awakened by smoke in the early morning hours. Most of the girls slept in the den and it was easy to alert everyone and get them out of the house. They run next door and call the fire department. Now the house is really burning. Susan remembers two friends who wanted to sleep upstairs in the bed. Susan starts to run back in the house to get them out, but everyone tells her to wait on the firefighters to get there.

Focus Question: Should Susan get her friends out of the burning house?

Medicine

Tina is getting over a cold. It is nothing serious, but she stayed home from school for two days. Now she is back. Her cold is almost gone, but she is still coughing. At lunch, Tina sits with her friend Pam. Pam has been taking medicine for an infection that she has. "It's real good stuff," Pam says to Tina. "I'll bet it would make your cough go away just like that. Why don't you try some?"

Focus Question: What should Tina do?

Building a Fire

Brian's parents have gone out to buy groceries. Brian is home by himself. It is a cold winter day and there is a chill in the house. There is some wood next to the fireplace. He thinks that a fire would be nice. It would warm up the house. Brian knows that his parents don't want him to play with the fireplace, but he has seen them build fires many times. He is sure that he could do it, too. At least he is *pretty* sure. . . .

Focus Question: What should Brian do?

DRAMATIZATION

Disaster Drama

Divide the class into groups of five. After the earthquake that hit Mexico a few weeks ago, the students have talked about what happened. Each group of students must read all the newspapers that dealt with the earthquake. They must go to the library and either make a copy of the article or write a summary of it. Students can divide the number of articles by five, each person reading only her part. At the end of a two-week study, each group designates a spokesperson who must give an oral account of what was found.

School Bus Behavior

Students are in groups. Each group is given a situation that has happened on the bus and the students must decide what should be done.
Case 1—two students are fighting.
Case 2—two students are sitting on the same seat; one student wants the window up, the other student wants the window down.
Case 3—a student will not stay in her seat.

Looking for Hazards

Assign students to go to various rooms in the school and look for hazards: shop rooms, cooking and sewing classes, and gym classes. Students are to report the findings. In one week, the students return to the same classes and see if the hazard still exists.

Safety

Students are asked what they would do if the boat they were riding in stopped in the middle of the lake.

Proper Use

Students should bring in an appliance, tool, or other device and explain the proper use of it. They should also explain what could be done if something went wrong with the tool.

Phoning for Help

In many emergency situations, assistance can be obtained by telephoning the proper authority or agency. Stress the importance of knowing whom to call and what to say on the telephone. Have the students prepare a list of emergency telephone numbers, including those of the fire department, the poison control center, and so on. Then have them role play emergency situations. One student plays the part of the telephone operator or official. Another student then phones for help. Point out that information given over the telephone should be stated clearly and accurately. Let each student role play the part of an emergency caller at least once. Follow the activity with general discussion of proper use of the telephone.

Accident Pantomime

Assign various accident situations to individual students. These could include careless bike riding, improper use of tools or kitchen implements, and so forth. However, no props are used. Instead, each child must act out the behavior using mime techniques. The children should observe each performance and note how human error leads up to the "accident" that finally occurs.

The Hazard Family

Prepare a skit concerning the Hazard family—Harry and Harriet Hazard, and their four children Herbert, Honey, Hubert, and Hortense. This family just doesn't appreciate the benefits of safety. Mr. Hazard, for example, uses power tools without following safety procedures such as wearing safety glasses. Mrs. Hazard overloads electrical appliances. The children leave roller skates on the steps, play with matches, and so forth. Assign parts to students and have them act out the consequences of such hazardous behavior. Follow with a general discussion.

Safety Puppet Show

Have children make or use puppets to perform safety-related skits. Topics could include disaster situations, handling medical emergencies, fire safety, recreational safety, and safety in the home.

Commercials for Safety

Discuss public service safety messages that children may have seen on television. Then have students prepare individual 30-second or one-minute scripts that offer safety advice on specific safety hazards. Some children may want to work in small groups to dramatize the situation under discussion. Others may want to use props, such as an electrical appliance, to demonstrate a safety concept. Encourage imagination.

DISCUSSION AND REPORT TECHNIQUES

Safety Belt Debate

Choose two teams of students to research the use of seat belts in automobiles. One team should argue that wearing seat belts, even for short trips, can save lives and prevent needless injuries in case of an automobile accident. The other team should present reasons why many people don't bother or refuse to wear seat belts. Have the class decide which argument is more factually based.

Pedestrian Safety

Have two groups of students present panel discussions about pedestrian safety. The first group should emphasize the situation from the pedestrian's point of view, while the second group should discuss the problem from the driver's point of view. Follow with a general discussion that synthesizes the two points of view into one overall concept that pedestrians and drivers have mutual responsibilities and obligations toward each other.

Presentation by Safety Officials

Students select five representatives from the community to visit the class. Students are in charge of asking the officials to come. Officials could be fire, police, emergency personnel, etc.

Disaster Report

Students should contact a volunteer organization (such as Red Cross) and find out what services they offer in emergency situations.

Pedestrian Safety

Students write five rights and responsibilities of the pedestrian.

Accident Recall

Students talk about accidents that have happened to them in the past. The teacher writes down key words of the accident. The class then discusses how those accidents could have been prevented.

Individual Safety Reports

Students make a list of the unsafe practices in their home. Examples: items left on the staircase; oil slicks in the garage; and loose wires left lying around.

Safety Diary

Students should list the major holidays. Students make a list of accidents or safety hazards that occur more during that particular holiday. On another list the students write ways in which those accidents could be reduced or prevented.

EXPERIMENTS AND DEMONSTRATIONS

Tool Safety

Bring a variety of tools, appliances, and common implements to class and discuss the safe use of each. Demonstrate items that are appropriate to your age group. These might include scissors, knives, hand tools, small electrical appliances, gardening equipment, and kitchen equipment.

The Hug of Life

Demonstrate the proper use of the Heimlich maneuver if this knowledge is appropriate for your age group. Emphasize that you are only conducting a mock demonstration, and be careful not to apply too much pressure.

Resuscitation Annie

If you have a Resuscitation Annie model available, demonstrate the proper technique for mouth-to-mouth resuscitation. Contact your local chapter of the American Red Cross for assistance in presenting this demonstration.

First Aid Procedures

Each student should have bandages (or strips of cloth) and have a small first aid kit to work with. Create this case study: A person has been hurt. Give all the details and the students can explain or act out what they would do.

First Aid Kits

Each student makes her own first aid kit and brings it to class. Students should explain how they would use the items in their kits. They should explain what kind of accident or injury would require those items in their kit.

Fire Extinguishers

Students should be familiar with the operation of the extinguisher and able to use it if necessary. Students should be able to identify the different classes of extinguishers.

Class A—used for wood, paper, or textile fires
Class B—used for oil, grease, or paint fires
Class C—used on electrical equipment

Bicycle Safety

Have a general inspection of bicycles used by your children. Develop a checklist and use it to inspect each bicycle. Is the chain well-oiled and tight? Are the spokes straight and undamaged? Are the brakes in good working order? Does the bike have a light and a rear reflector? Is the seat properly adjusted for the rider? Are the tires in good shape and properly inflated? Suggest that repairs be done immediately if any bicycle is not in a safe condition.

Special Safety Equipment

Bring in, or have students bring in, various pieces of safety equipment used in different activities, including sports, games, home repair work, and industry. Items could include safety glasses or goggles, helmets, knee pads, gloves, masks, and dust masks. Demonstrate or discuss the use of each and explain how such equipment contributes to safety.

PUZZLES AND GAMES

Know Your Bike

Prepare a student worksheet as shown in figure 16.1. Have the students neatly cut out the parts of the puzzle and paste them in the correct order on a sheet of construc-

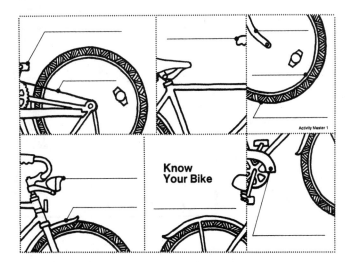

Figure 16.1
Bicycle safety puzzle worksheet.
Source: *A bicycle built for you*, U.S. Consumer Product Safety Commission, Washington, D.C.

tion paper. Next, ask the students to label the parts of the bicycle indicated. Afterwards, discuss the parts of a bicycle and the importance to safety of each part.

Spot the Hazards

Prepare a student worksheet as shown in figure 16.2. Before you distribute the worksheet, discuss the following poor bicycling habits:

1. Riding while wearing floppy, wide-leg pants: To avoid having pants fabric become entangled in a bicycle's moving parts, pants should be secured close to ankles with bicycle clips or rubber bands.
2. Riding double: A bike is built for one driver. A passenger reduces the driver's ability to control the bike and to see obstacles. Riding double is a leading cause of bike accidents.
3. Carrying large packages: A bicycle driver needs two hands to operate a bicycle safely. Any object that impairs vision or control is dangerous.
4. Turning without signalling: A bicycle driver who makes turns without signalling can cause accidents. Signalling helps others know where the bicyclist intends to drive his bike.

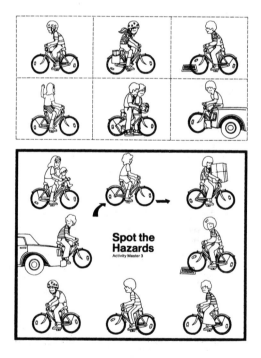

Figure 16.2
Spot the Hazards worksheet.
Source: *A bicycle built for you*, U.S. Consumer Product Safety Commission, Washington, D.C.

5. Driving on the wrong side of the road: Always drive with the flow of traffic (i.e. on the right side of the road), never against it. Bicycles are subject to the same rules of the road as cars.

6. Not watching out for obstacles: Drain grates, soft shoulders, loose sand or gravel, and potholes can cause loss of control. Bike drivers should be alert at all times.

Next, hand out the activity sheet. Instruct students to examine the illustrations and to find examples of the poor habits you have been discussing. Then ask students to cut out the "patches" at the top of the page and paste each patch over the appropriate portion of the picture to "correct" the picture. Discuss the corrected sheet.

Halloween Safety Crossword Puzzle

Discuss safe Halloween behavior before passing out the crossword puzzle shown in figure 16.3. Correct answers have been filled in.

Safety Slogan Puzzle

Prepare a safety slogan puzzle sheet as shown. Children should guess the correct answer to each clue and then write the word in the blanks. A safety slogan, as in this completed example, will result.

```
W A S T E B A S K E T
        B E D
    P O I S O N O U S
      L A D D E R
        F A L L
      H E L M E T
  C H I L D R E N
        S T O P
I N T E R S E C T I O N S
      M O U T H S
        C O R D S
    S T A I R W A Y S
    F L O O R S
      P L A Y G R O U N D
```

1. All litter should be deposited in the
2. No one should smoke in
3. Be alert for plants that are
4. When changing a light bulb, use a
5. Leaving toys on the stairs can cause a
6. Everyone who rides a motorcycle should wear a
7. Most home accidents happen to
8. When riding a bicycle, be sure to _____ at each intersection.
9. Many pedestrian accidents happen at
10. Many babies are poisoned because they put the wrong things in their
11. Electrical fires happen when _____ are frayed
12. Never leave shoes or books on
13. One cause of falls is cluttered
14. Always obey the rules of the game on the

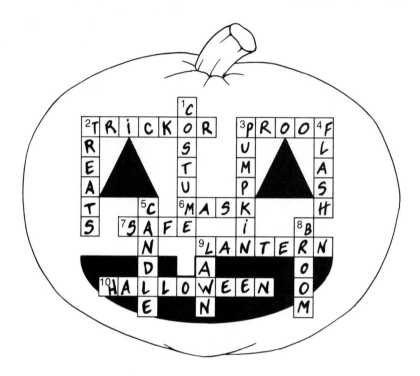

Across

2. " ? - ?-treat" with safety in mind!

3. Try to find a costume which is flame-resistant. But remember, even if labeled "Flame- ? ," a costume can still catch fire.

6. Make sure that this covering for the face has large eyeholes so you can see clearly.

7. This long strip will stick right on. Use the reflective kind to decorate costumes and make them "glow" in the dark.

9. A Jack-O- ? should be kept away from the door so no one trips over it.

10. This October holiday is a time for costumes, treats, and safety tricks.

Down

1. When you dress up in this disguise, make sure you can still move freely.

2. These collected goodies must be checked over before they are eaten.

3. Carve a face on this orange fellow, and light him safely with a flash-light.

4. Here's a kind of light that runs on batteries and helps trick-or-treaters to see in the dark.

5. This is made from wax and a wick and then lit with a flame, so it must be kept away from curtains and carpets and things that burn.

8. Witches ride this, people sweep with it, and kids move it off the stairs so that no one trips over it!

9. Better not run across this patch of grass around the house—clotheslines and statues are hard to see in the dark.

Figure 16.3
Halloween safety crossword puzzle.
Source: *Halloween safety: Teachers guide,* U.S. Consumer Product Safety Commission, Washington, D.C.

Safety Puzzle

Arrange the words in the right order.

			Answers
1.	FFTRAIC/GHTIL	a.	oil
2.	LMTEEH	b.	poisonous
3.	ESOKM	c.	smoke
4.	CCIAENSTD	d.	traffic light
5.	OISPNOUSO	e.	first aid
6.	RAC	f.	safety
7.	LOI	g.	car
8.	GNEINE	h.	helmet
9.	GGGLESO	i.	home
10.	STYAFE	j.	engine
11.	MHOE	k.	accident
12.	RSTIF/DIA	l.	goggles

BULLETIN BOARDS

Pool Safety

Discuss safety when swimming in a pool. Note the potential danger of running alongside the pool because of the slippery surface, the hazards of diving when others may be under the board, and so on. Have each student prepare a drawing that can be used as a bulletin board display showing how these dangers can be minimized or prevented.

Hazards Collage

Have the students search through old magazines to find pictures that represent possible safety risks. For example, a person walking in the woods might encounter poisonous plants or a poisonous snake. The pictures do not have to show obvious hazards, but each child's choice of a picture should suggest some hazard to that child. Have the students make a collage from the entire set of pictures. Then have them try to guess which hazards are suggested by each picture in the collage. If any picture stumps the class, have the student who chose that picture explain the safety risk involved. Encourage subtlety in picture choice, pointing out that potential hazards in the environment are not always obvious either.

First Aid Posters

Assign a particular first aid procedure to each student. Then have the students prepare posters illustrating the correct method of providing that aid in the accident situation.

Safety Slogans

Ask each student to come up with his or her own safety slogan, such as "Playing baseball means getting to first base safely." Have the class vote for the three best slogans. Then prepare a bulletin board display illustrating each one.

Traffic Accidents

Students are to cut out pictures or articles from their newspaper on traffic accidents. Students put these pictures on the bulletin board. The class then discusses the pictures.

Sports

Students are to list some of the sports they play. Opposite the sports they are to write the potential hazards of participation in that sport. Example: Football—broken bones, knee injuries

OTHER IDEAS

Fire Escape Plans

Ask students to draw a basic plan showing the layout of their residences. Have the students discuss a fire evacuation route and an alternate route with their parents, and then ask them to show these routes on their drawings, using different colored arrows for the two routes. Each student should be able to explain why the routes are the best ones to use in case of a home fire.

Traffic Safety Obstacle Course

Set up a simulated "obstacle course" on the playground illustrating such traffic hazards as busy intersections, unmarked intersections, and so on. Mark each potentially hazardous part of the course with traffic safety signs, including speed limit signs, yield signs, and pedestrian signals. Have some children go through the course on their bicycles, while others play the part of pedestrians. Discuss the importance of following traffic safety signs, signals, and regulations.

Field Trips

If feasible, take the class on a field trip to the local fire station or other safety agency outlet. Prepare the class thoroughly for what they will see and have them write down a list of questions they wish to ask those in charge.

Fires

Students should make a list of five reasons how fires start and at what time of the day they usually start.

Speakers

Ask a state highway patrol or city police officer to talk to the class about why traffic accidents happen.

17. Alcohol, Tobacco, and Drugs

. . . . Now I know that drug abuse problems are not so mysterious or special, except sometimes in the ways they work themselves out in people's lives. . . . Drug abuse prevention depends on many things, but it seems to me that primarily it depends on helping people work things out without turning to artificial experiences or supports. People can help people best, if they learn how to relate effectively, interact compassionately and honestly, and draw strength from the relationships they build with each other. . . . The first step towards drug abuse prevention is not much of a step at all, and it is everything. It is the hand that reaches out to touch another.—Art Linkletter, *Questions and Answers About Drug Abuse*

SUBSTANCE USE AND ABUSE

For many people, the word *drug* is an emotionally charged term associated with such substances as heroin, marijuana, and LSD. These substances are drugs, of course, but so are antibiotics, aspirin, the caffeine in a cup of coffee, and the alcohol in a glass of table wine. All of these substances have in common the ability to bring about a change in bodily functioning, and that is the definition of a drug (Lingeman, 1969).

Drugs can either be used or abused. For example, a tranquilizer taken under a physician's orders can help to combat stress in a specific situation. However, if a person relies on tranquilizers as an emotional crutch, use turns into abuse. In the same way, many people enjoy a glass of wine with a meal, but drinking a gallon of wine a day constitutes abuse.

To some degree the difference between use and abuse is a value judgment. More objectively, drug abuse can be defined as the ingestion of any substance that leads to deleterious effects, either physically, psychologically, or both.

Drug education is one of the more controversial aspects of health education. There are many differences of opinion as to how the subject should be approached. In fact, some parents would prefer that the subject not be approached at all.

In this chapter, we will examine those substances that are commonly abused or misused. Some of them, such as alcohol and tobacco, have little or no therapeutic value but can be purchased by adults for their personal use. Over-the-counter drugs, such as cough medicines, can have beneficial effects when used carefully. Because many individuals wrongly consider these drugs to be essentially harmless, however, misuse and abuse are common. Prescription drugs, such as tranquilizers, are more closely controlled, but these substances are also widely abused. Finally, we shall look at illegal substances, such as heroin, hallucinogens, and marijuana.

Reasons for Drug Abuse

Individuals misuse or abuse drugs for a variety of reasons. Young people are especially likely to do so for the following reasons:

Low Self-Esteem.   Many individuals have poor opinions of themselves. By using drugs, these individuals attempt to avoid coming to grips with their own feelings of inadequacy. Drugs thus serve as a coping mechanism.

Peer Pressure.   Particularly during adolescence, individuals have a strong need to belong to "the group." If peers are abusing drugs, there is strong pressure on the part of all members of the group to do likewise.

Adult Modeling.   Young people want to feel grown up and view drug-taking as a form of adult behavior to be emulated. Smoking tobacco or marijuana, drinking alcohol, or taking pills may all result from adult modeling.

Mood Alteration.   Some people take drugs simply to change their psychological state. The mellow feeling or the excitement produced is the motivation for this behavior.

Boredom and Curiosity.   Many young people, especially during the teenage years, are at loose ends about their place in society. The activities of childhood no longer interest them, but they are not yet able to engage in adult activities. As a result, they feel bored with life. At the same time, they are curious about new experiences. They want to try something different, and "experimentation" with drugs may follow.

Alienation.   Some individuals feel that they have little or no power to control their destiny. They may also feel unwanted and unloved. Often, such individuals have few friends and view themselves as misfits in society. Drugs provide an outlet for the expression of such feelings of alienation.

EFFECTS OF DRUGS ON THE BODY*

Drugs are chemicals that work in predictable patterns. First, a drug either mimics, facilitates, or antagonizes the body's normally occurring functions. Second, a drug can have one of four effects on a cell: it can increase activitiy, decrease activity, increase sensitivity, or disrupt the cell so that normal activity is sporadic. Third, the effect obtained from a drug depends on the concentration of the drug at the site of the

---

*This section is taken from *Health* by Michael Hamrick, David Anspaugh, and Gene Ezell (Columbus: Merrill, 1986).

action (Ray, 1983). The effects of drugs result from their biochemical actions. This action depends both on the drug reaching the desired site and on the body's chemistry. Other factors include the route of administration, distribution, dosage, expectations of the user, and frequency of use.

Route of Administration

Drugs can be taken orally in the form of pills, capsules, or liquids. They may be injected *intravenously* (directly into the bloodstream through a vein), *intramuscularly* (injected into a muscle), or *subcutaneously* (under the skin). Another method of administering a drug is *topical administration,* which is the application of the drug to the skin or mucous membranes.

The faster a drug reaches its intended site, the more quickly the intended effect can take place. The fastest, yet most dangerous method is intravenous injection, since their risk of infection, vein collapse, or overdose is extremely high. Overdose is a significant problem because chemicals can enter the circulatory system so rapidly. Intramuscular injection works most rapidly in the deltoid muscle and least rapidly in the buttocks since the poorest blood supply is found in the buttocks. Subcutaneous injection can be extremely irritating to the tissue. Topical administration is usually short acting and may damage the skin or mucous membranes since this form of administering a chemical can serve as an irritant. A danger of taking a drug orally is that the liver may metabolize the drug so quickly that the chemical is not in the bloodstream long enough to be effective.

Distribution

Drugs are carried to body parts through the bloodstream. Some drugs are absorbed and then excreted quickly. Asprin is an example of a drug that is excreted within a few hours. Other drugs are cumulative and are excreted very slowly. It may take several days to build up the level of the drug in the body to produce the desired therapeutic effect. Once built up, only maintenance doses are needed to maintain the drug's level. Certain heart medications are of this type.

Dosage

This is the amount of a drug given and serves to determine the effect of the drug on the body. The term to describe this is *dose-response relationship*. The larger the amount taken, the greater the probability of several different effects. The *threshold dose* is the minimum amount required to produce a therapeutic effect. The dose in which maximum effect is obtained is called the *maximum dose*. The *effective dose* is the dose needed to produce a desired effect. A *lethal dose* is the amount that will produce death. The ratio between the effective dose and the lethal dose is the therapeutic index. This is obtained by dividing the amount of a lethal dose by the amount required for an effective dose. The higher the index, the lower the chance of a given dosage being lethal.

Another important concept concerning dosage is the *potency,* or the difference in effective doses between drugs that are used for the same purpose. For example, drug

A may require twice the dosage to achieve the same effect as drug B. Therefore drug B is a more potent drug. The time required for the drug to produce an effect after the body receives it is called the *time-action response*. As a general rule, the more quickly an effect appears, the shorter its effectiveness. The presence of other drugs can produce what is called *synergism*, or an effect that neither drug could produce when used alone. For example, some drugs *potentiate* or increase the effect of another drug. The effect of one drug may be enhanced because of specific enzymes, or formation of more potent metabolites, or for unknown reasons. It is frightening that pesticides, traces of hormones in meat and poultry, traces of metals in fish, nitrites, nitrates, and a wide range of chemicals used as food additives have been shown to interact with and potentiate some drugs. The classic example of dangerous potentiation is that a safe dose of alcohol mixed with a safe dose of a barbiturate can become lethal by causing repressed respiration.

Expectations of User

The mood of the user and the setting in which the drug is taken may also effect the reaction to the drug. If we expect the drug to help us or produce an effect, then the probability of that effect is greater. The effect may occur even when the substance administered is only a *placebo*. The placebo effect is quite common. If the environment is such that results are expected from the drug, then the desired behavior will probably occur. Friends, soft lights, and music may help create an environmental setting for particular drug effects. In addition, placebos are often effective against pain. This effect was not understood until the endorphins and enkephalins were discovered. Both are peptides produced by the body and have an action similar to morphine. Enkephalins were first isolated from the brain and endorphins from the pituitary gland. Reserarch has shown that endorphins and enkephalins alleviate pain. Physicians are just beginning to realize the importance of the mind in controlling disease and pain, but it is clear that placebos can affect the release of biochemical substances already present in the body if the mind believes a desired effect can be achieved.

Frequency of Use

A general rule is that when some drugs are used frequently, larger dosages are required to maintain the effect. This is called *tolerance*. There are several forms of tolerance: disposition tolerance, cross-tolerance, parmacodynamic tolerance, and reverse tolerance. Disposition tolerance refers to the rate at which the body disposes of a drug. Certain drugs tend to increase the rate of action enzymes in the liver and consequently the deactivating of the drug. Alcohol and barbiturates are examples of drugs that cause the liver to produce the metabolic enzymes. Another important point is that these enzymes are not very discriminating; therefore, tolerance to one drug may lead to tolerance of other drugs that are pharmacologically similar. This effect is called cross-tolerance. Usually a heavy drinker will exhibit tolerance to barbiturates, tranquilizers, and anesthetics.

Evidence indicates that a considerable degree of central nervous system tolerance to certain drugs may develop independent of changes in the rate of absorption, metabolism, or excretion. This is called pharmacodynamic tolerance, whereby the nervous tissue or other target tissue adapt to the drug so that the effect of the same concentration of a chemical decreases. In the case of reverse tolerance, users will have the same response to a lower dose of a drug that they had with initial higher doses. Reverse tolerance is believed to be primarily a learning process and does not result from a physiological response. However, it is possible for some drugs, such as marijuana, to be stored in the fat cells and released later as the fat cells are broken down. The fact that drug products remain in the body for extended periods of time may account for some of the reverse tolerance effect (AMA Council on Scientific Affairs, 1981). Usually, tolerance to a drug that requires increasing amounts of a chemical to maintain normal body functioning will lead to a physical dependence. Some drugs, such as aspirin, cause neither tolerance nor dependence. *Psychological dependence,* or habituation, occurs when taking a drug becomes a habit and there is a feeling of satisfaction or psychic drive that requires repeated administration of the drug to produce an effect or avoid discomfort (World Health Organization, 1964). *Addiction* is a term that has various meanings. It is sometimes used interchangeably with dependence, either physiological or psychological, yet at other times appears to be synonymous with drug abuse. The model of addiction-producing drugs is based on the opiates, which require the development of tolerance, along with physical and psychological dependence. Opiates, alcohol, and barbiturates are examples that fit the traditional addiction model.

ALCOHOL

Ethyl alcohol is the active ingredient in beer, wine, and distilled beverages such as whiskey. Ethyl alcohol is not highly toxic as are some other forms of the chemical, such as methyl alcohol, used as rubbing alcohol. In this discussion, we will use the term *alcohol* to refer to ethyl alcohol.

Alcohol is a colorless, flammable liquid formed by the fermentation of fruits, juices, or cereal grains. Alcoholic beverages contain varying amounts of alcohol, depending upon the type of beverage. Beer usually contains from 5 to 7 percent alcohol. Wines may vary from 11 to 20 percent. Distilled beverages have the highest alcohol content. This content is measured by the proof of the beverage, which is a number that is twice the alcohol content. For example, a 100 proof whiskey contains 50 percent alcohol, while a 90 proof one contains 45 percent.

Effects of Alcohol

Alcohol is a central nervous system depressant. In small doses, the drug has a mellowing or tranquilizing effect. The individual may feel relaxed and free from tension. As a result, behavior may become less inhibited, leading to the misconception held by some that alcohol is a stimulant. Actually, what appears to be stimulated, or at least animated, behavior results from the anesthetic, depressant effect that alcohol has on the cerebral cortex area of the brain.

In large amounts, alcohol impairs brain activity, muscular control, coordination, memory, reaction time, and judgment. Heavy intake over a short period of time can

Table 17.1
Effects of Alcohol on the Body

Percentage in bloodstream	Effects
0.05	Careless behavior; Some loss of self-control; Some loss of judgment
0.10	Poor judgment; Greater loss of self-control; Serious loss of coordination
0.20	Very drunk; Slurred speech; Staggers when walking
0.40	Unconsciousness—passes out
0.70	Death occurs

bring about a dulling of the senses. Continued heavy drinking can result in coma and death. Table 17.1 summarizes the effects of alcohol by percentage in the blood-stream.

Consumption of alcohol over a long period of time can result in damage to the brain and liver. The brain may be damaged to the extent that memory, judgment, and learning deteriorate. Cirrhosis of the liver is a fatal condition caused by damage to that organ by alcohol.

Recently, the harmful effects of even moderate amounts of alcohol consumed by pregnant women have become known. The alcohol can have a deleterious effect on the developing fetus, resulting in a condition known as *fetal alcohol syndrome*. A child born with this condition may suffer permanent impairment. Characteristics of the condition include low birth weight, abnormal formation of the nose, small finger-nails, poor joint movement, ear abnormalities, and mental retardation.

In moderation, alcohol does not seem to permanently harm the body. However, if an adult decides to partake of alcoholic beverages, care should be exercised. Alcohol should be consumed slowly, with adequate food in the stomach. Individuals should also recognize that tolerance to alcohol builds up. More of the drug may be required to produce the pleasant, mellow effect associated with its use. Drinking without recognizing the potential dangers of alcohol can lead to tragedy.

Who Drinks?

Consumption of alcohol in the United States is widespread. An estimated 77 percent of adult males and 66 percent of adult females regularly drink alcoholic beverages (Ray, 1978). The total number of drinkers in the United States is estimated at 96 million, with each drinker consuming an average of four gallons of alcohol per year (Hafen, 1977). Not only adults drink. By grade 7, 63 percent of boys and 54 percent of girls have tried alcoholic beverages. By grade 12, 93 percent of boys and 87 percent of girls have tried alcohol (HEW, 1974, p. 9).

Drinking and Accidents

Alcohol is involved in 50 percent or more of all fatal traffic accidents. Without question, drinking and driving don't mix. Nearly 8,000 teenagers are killed each year in accidents involving alcohol. It is estimated that another 40,000 teenagers are disfigured each year in accidents involving alcohol. Young people are especially at risk from alcohol-related accidents because of their low tolerance to the drug.

Alcoholism and Alcohol-Related Problems

The misuse of alcohol can lead to many personal and social problems. One of these is alcoholism. Definitions of this term vary from source to source. In general, an alcoholic can be described as a person who is unable to choose whether he or she will drink and is unable to stop drinking. Alcoholics use the drug in such a way that their personal, social, and occupational behavior is interfered with or totally disrupted.

The common image of an alcoholic is that of a skid row derelict. In actual fact, however, only 5 percent of alcoholics are skid row types. The other 95 percent come from all walks of life and include businesspeople, physicians, teachers, ministers, homemakers, politicians, factory workers, musicians, police officers, and retired people. Both rich and poor, young and old, are susceptible. As many as 10 million Americans have a serious drinking problem.

Health Highlight: Facts on Alcoholism

Alcohol is America's favorite recreational drug. It is also the nation's number one drug of abuse. Alcohol is a mood changer, as are tranquilizers, heroin, cocaine, barbiturates, and amphetamines. The chronic alcoholic is physically and psychologically addicted.

In 1956, alcoholism was recognized by the American Medical Association as a disease with identifiable and progressive symptoms. This position is endorsed by the American Hospital Association, the American Bar Association, the American Psychiatric Association, and the World Health Organization. Of all male admissions to state mental hospitals, 52 percent suffer from alcohol-related problems. There are an estimated 12 million alcoholic persons in America today. Of the 100 million persons in this country who drink, one in ten is prone to alcoholism.

Alcoholism is one of the top three killer diseases, along with cancer and heart disease. Persons afflicted with alcoholism are sick, as are people who suffer from heart disease or cancer. If not treated, alcoholism ends in permanent mental damage, physical incapacity, or early death. The average alcoholic is in his or her 40s with a responsible job and a family. Fewer than 5 percent of all alcoholics are found on Skid Row. Around 95 percent are employed or employable, like many people you see every day.

About 50 percent of all fatal accidents occurring on the roads involve alcohol, and half of these involve an alcoholic. Alcoholism involves both sexes and crosses all ethnic, religious, economic and sociocultural groups. While there are as many women alcoholics as there are men, only 25 percent of the women receive treatment.

About 31 percent of those who take their own lives are alcoholics. The suicide rate among alcoholics is 58 times that of the general population. Alcoholism costs the nation $54.1 billion annually. Industry alone picks up a $25.2 billion tab for lost work time, health and welfare service benefits, property damage, medical expenses, and overhead costs of insurance and wage losses. Around 80 percent of all violence in the American home is alcohol-related. Children of alcoholic parents are 50 percent more likely to marry an alcoholic person. Alcoholism is a treatable disease.

Education, early detection, and community treatment facilities are the greatest forces operating today for the control and reduction of alcoholism. Prevention and intervention through programs of information and education have been primary objectives of the National Council on Alcoholism since its founding in 1944.

Source: From material published by the National Institute on Alcohol Abuse and Alcoholism (NIAAA) 1977–1978.

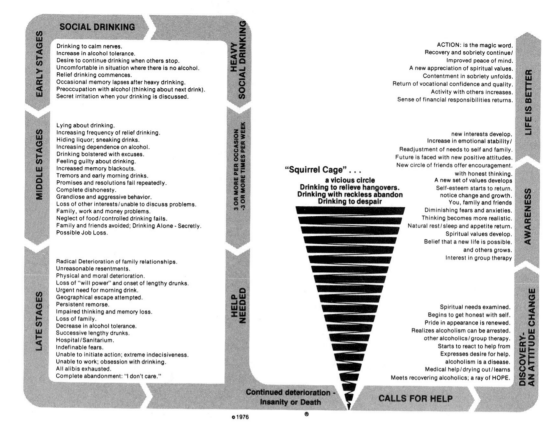

Figure 17.1
Alcoholism and recovery.

Alcoholism is considered to be a disease. The causes of alcoholism are not completely understood, but Ray (1978) notes:

> It is fairly well accepted now that there is a genetic component, a predisposition to alcohol addiction. The exact nature of the contribution from heredity is not known, but some of the relevant evidence is very suggestive.

Regardless of how important the heredity factor is, social and psychological factors also influence the development of alcoholism. Because alcohol use is generally accepted in our society, many individuals feel free to use it. Too often however, use leads to misuse and alcoholism is the result. The drug becomes a crutch for dealing with everyday problems until the individual can no longer get along without it.

Alcohol-related problems are all too well known in our society. Aside from the thousands of traffic deaths and injuries that occur each year because of alcohol abuse, alcohol is also related to the high divorce rate, job absenteeism, crimes of violence, suicide, and social disorder.

Treatment of Alcoholism

Alcoholism, like many other diseases, can be treated successfully. There are three phases to any program that seeks to help the alcoholic. The first phase is *detoxification*. This involves helping the individual withdraw from the drug. The second phase is *treatment*. This involves helping the alcoholic work through personal problems, build greater self-esteem, learn more effective methods for coping with life, and stop destructive drinking. The third phase is *aftercare*. This involves helping the alcoholic stay sober. Alcoholics can never return to even social drinking or they will fall back into their devastating former lifestyle. Figure 17.1 outlines the progress of alcoholism and the steps necessary for recovery.

Alcoholics and their families can receive help from many sources, including such nonprofit groups as Alcoholics Anonymous. Al-Anon and Al-Ateen are groups specifically established to assist the families of alcoholics. There are also many commercial alcoholic treatment programs. These can be expensive, but many insurance companies now pay for such treatment.

TOBACCO

Tobacco has been known and used for hundreds of years. It can be snuffed, chewed, placed between the gum and lips, or smoked. The most popular method of tobacco use is smoking. Cigarettes became popular in the early 1900s. Before then, tobacco was usually chewed or smoked in a pipe.

Cigarettes were provided free to soldiers in both World Wars I and II. This only served to help further or start the tobacco habit. Although the dangers of tobacco smoking are now much better known, an estimated 42 percent of adult men and 31 percent of adult women still smoke. Teenage girls constitute the fastest growing group of smokers.

Effects of Tobacco Smoking

The primary drug in tobacco is nicotine. A typical filter cigarette contains between 1 and 2 mg of nicotine, with about 90 percent of this amount being absorbed when inhaled.

Smoking results in the constriction of the blood vessels, which decreases the skin temperature. Nicotine acts as a stimulant on the heart and nervous system, causing an increased heart beat and elevated blood pressure. In addition, the blood decreases in its ability to carry oxygen because of the carbon monoxide in tobacco smoke, which is more easily picked up by hemoglobin.

Cigarette smoke also contains chemicals known collectively as *tars*. These substances have been identified as *carcinogens,* or cancer-causing agents. Smoking is a major cause of lung cancer and may contribute to other forms of malignancies as well.

Smokers run not only an increased risk of developing cancer, but they also have much higher rates of coronary heart disease. *Emphysema*, a breathing disorder that results from deterioration of lung tissue, is also associated with cigarette smoking, as are many other respiratory diseases. Russell, Taylor, and Law (1969) report that smoking during pregnancy increases by 200 to 300 percent the chance of having a premature or stillborn baby or of having the fetus abort.

In 1979, the U.S. Surgeon General released a comprehensive report on smoking and health (HEW, 1979). The report noted that cigarette smokers spend a third more of their time away from their jobs because of illnesses than do nonsmokers. Women who smoke are sick in bed 17 percent more often than women nonsmokers. The death rate of all age groups is almost 70 percent higher for cigarette smokers than for nonsmokers.

Although cigarette smokers run the highest risk, use of tobacco in other forms can also lead to serious problems. For example, pipe smoking is related to cancer of the lip. Both pipe and cigar smokers run a higher risk of developing cancer of the mouth, larynx, and esophagus. Snuff dippers have a higher incidence of cancer of the gums than do nonusers.

Why People Smoke

Individuals begin smoking for some of the same reasons that apply to drinking. Adult modeling and peer pressure are certainly factors. The appeal produced by cigarette advertising also plays a part. According to Horn (1973), once a person has developed a smoking habit, one or more of the following reasons may apply:

Stimulation. Smokers claim that smoking helps wake them up, organize their intellectual activity, and enhance their energy level.

Relaxation. Smokers say that smoking helps promote and enhance pleasant feelings. Smokers also believe that smoking reduces negative feelings.

Crutch. Smokers use cigarettes in times of stress or personal discomfort. Smoking is seen as a tranquilizer, again helping to reduce negative feelings.

Handling. Smoking gives the individual something to occupy his or her hands. Handling the cigarette is satisfying in itself.

Craving. The smoker is dependent upon cigarettes; there is a psychological and possibly physical dependence upon cigarettes.

Habit. Smoking is done simply out of habit, although the smoker gets very little pleasure from smoking. The person may have minimal awareness of the act of smoking, sometimes lighting one cigarette while another one is still burning.

Reducing the Hazards of Smoking

The best way to avoid the hazards of smoking is simply not to smoke. This means not beginning in the first place or giving up the habit if smoking has already begun. Individuals who smoke should also recognize the possible harmful effects of "second-hand" smoke upon others. Inhaling smoke produced by a smoker can aggravate respiratory conditions and may even be the cause of such conditions in a nonsmoker.

Those who refuse to stop the smoking habit can lower the risk they run by choosing a brand of cigarettes with less tar and nicotine, by smoking fewer cigarettes, by taking fewer puffs and not inhaling so deeply, and by not smoking the cigarette all the way down to the end.

OVER-THE-COUNTER DRUGS

Drugs that can be purchased without a prescription and that are used for self-medication are called *over-the-counter* (OTC) drugs. There are thousands of OTC drugs. These include aspirin and other analgesics, cold remedies, antihistimines and allergy products, vitamins, laxatives, antacids, and mild sedatives.

Most OTC drugs are somewhat effective in relieving the symptoms of the mild illnesses and disorders for which they were developed, as long as they are used according to directions. However, despite regulation by the Federal Trade Commission and other government agencies, advertising claims for many OTC products are often misleadingly optimistic. As a result, when the product fails to produce instant relief, some individuals may be tempted to exceed the recommended dosage in hopes of additional or faster aid. This sort of misuse can create health hazards.

Individuals should also recognize that there is some risk involved in using *any* medication, including aspirin, even when the directions are carefully followed. First, there is a possibility of allergic reaction. In rare cases, such reaction can be fatal. Second, relief provided by an OTC drug may mask symptoms of another illness or underlying disorder. For this reason, self-medication should only be attempted when the problem is minor and obvious, as in the case of a mild cold.

Another risk in using OTC drugs comes from the phenomenon called *synergism.* If two or more drugs or medications are taken at the same time, one substance can cause an increase or decrease in the potency of another. This synergistic reaction can have harmful and even fatal results.

As with any drugs, OTC drugs can have a stronger effect on children than on adults. Recently, for example, children's aspirin, formerly thought to be safe, has been identified as a cause of a severe reaction that can lead to death under certain conditions.

DEPRESSANTS

Drugs that slow down, inhibit, or depress the nervous system are classified as depressants. The most commonly used depressant drug is alcohol. There are dozens of other depressants, most of which are prescription drugs. Whether obtained legally or illegally, however, depressants are among the most common of misused and abused drugs.

Depressant drugs have four main effects on the body. As *sedatives,* they can produce relaxation. As *tranquilizers,* they can reduce anxiety and act as muscle relaxants. As *hypnotics,* they can promote sleep. As *anesthetics,* they can create a loss of sensation. Various depressant drugs differ in their potencies, but in sufficient amounts they can all produce these four effects.

The sedative-hypnotics include barbiturates and tranquilizers. Examples of barbiturates by trade name include Amytal, Nembutal, and Seconal. Commonly prescribed tranquilizers include Valium, Librium, and Miltown. Both of these types of drugs are usually taken orally, although some can be given intravenously as a general anesthetic.

Barbiturates

Barbiturates represent one of the nation's biggest drug abuse problems. Generally known as "downers," barbiturates are often taken as a way of escaping from the problems of daily living. Abusers of this type of drug "fog out" and feel removed from the cares of existence. The potency of such drugs is increased by combining them with alcoholic intake, which often results in fatal overdoses that cause cardiorespiratory failure. More commonly, barbiturate abuse results in mental confusion, dizziness, and loss of memory.

Barbiturates are highly addictive and physical as well as psychological dependency can quickly develop. Withdrawal from barbiturate dependency can be life-threatening and should be done under close medical supervision.

Tranquilizers

Tranquilizers are classified as major and minor. The major tranquilizers, such as Thorazine, are used to treat psychosis. Minor tranquilizers, such as Valium and Librium, are prescribed for stress and anxiety. They are also useful as muscle relaxants. However, partly because they are so widely prescribed, such tranquilizers are often abused. Physical and psychological dependency can result. Symptoms of physical dependency include drowsiness and slurred speech. Psychological dependency may be characterized by increased irritability and irrational fear. As in the case of barbiturates, withdrawal from tranquilizers can be highly traumatic.

Cross Tolerance

Tolerance to depressant drugs can be developed fairly quickly. Then higher and higher doses of the drug must be taken to produce the desired relaxing effect. Tolerance to one kind of depressant drug also produces tolerance to other types that are not even being taken. This phenomenon is known as *cross tolerance*. The danger of cross tolerance may not be as obvious to drug abusers as it should be. Once tolerance to one depressant drug has developed, the individual may decide to switch to another depressant in hopes of achieving the same desired effect. However, because of cross tolerance, the outcome is not as hoped. A higher dose may them be resorted to. If the new drug is more potent, a fatal overdose may result.

NARCOTICS

Narcotic drugs are produced for the most part from opium and its derivatives, although some are synthesized substances. Such drugs act on the central nervous system and gastrointestinal tract. They are excellent painkillers, but they can be highly physically and psychologically addictive.

Opium is derived from the opium poppy. Morphine, codeine, and heroin also come from this source. Of these drugs, only codeine is much used for medicinal purposes today. It is used to kill pain and to suppress coughing. Morphine is still used as a painkiller, although to a lesser extent than in years past because of the danger of addiction involved.

Heroin is one of the most dangerous drugs abused. Much heroin is produced illegally in foreign countries in Asia and smuggled into the United States. The drug can be smoked, swallowed, injected under the skin, or injected directly into a vein. The latter method is used most often by heroin addicts because the drug reaches the bloodstream most quickly this way.

The desired effect is a sudden rush of euphoria, followed by a dreamy state of complete relaxation. This period may last up to several hours, depending upon a variety of factors including the strength of the dosage. "Street" heroin is always sold in an adulterated state, usually mixed with milk sugar so that the actual percentage of heroin is small.

Although considered physiologically "clean," in the sense that it does not damage organs, heroin is extremely addictive, and a user soon may live for no other reason than to inject more heroin. Tolerance also quickly develops, leading to a need for higher and higher or more frequent doses of the drug. The result is too often a fatal overdose, which results in death because of cardiorespiratory failure.

Withdrawal from heroin is agonizing. It is characterized by chills, fever, diarrhea, and vomiting. However, painful though it is, heroin withdrawal is seldom life-threatening. Still, most heroin addicts, even when they would like to quit, find it almost impossible to do so because of the craving they have developed for the drug.

The dangers from heroin use are manifold. Aside from weight loss, lethargy, sexual inadequacy, and the constant problems of withdrawal that require regular doses of the drug, injection of heroin can lead to other health problems, including hepatitis and AIDS due to dirty needles and anemia due to disregard for proper nutrition. Toxic adulterants in heroin sold on the street can also kill.

Heroin was once considered to be a drug used only by the socially desperate, for whom no price was too much for a chance of psychological escape. However, more and more middle-class individuals have been using the drug in recent years, perhaps with the feeling that they have the socioeconomic options to experiment with heroin in relative safety. This is a sad and dangerous misconception.

STIMULANTS

Stimulants are drugs that stimulate, or speed up the nervous system. Physiologically, the stimulant drugs increase heart rate, blood pressure, and amount of blood sugar. They also constrict the blood vessels and dilate bronchial tubes and the pupils of the eyes. Some can produce a temporary euphoria.

Caffeine

The most common stimulant is caffeine, which is contained in coffee, tea, cola drinks, and even chocolate. Caffeine is a mild stimulant that is often abused. Nonetheless, it is a drug and should be recognized as one that can lead to health problems.

Caffeine is absorbed rather quickly into the bloodstream and reaches a peak blood level in about 30 to 60 minutes. It increases mental alertness and provides a greater feeling of energy. However, high doses of caffeine can overstimulate and cause nervousness and increased heart rate. Caffeine can also cause sleeplessness, excitement, and irritability. In some cases, high doses of caffeine can induce convulsions.

Coffee or cola drinking, let alone chocolate eating, cannot be considered drug abuse by most commonly accepted standards, but some individuals seek out caffeine for its own sake, in OTC products and in illegal substances, to produce a caffeine "high." Because it is not considered a dangerous drug, the opportunities for caffeine abuse are often overlooked.

Amphetamines

Amphetamines represent more serious stimulant drug abuse problems. These drugs have limited legitimate and useful medical applications, but because of their wide availability they are often abused. Examples of commonly prescribed amphetamines include Benzadrine, Dexadrine, Methadrine, Ritalin, and Narodin. Because of the possibility of dependency, the uncertainty of side effects, and the questionable nature of some applications, use of amphetamines has come under closer scrutiny in the last few years. For example, although amphetamines do suppress hunger, they are no longer recommended as "diet pills" by most doctors. Treatment of hyperactive children with Ritalin, which curiously seems to act as the opposite of a stimulant among such individuals, has also been called into question.

Still, stimulant drugs are fairly easy to obtain, and this has resulted in continued drug abuse problems. The general street name for such drugs is "speed," because of the way these substances seem to speed up the nervous system. Amphetamine pills are also known as "uppers." Abusers of amphetamines pass into an extremely excited state and may feel omnipotent until the drug begins to wear off. A depressed period, called a "crash" by abusers, then follows, leading to a craving for more amphetamines.

As with many drugs, a craving for amphetamines often undermines a person's regard for good personal health practices. Because appetite is inhibited by such drugs, poor nutrition leading to weight loss often results. An amphetamine user soon becomes a physical wreck, often looking five or more years older than is the case (Pawiak, 1976).

There is debate as to whether amphetamines result in true physical dependency, but there is no doubt that strong psychological dependency soon develops. Long-term use of these drugs can result in heart, liver, and kidney damage. Speech problems and facial twitches may also be apparent. In high doses, amphetamines can cause hallucinations, delusions, and disorganized bahavior.

Withdrawal from amphetamines is not life-threatening, but the process does result in depression and anxiety. Professional treatment is often necessary.

Cocaine

Known on the street as "snow" or "coke," cocaine is an expensive illegal drug that produces strong psychological, if not physical, dependency. It is taken to produce a feeling of euphoria and boundless energy, which it often does. The drug, which is in the form of a white powder, is usually sniffed directly up the nostrils, where it enters the bloodstream through the nasal membranes. Its effect is first to anesthetize the nerves of the nose, then to relax the bronchial muscles and increase the heart rate and blood pressure. Mental awareness and euphoria then result as the drug reaches the brain, but the effects of cocaine are short-lasting, usually wearing off in 10 to 15 minutes.

Tolerance to cocaine develops quickly, so that higher and higher doses are often necessary to produce the desired effect. Very high doses can cause toxic psychosis. Overdose can result in respiratory failure, convulsions, and death. Even if such extremes are avoided, chronic users often develop holes in the nasal septum caused by damage to tissue resulting from lack of oxygen.

Cocaine was until recently thought of as an "upper class" drug because of its high price. However, the drug is now more readily available, and, consequently, more and more people have tried it.

When heated to high temperatures, a refined, purer form of cocaine results. This process is called free-basing, and the mixture that results is smoked in a water pipe. The vapors from the process are inhaled and results are immediate. The free-base mixture is highly explosive, and people have been seriously injured from this preparation of the drug.

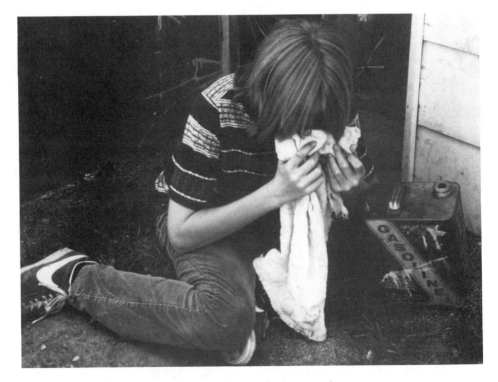

Inhalants are one of the most dangerous forms of substance abuse.

INHALANTS

If cocaine is the drug of the affluent adult, then the inhalants must be seen as the drug of children with little money to spend. An incredible variety of substances can be inhaled to produce a drug "high," including toluene-based glues (plastic cements), gasoline, paint products, and various aerosols. Claims of liver, brain, and bone and blood cell damage from abuse of such products seem to have been exaggerated, but the dangers of inhalation abuse are still very real.

Because a great deal of the inhalant is often required to produce the desired mood-changing effect, some abusers will put a plastic bag over their heads to concentrate the fumes while inhaling. Unconsciousness that may result from inhalation can be fatal because of the plastic bag. Even without such practices, inhalation can result in heart stoppage and lung collapse. The oily base of some inhalants can coat the lungs and prohibit the exchange of gases.

HALLUCINOGENS

Hallucinogens are substances that occur naturally or are produced synthetically that distort the perception of reality. Such drugs cause sensory illusion that makes it difficult to distinguish fact from fantasy.

Perhaps the most widely known hallucinogen is LSD (lysergic acid diethylomide), which was first synthesized in 1938. Although still occasionally used in medical research, the drug has no commonly used therapeutic applications. Even a tiny amount is enough to cause hallucinations, which manifest themselves in intensified colors, individualized sound perceptions, and bizarre visions, which may be pleasant or extremely frightening.

In mentally unstable individuals, LSD can produce psychotic reactions. There is also a danger of so-called "flashbacks," where an individual will suddenly have hallucinations even weeks after having last ingested the drug. LSD does not cause physical dependency or seem to result in brain damage or birth defects, as once supposed. However, a "bad trip," or unpleasant experience while under the influence of the drug, can have long-lasting psychological effects.

Other hallucinogens are either derived from peyote, a kind of cactus that grows in Mexico and the American Southwest, or made synthetically. Most have effects similar to those produced by LSD, but some are particularly dangerous because of unpredictable side effects. One of the more common of these illegal drugs is PCP (phencyclidine hydrochloride), known as "angel dust." Originally synthesized as an animal tranquilizer, PCP is a relatively easy chemical compound to manufacture illegally. The drug is usually mixed with tobacco or marijuana and ingested by smoking.

PCP produces perceptual distortions, feelings of depersonalization, and changes in body image. Apathy, sweating, and auditory hallucinations may also result. High doses produce a stupor and overdose coma that can last for several weeks. This period can be followed by weeks of confused mental state. In some individuals, PCP also has also been reported to precipitate extremely violent behavior, including random murder.

MARIJUANA*

After alcohol and nicotine, marijuana is the third most popular recreational drug in the United States. Marijuana, sinsemilla, hashish, and hashish oil are all derived from the Indian hemp plant cannabis sativa (or just cannabis). Marijuana is the dried leaves and flowers of the plant that are used for smoking. Sinsemilla is the most potent version of marijuana used for smoking. Sinsemilla is taken from the female plant. The unfertilized female plant is the most potent. The male plants are harvested and removed before they can pollinate the female plants. Often the remaining female plants are covered so that they will not be contaminated by any stray male spores. Because the small leaves contain more potency, the larger leaves are often picked off (Mann, 1985). Hashish, or hash, is a more potent resin derived from the plant. Although there are 421 known chemical compounds in the cannabis plant, the active ingredient in marijuana, sinsemilla, and hashish is delta-9 tetrahydrocannebinol, which scientists often refer to as delta-9 or THC. Marijuana is a hard drug to classify. Depending on various factors, including the amount of drug taken, the type of drug, the setting, and the mood of the user, cannabis intoxication may resemble alcohol, a sedative, a stimulant, or a hallucinogen. In average doses, it acts much like alcohol. In addition, there is distortion of time, increased heart rate, increased appetite and thirst, dilation of the blood vessels in the eyes, and perhaps muscular weakness. Some individuals may act emotionally unstable or anxious or experience sensory distortions. The ability to think seems to be reduced in terms of short-term memory. The ability to drive a car effectively is hindered because of the lessening of perception and motor coordination.

There appear to be several serious long-term effects of marijuana use. When it is smoked, nearly 70 percent of the suspended particles remain in the lungs. In addition, marijuana produces up to 50 percent more tar than does an equivalent weight of tobacco. This tar causes the lung tissue to undergo precancerous changes (Jones, 1980). It is believed that tar from tobacco and from marijuana has damaging effects. It is not known whether use of both products causes a synergistic effect.

The National Academy of Science's Institute of Medicine recommends that people with cardiovascular disease avoid the drug. In healthy users, slight changes in heart rhythms occur, but these appear to be insignificant and transitory in nature. In people with angina pectoris, the increased oxygen requirement can cause pain more readily. The effect of marijuana on heart irregularities is not known. There is some evidence that marijuana smoke impairs the antibacterial defenses within the lungs and thus increases the risk of infection (AMA, 1981).

Marijuana affects the reproductive system in various ways. It affects the sympathetic nervous system, increasing vasodilation in the genitals and thus delays ejaculation. High doses over a period of time can lead to a lessening of sexual desire along with impotence. This probably occurs because of decreased testosterone, which is the result of THC affecting either the hypothalamus, pituitary, or perhaps both glands. The number of sperm ejaculated decreases, the proportion of abnormal

---

*Source: This section is taken from *Health* by Michael Hamrick, David Anspaugh, and Gene Ezell (Columbus: Merrill, 1986).

sperm is greater, and the motility of the sperm is reduced in marijuana users. Although studies have reported that female users experience problems with the reproductive cycle, this information is not conclusive. It is known that THC is excreted in the milk of lactating females, although the effect on infants has not been determined.

The effects on adolescents in the 12 to 15-year range has raised many questions but provided few answers. The effect it has on the reproductive system, as well as psychological and sociological development, is unknown. However, even the advocates of more liberal marijuana laws agree that its use should be limited to those over a particular age.

Although marijuana tolerance can develop, the frequent user may actually over time require less to gain the effects of the drug. Physical dependence seems to be rare. There is a danger of psychological dependence, however.

For some time, marijuana has been under investigation for possible medical use. Dr. Sidney Cohen of the Neuropsychiatric Institute at UCLA has summed up the state of marijuana's therapeutic use in these words (cited in Mann, 1985):

> *For cancer chemotherapy patients:* I think we can say the THC is at least as good as Compazine. It also helps people that Compazine does not help, and therefore we should have it around. But I predict that THC will turn out to be a transitional drug for this purpose. Other more effective chemicals will replace it. Consequently, within a few years there should be no need for THC capsules or smoked marijuana for this purpose.
>
> *For glaucoma patients:* Although THC eyedrops do reduce intraocular pressure, at this point it looks as though the THC molecule is too irritating to the eyeball; therefore, use of THC eyedrops may not be possible. As far as smoked marijuana goes, it does appear to improve—though not to cure—the condition. However, glaucoma is particularly common among the elderly, many of whom cannot tolerate the intoxicating and disorienting effects produced by the drug.
>
> *Antiasthmatic:* As Dr. Donald Tashkin's studies clearly show, although marijuana smoking does cause initial brief bronchodilation, on continued smoking the irritant effects worsen the condition and since asthma is a temporary constriction of the bronchial tubes, smoking marijuana is definitely contraindicated. The ideal solution would seem to be a THC aerosol, but THC researchers in Boston and Los Angeles have indicated that THC is so insoluble in fluid that it precipitates out; it doesn't stay in solution. Tiny globs of THC are deposited in the throat and are therefore ineffective in treating the bronchial passages in the lungs. Researchers have tried to develop a microspray with extremely small THC globules, which would penetrate into the bronchial tubes, but this was unsuccessful. No further work is being done in this area.
>
> *Pre-anesthetic:* There is no evidence that supports THC for this use. This has therefore been abandoned on a research basis.
>
> *Appetite enhancer:* Users report appetite is increased by cannabis (the "munchies"), yet studies only partially confirmed this.
>
> *Treatment for anorexia nervosa:* In a study conducted by the National Institute of Health, THC was no better than diazepam in treating anorexia in a small number of patients, and some reported feeling paranoid with THC. (It should also be noted that diazepam has not been shown to be effective for this condition.)
>
> *Withdrawal from alcohol and opiates:* Antabuse is a drug that produces a severe reaction when taken with alcohol. It is therefore sometimes used to discourage alcoholics from drinking. Marijuana, unlike some other drugs, can be taken with Anta-

buse; the two appear to be compatible. However, marijuana seems to play no role in alleviating the problems of withdrawal from alcohol. Nor have studies shown that it is effective in use for opiate withdrawal.

Epilepsy treatment: When you ask epileptics what smoking pot does for them, the reports are highly inconsistent. Some say that it brings on a seizure. Some say there is no improvement, and some say that it improves the condition. However, one of the cannabinoids, cannabidiol, has been found to be helpful in grand mal epilepsy. It elevates the seizure threshold. Studies have been done in Salt Lake City, Brazil, and in Israel. This is a promising area for research—especially since cannabidiol is nonpsychoactive.

Muscle relaxant: Several studies done in the United States seemed to indicate that marijuana or THC was effective as a muscle relaxant, though neither did better in this area than standard muscle relaxants such as Baclofen. These were not double-blind studies. However, a more recent double-blind study completed in 1983 failed to show any effectiveness of marijuana or THC in this area.

Tumor growth retardant: Some animal work done at the University of Virginia during the mid-seventies indicated that THC had some tumor-suppressant effects. This, however, did not compare favorably with tumor-suppressant effects of cancer chemotherapy drugs. In fact, one cannabinoid, cannabidiol, has been found to enhance tumor growth to a moderate degree. When marijuana or THC is given for control of nausea or vomiting, it cannot be assumed that it has any cancer-controlling effects whatsoever. When marijuana is smoked, the cancer-enhancing effects of cannabidiol are probably neutralized by other cannabinoids, although no work has been done on this yet.

Should marijuana become an accepted drug?: Marijuana is an unstable substance. It has a poor shelf life. It will be found to contain over a thousand chemicals—we only know of about four hundred–odd now but that's because we haven't been researching it very long—and it contains dozens of things that may not contribute to what we want it to do.

I can't think of very many drugs in the pharmacopoeia that are crude drugs any more (the whole plant, rather than the essential active ingredients). We seem to have moved beyond the crude drug stage to extracting from them items we want to use, and then we have fewer problems with them.

At best, marijuana is a controversial drug. While it may not be as harmful as some researchers report, it certainly is not harmless. Any use of THC for medical purposes does not stand as an endorsement for the recreational aspects of the drug.

TERMS AND SYMPTOMS OF DRUG ABUSE

Drug abuse, unfortunately, is all too prevalent in our society today. As a teacher, you must become aware of the drugs that are commonly being abused in your community so that you can act and react appropriately. Your knowledge of abused drugs should include street names of the substances, symptoms of their use, and possible consequences of abuse.

What should you do if you realize that you have a drug problem in your school? There are no definitive answers for this question, but you must begin by having a solid informational base about just what drugs do and do not do. Then you can take action based upon the facts.

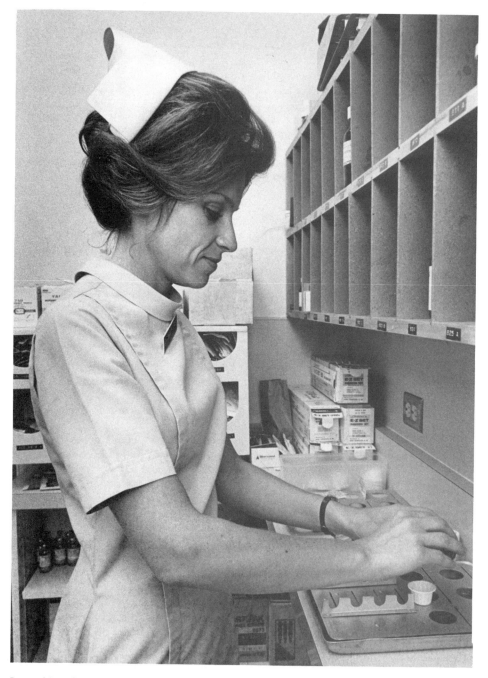

In teaching about drugs, it is important to let students know that there are positive aspects of drug use.

DRUG EDUCATION

A drug education program is not an easy undertaking. For every strategy that has been proposed there have been critics with good and plausible arguments as to why that strategy is the worst one possible. There are even those, including many parents, who feel that the best approach is no approach at all. Don't mention drugs and then the problem won't exist is the basic feeling here.

This latter view seems out of touch with reality, and yet it is understandable considering how so many drug education programs have led to unfortunate results. For example, one approach in the past was to provide students with complete information about all the possibilities of drug abuse, from the names of every street drug, to how the drugs are usually ingested, to detailed descriptions of possible effects of the drugs and possible consequences of an overdose. Given the inquiring and curious nature of children, such an approach could well amount to a primer on how to take drugs, not how to avoid them.

Scare tactics are equally counterproductive. Children soon learn to recognize the difference between fact and possible fiction. Attempts to equate the dangers of marijuana with those of heroin, suggestions that any drug can kill or permanently impair an individual, and other dire warnings—no matter how true—are often disregarded as propaganda.

The only effective approach to drug education is one in which children come to see that drug-taking constitutes unnecessary and self-abusive behavior. Certainly, you must provide factual information about the consequences of drug abuse. But that in itself will not influence behavior. You must provide alternatives—and realistic ones. Too often, the real appeal of such drugs as marijuana or alcohol is dismissed by asking children to take up a sport or go bike riding or learn to play a musical instrument. Such suggestions are fine as far as they go, but they often fail to take into account the personal problems that children are experiencing that may tempt them into drug abuse.

Never lie about the dangers of drugs, either one way or the other. But never play down the problems that children are facing that may make drugs seem to be an appealing way to cope. Effective drug education walks a fine line, one that requires sensitivity on your part to the environment in which your children must live and function. But always point out that, no matter what the circumstances, each individual has a choice—and must make a choice—about drug use or abuse. Drug education must be a part of mental health education. Only when children realize that drugs are not the answer to a problem but part of the problem can you be successful in your instruction.

SUMMARY

A drug is any substance that alters bodily functions. Drugs can be used or abused. Reasons for drug abuse include low self-esteem, peer pressure, adult modeling, mood alteration, boredom, curiosity, and alienation.

Drugs act on the body by stimulating or depressing cellular activity. Even when drugs are prescribed for medical purposes, there is a possibility that drug abuse can result.

Alcohol is one of the most commonly used and abused drugs. In small or moderate doses, this drug has a tranquilizing or mellowing effect. But alcohol can easily lead to psychological and physical dependency, sometimes resulting in alcoholism, a disease that can wreck lives.

Smoking tobacco is also a serious health problem. Smokers often become psychologically and perhaps even physically dependent upon tobacco. Smoking is a difficult habit to break, but failure to do so can lead to a variety of serious diseases, including cancer and emphysema.

Over-the-counter drugs are usually safe when taken as directed, but ingestion of any drug, no matter how mild, can cause health hazards. Advertisements for OTC drugs can often lead people to believe that they are safer and more effective than they actually are.

Particularly dangerous drugs include barbiturates and amphetamines, known commonly as "downers" and "uppers." Barbiturates are depressants, while amphetamines are stimulants. Both, if abused, can cause serious health problems or death.

Narcotics are in some ways much more dangerous than barbiturates. This class of drug includes opium, morphine, and heroin. Heroin is extremely addicting and can lead to many related health problems. As with any street drug, the user can never be sure of just what is contained in the dose sold.

The hallucinogens include such drugs as LSD and PCP. Although not physically addictive, such drugs can lead to psychological breakdowns and irrational acts.

Marijuana, for various reasons, is in a class by itself. While not particularly dangerous, its use can lead to personal and social harm. The stronger derivatives of the cannabis plant, including hashish and hashish oil, are more potent and can lead to even greater harm.

Drug education is a difficult topic, one where there are no easy answers as to the correct course. Factual information must be provided, and yet drug education must not be allowed to become a primer on *how* to take drugs. Community mores and life styles must be considered so that information and advice given are realistic and practical. The best course is to build self-esteem in students so that drugs are not seen as a viable alternative for coping with personal problems.

DISCUSSION QUESTIONS

1. What is the definition of a drug? Give examples of substances that qualify as drugs under this definition.

2. List six common reasons for drug abuse, especially as these reasons apply to young people.

3. Discuss the physiological, psychological, and sociological effects of alcohol.

4. List six reasons that contribute to the habit of smoking tobacco.

5. What factors contribute to the misuse and abuse of OTC drugs?

6. What effects do barbiturates have on the body? Discuss the consequences of physical and psychological dependence on these drugs.

7. What is cross tolerance? What are the dangers of this phenomenon?

8. Why is heroin dependence so difficult to overcome?

9. What effects do stimulant drugs have on the body? Discuss the consequences of psychological dependence on these drugs.

10. Discuss the dangers of using hallucinogenic drugs.

11. How can marijuana use lead to personal and social harm?

12. Why is drug education such a controversial topic? Discuss what the goal of an effective drug education program should be and how this goal can be achieved.

REFERENCES

AMA Council on Scientific Affairs. "Marijuana: Its health hazards and therapeutic potentiates." *Journal of American Medical Association 246,* (October 16, 1981): 1,823–1,827.

Andersen, Kurt. "Crashing on Cocaine." *Time, 121* (April 11, 1983): 22–31.

Hafen, B. *Alcohol: The crutch that cripples.* St. Paul, Minn.: West Publishing, 1977.

Horn, D. *Smoker's self-testing kit.* Washington, D.C.: National Clearinghouse for Smoking and Health, 1973.

Jones, R. "Human Effects: An overview." in *Marijuana research findings: 1980,* ed. R. Peterson. Washington, D.C.: National Institute on Drug Abuse, 1980, 54–80.

Lingeman, R. *Drugs from A to Z—A dictionary.* New York: McGraw-Hill, 1969.

Mann, Peggy. *Marijuana alert.* New York: McGraw-Hill, 1985, 85.

National Institute on Alcohol Abuse and Alcoholism. *Alcohol and health.* Second Special Report to the U.S. Congress. Washington, D.C.: Department of Health, Education and Welfare, 1974, 9.

National Institute on Drug Abuse. *For parents only: What you need to know about marijuana.* Rockville, Md.: National Clearinghouse for Drug Abuse Information, 1980.

Pawiak, V. *Drug abuse: A realistic primer for parents.* Phoenix: Do It Now Foundation, 1976.

Ray, Oakley. *Drugs, society, and human behavior.* St. Louis: C. V. Mosby, 1978.

Russell, C., Taylor, S., & Law, C. "Smoking in pregnancy, maternal blood pressure, pregnancy outcome, baby weight and growth, and other related factors: A prospective study." *British Journal of Preventive Social Medicine,* 1969, 22, 119–26.

United States Department of Health Education and Welfare, Public Health Services. *Smoking and health,* report by the Surgeon General, January, 1979.

World Health Organization Expert Committee on Addiction-Producing Drugs. *Terminology in regard to drug abuse,* 1964, 9–10.

18. Techniques for Teaching About Alcohol, Tobacco, and Drugs

Nothing is of itself good or evil; only the manner or usage makes it so.—Latin saying

THE CHALLENGE OF DRUG EDUCATION

Elementary school children need to be provided with learning experiences that will help them to develop attitudes and values that build self-esteem and respect for the body so that drug-taking is not seen as a way of coping with life. They must be taught to accept responsibility for their own behavior so that they will know how to deal with the problem of drugs in society.

The challenge of drug education is not to make every child a drug expert, nor to frighten children with scare tactics. Instead, it is to help children recognize that there is no need for them to misuse or abuse any drug, regardless of what reason they may have for being tempted to do so.

As a teacher, you must realize that there are almost as many reasons for drifting into drug-taking as there are different kinds of drugs. A youngster may wish to start smoking for an entirely different reason than would be the case for amphetamine abuse. The temptation to take a particular drug may not stem from any self-destructive impulse, although this is sometimes the case. But the resultant behavior is self-destructive, regardless of the motivation. If children recognize this fact, and if they are on their way to building a strong self-image, then drug abuse is far less likely to occur in later years.

Concepts to be Taught

- Dealing effectively with personal problems is important in preventing drug abuse.
- Poor self-image increases the potential for drug abuse.
- Drugs should be taken only when a doctor prescribes them and only in the amount prescribed.

- People use and abuse drugs for physical, emotional, and social reasons.
- Certain drugs can be legally purchased only with a doctor's prescription.
- Some drugs, called over-the-counter drugs, can be purchased without a doctor's prescription.
- Smoking is dangerous to health.
- Tobacco smoke can be harmful to those who do not smoke as well as to smokers themselves.
- Alcohol is a drug.
- Misuse of alcohol can cause physical, emotional, and social problems.
- Alcoholism is a disease.
- Alcoholism can lead to many health problems.
- Barbiturates can cause both physical and psychological dependency.
- Amphetamines, like barbiturates, can be dangerous if abused.
- Illegal drugs, including narcotics and hallucinogens, can have unpredictable and serious health consequences.

Cycle Plan for Teaching Topics

Topic	Grade Level						
	K	1	2	3	4	5	6
Drugs and Decision-Making	**	**	**	**	***	***	***
Drugs for Beneficial Use	**	**	**	**	**	*	*
Commonly Abused Drugs	*	*	*	*	**	**	***
Alcohol	*	**	*	***	*	*	***
Smoking	*	**	***	**	**	**	***
OTC Drugs	*	*	*	**	**	***	***

Key *** = major emphasis, ** = emphasis, * = review.

VALUE-BASED ACTIVITIES

Smoking and the Law

After you have discussed the definition of a drug, point out that tobacco qualifies under the definition. Note that although smoking is known to be hazardous to health, tobacco products can be purchased legally by adults. Ask students to consider the implications of this fact. Point out that smoking is a decision that each individual must make. Then have the students consider the following questions:

- Should laws be passed that prevent people from smoking in certain public places?
- What are some reasons to be considered in making such laws?
- Should cigarettes be made illegal? Why or why not?

- What legal rights should smokers have?
- What legal rights should nonsmokers have?
- How do you feel about laws regulating smoking?

Smoking and You

Have each student prepare a list with two columns. In the first column, ask the students to write reasons why they think a person might want to start smoking. In the second column, have them list reasons why a person might decide not to start smoking. Talk over the various reasons that the students list in a general discussion. Which reasons in each column are rational ones? Which are irrational ones?

Drugs and You

Repeat the activity just described for any drug discussed in class. Include alcohol, depressants, stimulants, and so forth or have the students prepare their lists for drug-taking in general.

Change Agents

This activity is adapted from *Tribes: A Process for Peer Involvement* by Jeanne Gibbs and Andre Allen, Center Source Publications, Oakland, California. It can be especially useful in helping older elementary school students consider their developing values.

Prepare individual sheets describing the following 15 change agents. First, have the students read the sheet. Then proceed with the activity as directed.

A group of 15 experts, each capable of bringing about change in a person's life, have agreed to offer their services to members of this class. You must decide which of these experts can best provide the change you want in your own life.

J. Paul Gettrich—Will teach you how to handle money successfully. Become a millionaire in weeks.

Dr. I. Q. Brainey—Guarantees to make you a genius. You will be able instantly to master any mental task you attempt.

Ma Thusela—Is a sorceress whose herbs and potions will increase life expectancy to as much as 500 years of vital, productive life.

Atlas Armstrong—Provides a course of diet and exercise guaranteed to make you ten times stronger, with no loss of agility or distortion of body image.

Madame De Bonaire—Teaches you to be poised and at ease in any social situation.

Dr. Mae Q. Gorgeous—Through plastic surgery and hormones, provides you with the face and figure of your choice.

Lotta Chuckles—Helps you develop your sense of humor. You will be able to laugh at your own mistakes and to see the funny side of many things that used to bring you down.

Dr. Will B. Charming—Instructs you in the art of winning and keeping friends. People will find you charming and lovable; you will never again be lonely.

B. A. Superjock—Trains you to achieve superstar status in the professional sport of your choice—baseball, football, soccer, tennis, golf, and so on.

Ina Mirror—Enables you to see yourself objectively to understand yourself, your values, and your motives for everything you say and do.

Ms. Mary Selfworth—Will help you increase your self-esteem, self-respect, and self-confidence. Ms. Selfworth will enable you to become your own best friend.

Prof. Sven Galley—Teaches you ways of increasing your persuasive powers over people. You will be able to influence others to do virtually anything you want them to do.

Dr. Feelgood—Teaches you how to "get high" naturally; to feel good all the time without drugs.

Ralph Radar—Helps you become an effective political reformer and consumer advocate. You will be able to make government and industry more responsive to the needs of the citizen and consumer.

Dr. I. Hugalot—Will teach you to be an ideal companion and loving person. By doing so, you will bring pleasure and fulfillment to yourself and others.

Have each student decide which five of these change agents could best fulfill his or her needs by writing the letter A next to the top five. Then have the students decide which of the next five experts would be next best by writing the letter B by their names. Have them indicate the least useful of the five remaining change agents with the letter C.

Divide the class into small groups of five or six students. Ask each group to discuss its individual choices for ten minutes. Each group should try to reach a consensus as to which of the five change agents would be most helpful. Ask each group to share its consensus choices with the class. Compare and discuss the choices made. If time allows, ask volunteers to role play the different change agents. Each student should argue that what he or she has to offer is the most valuable.

After the group activity, ask each student to consider these questions:

- What seems to link together the five most desirable change agents on your list? What do the five least desirable change agents have in common?

- What values are behind the choices you made?

- What are you doing now to achieve any of the changes that your top five change agents offer?

Where Do You Stand?

Draw a chalk line on the floor. Explain to your class that the line is a continuum on how they feel about various decisions. One end of the line represents complete disagreement with a position, while the other end represents complete agreement. Or the line could represent degrees of willingness or unwillingness.

Then ask for volunteers to demonstrate where they stand on a variety of questions that you put forward. Try to keep the questions nonthreatening and nonincriminating. Questions that you might ask include the following:

- Where do you stand on smoking cigarettes?

- Where do you stand on drinking alcohol?

- How willing would you be to tell a friend who takes drugs that you do not approve of that behavior?

- How dangerous do you think it is to take a drug that you don't know anything about yourself?

Sentence Completion

Ask the students to complete statements such as the following with values-related answers:

1. For me, smoking is _____ .
2. If I saw another student using drugs, I would _____ .
3. Some people start drinking alcohol because _____ .
4. Drugs are _____ .
5. To me, drug abuse means _____ .
6. The best reason for not taking any drugs is _____ .
7. One thing I don't believe about drugs is _____ .
8. If I made the laws about drugs, I would _____ .
9. I was surprised to learn that drugs _____ .
10. People who take drugs _____ .

Decision Stories

Present decision stories such as the following, using the procedures outlined in chapter 5.

Want a Smoke?

Mark always walks home from school with a group of friends. One day, two of his friends light up cigarettes. Mark is surprised because he didn't know that they had started smoking. "Want a smoke?" his friend Jim asks. "They're real mild," his other friend George says. "Try one." Mark can see that his friends Jim and George are trying to look grown up. He wants to look grown up, too. The other two boys in the group are not smoking, however, Mark wonders what he should do.

Focus Question: What should Mark say to his friends?

Problems at Home

Michael's problems at home were getting worse, and he felt that he had nowhere to turn. He was very lonely and frightened about what was happening in his life. His parents were always fighting. They didn't seem to have any time for him anymore. He wanted so much to have someone show him love and concern. He also wished that he could just leave his problems behind him.

Focus Questions: What are some methods of coping that Michael might try? What might be the consequences of each of these methods?

Slumber Party

Sally is throwing a slumber party at her home. Her parents respect Sally's judgment and ask her to make sure that the party does not get out of hand. Sally doesn't think it will. But after her parents have gone to bed, some of Sally's friends start passing some pills around. They tell her that these pills are fun to take and are not dangerous. They also say that Sally doesn't have to try the pills if she doesn't want to. But they ask her not to spoil the party for them.

Focus Question: What should Sally do?

Drugs in the Neighborhood

Darlene knows that some of the older kids in her neighborhood are using and selling drugs. They don't seem to care that Darlene sees what they are doing.

"It's none of your business," one of them told her. But Darlene is not so sure. A couple of her friends bought some of these drugs and have started using them. Darlene doesn't know what will happen in the neighborhood next.

Focus Question: What can Darlene do about the drug problem in her neighborhood?

DRAMATIZATION

Drug Court

Have the students role play various drug-related court actions. In this court, the class acts collectively as judge and jury. Various students come before the court acting the part of the arresting officer. They explain to the court that they have arrested an individual on a drug charge and then describe the offense. In each case, the defendant has already pleaded guilty to the charge. It is up to the court to decide what sentence or decision to make. The class must come up with a consensus on each offense. Follow each decision with general discussion. Also note to the students what the penalty might have been in an actual court.

Public Service Messages

Divide the class into small groups. Have each prepare a 60-second public service message for television broadcast about drug education. Encourage imagination. Some students may wish to write and sing a song bearing their message. Others may wish to act out a skit. Still others may opt for a panel format. Have each group give its "televised" presentation in front of the class. Each presentation must be one minute long. After the presentations, have the class discuss each. You may wish to have the students vote for the most effective presentation.

What Would Happen If . . . ?

After discussing the effects that various kinds of drugs can have on the body and brain, have students role play situations in which a person attempts an activity while under the influence of a certain kind of drug. For example, what would happen if an airline pilot tried to land a plane while under the influence of alcohol? What would happen if a surgeon tried to operate while under the influence of a hallucinogen? Have one student play the affected person. Another student, at the last minute, steps in and saves the day. After the activity, emphasize to the class that sometimes no one can keep a tragedy from happening. Bring this point home by discussing drunk driving statistics or other examples from the news.

I'm No Dummy

Have the students use hand puppets to act out skits about drug use and abuse. One puppet, for example, might be offered drugs by other puppets. "I'm no dummy," the first puppet replies, and then gives reasons for refusing.

DISCUSSION AND REPORT TECHNIQUES

Presentation by Health Professionals

With the permission from your school administration, invite an official from a drug abuse program to speak to your class about substance use and abuse. Talk with your guest alone before the presentation and emphasize that no scare tactics should be used. Presentation should be factual and objective. Allow time for a question and answer session afterwards.

The Question Box

Have students write on an index card a problem they are concerned about personally. No names or other means of identification should be included. Then have the students place their cards in a large ballot box. Allow them to place questions in the box for a week. After class, open the box and screen out any cards that inadvertently reveal any problems that would lead to identification of the student involved. The next day, distribute the remaining cards to the students on a random basis and have them tell how they would deal with the problem. Allow other students with different opinions to add comments.

Sharing

Have the students be seated in a large circle on the floor. Each student then shares one positive experience that happened to him or her in the last month. Sharing may relate to home, school, athletics, play, and so on. No one is to interrupt or ask any questions until every student has had an opportunity to share. Follow the activity with a discussion. Ask the following questions: Was it hard to find something to share? What were the similarities among the things shared? Did people share more as the activity progressed? What does this indicate?

The Space Colony

Tell the class that they are about to travel to a new planet by spaceship. On this planet there are as yet no governments or laws. As a group, the class must decide on the drug policy and drug laws for the new planetary settlement. The class, acting as a committee, must decide what drugs, if any, are to be taken to the new planet and how such drugs will be distributed or made available. Have the class keep in mind that drugs include useful medications, but that such medications can be abused. Laws relating to the misuse of drugs on the new planet must also be discussed. After thorough discussion, have the class come to a consensus about drug policy on the new planet. Write their conclusions on the chalkboard. Then have each student prepare an individual report, including any dissenting opinions. Such opinions must be backed up with reasons.

Buy Me, Try Me

Ask students to find adveretisements in magazines and newspapers for tobacco, alcohol, and OTC products. Each student should bring in three such advertisements. After the material has been collected, have the class analyze the content. Sort the advertisements into categories and subcategories. Categories can include the different types of products, such as cigarettes, beer, cold remedies, mouthwashes, and so on. Subcategories can be based on the different audiences the ads are intended to appeal to. For example, are some cigarette ads slanted toward women? Are others slanted toward men? Ask students to consider what the basic appeal of each ad is. Is the appeal for the product itself or some intangible associated with the product, such as a macho image? How does each advertisement try to manipulate the consumer?

Individual Reports

Ask students to do further research on a drug-related problem and prepare individual reports on what they find? Topics can include Smoking and Health, Alcohol Abuse and Accidents, Drugs and the Law, and Dangers of Drug Abuse.

EXPERIMENTS AND DEMONSTRATIONS

Smoking Machine

The purpose of this demonstration is to demonstrate the effect of cigarette tars on the human body by way of analogy. You will need a large glass bottle, a two-hole rubber stopper, glass delivery tubes, a cigarette holder, cigarettes, and a small hand pump. Most of this equipment can be found in a school chemistry lab or can be obtained from a scientific supply house. Set up the apparatus as shown in figure 18.1.

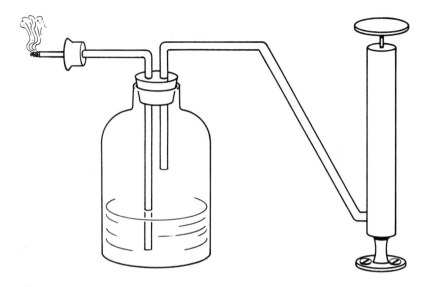

Figure 18.1
Smoking machine apparatus.

Fill the bottle halfway with water. Place a cigarette in the holder and light it. Operate the pump to draw smoke from the cigarette into the bottle and water. Continue to pump until the cigarette is burned completely. Burn additional cigarettes as necessary until tars can be seen in the water. Then have the students examine the water and note the distinct smell. Tars may also collect in the glass tubing. Ask students how this demonstration illustrates what happens when a person smokes a cigarette.

Effects of Smoking on the Body

For this demonstration, you will need the cooperation of an adult who smokes. Try to obtain the assistance of a nonfaculty member, who will not be so closely identified as a role model for the students. Have the smoker inhale from a lighted cigarette, holding the smoke in the mouth without allowing it to go into the lungs. Ask the smoker to place a white handkerchief over the mouth, stretching the fabric tightly, and then exhaling the smoke through the handkerchief. Students should note that the smoke causes a dark stain. Now, have the smoker inhale smoke into the lungs and then exhale into a different part of the handkerchief. The resulting stain will be lighter. Ask students to consider the implications of the demonstration.

Goldfish Demonstration

This demonstration illustrates the toxic qualities contained in cigarette smoke. Before you begin, explain to the class that there are more than 300 chemical substances in cigarette smoke. These substances include nicotine, cyanide, formaldehyde, lead, arsenic, and caron monoxide—all poisons. Set up a smoking machine apparatus like that shown in figure 18.1. This time, first add two or three goldfish to the water in the bottle. Then process three or more cigarettes by using the pump. The fish will begin to lose their equilibrium as they are affected by the chemicals in the cigarette smoke. As soon as this begins to happen, remove the fish by pouring the water into a net. Place the fish into a bowl of clean water. Do not pour the contaminated water into the clean water as you do this or the fish will die from continued exposure to the contaminants.

Influence of Alcohol Demonstration

Prepare a mixture of water and ethyl (not rubbing) alcohol by adding ½ ounce of alcohol to ¾ pint of water. This is approximately the amount in a 12 ounce bottle of beer. Then place a medium-sized goldfish in the solution and have the class observe what happens. In about 15 minutes, the goldfish will become so affected by the alcohol that it will float to the surface. Immediately remove the fish and place it in fresh water. It should revive in 5 to 10 minutes.

Breathometer Demonstration

Invite a local police officer to class to demonstrate how a breathometer works. This device is used to test the amount of alcohol in a driver's bloodstream. Have the police officer explain the dangers of drinking and driving. The person should note that even a small amount of alcohol has a deleterious effect on driving ability.

PUZZLES AND GAMES

Drugs Spell Trouble

Prepare individual worksheets as shown below. Have students write the name of the drug that answers each clue given in the letter spaces provided. The completed puzzle spells out vertically a message about drug abuse.

1. What cigarettes are made of.
2. The drug in beer, wine, and whiskey.
3. Three letters for a drug that causes hallucinations.
4. Drug made from the cannabis plant.
5. Street name for amphetamines.
6. Street name for barbiturates.
7. Street name for cocaine.

```
          T O │B│ A C C O
              │A│ L C O H O L
          L S │D│
M A R I J U A │N│ A
        U P P │E│ R S
        D O   │W│ N E R S
              │S│ N O W
```

Smoking Crossword Puzzle

Prepare individual puzzle sheets as shown in figure 18.2. After you have discussed smoking in class, distribute the sheets and have the students complete the puzzle. In this example, the correct answers have been filled in.

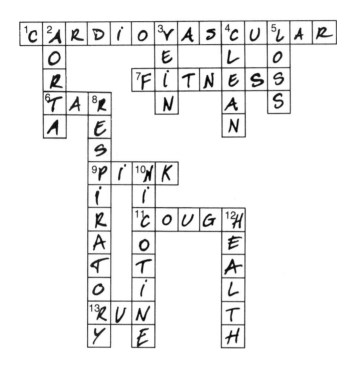

7. Cigarette smoking can lower your physical _____.
9. Normally, the lungs are a _____ color.
11. Many smokers awake every morning with a _____.
13. Cigarette smoking may cause you to be more breathless when you _____.

Down

2. The blood vessel which carries blood from the heart to the rest of the body is an _____.
3. The blood vessel which carries blood back to the heart from the body is a _____.
4. Non-smokers have a right to breathe _____ air.
5. When a person develops emphysema, there is a definite _____ of lung function.
8. Smoking is also bad for your _____ system.
10. A substance in tobacco that causes blood vessels to get smaller is _____.
12. Warning: The Surgeon General Has Determined That Cigarette Smoking Is Dangerous to Your _____.

Across

1. The _____ system contains the heart and blood vessels.
6. The cancer causing substance in tobacco smoke is _____.

Figure 18.2
Smoking crossword puzzle.

Drugs Crossword Puzzle

Directions: Use the words in the box to fill in the crossword puzzle. Clues are given below.

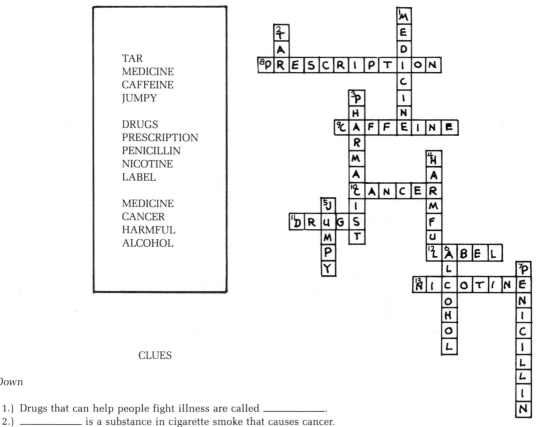

TAR
MEDICINE
CAFFEINE
JUMPY

DRUGS
PRESCRIPTION
PENICILLIN
NICOTINE
LABEL

MEDICINE
CANCER
HARMFUL
ALCOHOL

CLUES

Down

1.) Drugs that can help people fight illness are called _____.
2.) _____ is a substance in cigarette smoke that causes cancer.
3.) The prescription can be filled only by a _____.
4.) Drugs can be both helpful and _____ to your body.
5.) Too much caffeine can make a person feel _____.
6.) A person who has had some _____ to drink should not drive a car.
7.) _____ is a strong drug made from a mold.

Across

8.) The doctor's order for a special medicine is called _____.
9.) A drug called _____ is found in coffee, tea, and cocoa.
10.) Smoking may cause a very serious illness to the lungs called _____.
11.) Things other than food that can cause a change in a person's body are called _____.
12.} People should always read the _____ on medicine before using it.
13.) A drug in tobacco smoke that may cause damage to a person's heart is _____.

Figure 18.3
Drugs crossword puzzle.

The Magic Gumball Machine

Prepare individual sheets as shown in figure 18.4. Pass them out and have students complete the activity. Follow with a discussion of fun activities that your students enjoy.

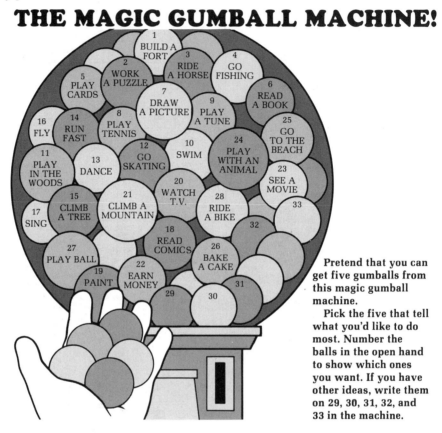

Pretend that you can get five gumballs from this magic gumball machine.

Pick the five that tell what you'd like to do most. Number the balls in the open hand to show which ones you want. If you have other ideas, write them on 29, 30, 31, 32, and 33 in the machine.

Figure 18.4
The Magic Gumball Machine

BULLETIN BOARDS

Natural High

Prepare a bulletin board display illustrating activities that can provide great pleasure and satisfaction—a natural high. An example is shown in figure 18.5. Ask the children for suggestions about natural high experiences that they have had. These might include whitewater rafting, a particularly exciting game or sports contest, hiking, going to an amusement park and riding a roller coaster, and so on. Discuss what a natural high means. Usually such an experience is associated with pleasurable excitement, clear-headedness, being in control, and a feeling of achievement.

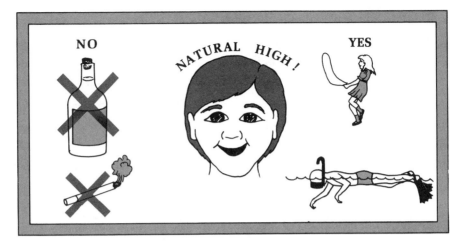

Figure 18.5
Natural high bulletin board.

Drugs Are Not a Solution

Prepare a bulletin board display emphasizing the fact that drugs do not provide real solutions to problems that we all face. Taking drugs does not solve these problems; they remain with us until better ways of coping are developed. An example of such a bulletin board display is shown in figure 18.6.

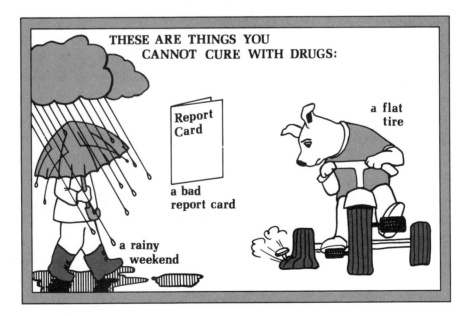

Figure 18.6
Bulletin board showing drugs as a poor coping mechanism.

Word Search

CAN YOU FIND THESE WORDS?

emphysema	stimulants	caffeine
cigarette	pharmacy	hallucinogens
cancer	dosage	narcotics
smoke	dependence	depressant
chemicals	withdrawal	overdose
incurable	tolerance	marijuana
hashish	hangover	alcoholic
counselor	tar	cirrhosis

Find each of the words and circle them. The words may read in any direction — up, down, across, or diagonally. The words may even intersect.

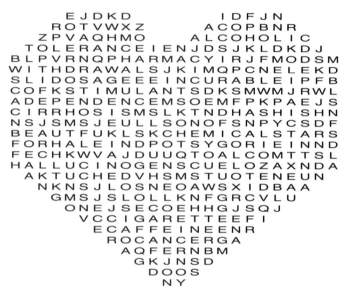

Figure 18.7
Word search.

Anti-Drug Display

The basic irrationality of drug-taking can be effectively illustrated in bulletin boards such as the examples shown in figures 18.8 and 18.9. This approach is often useful with younger children, where issues are often seen in either/or terms.

OTHER IDEAS

Dealing with Peer Pressure

Divide the class into groups of six to eight students. Have each group form a circle. Place pieces of candy in the center of each group. Give five members of each group a

People who take drugs for fun...

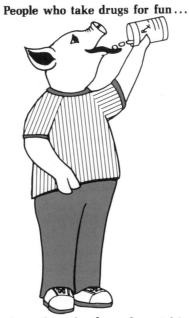

Can only make themselves sick!

Figure 18.8
Anti-drug display.

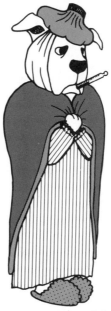

Only sick people need drugs!

Figure 18.9
Anti-drug display.

slip of paper stating that they are to eat the candy and attempt to get anyone not eating to do so. Give the remaining students in each group a slip of paper stating that they should not eat the candy and should resist all attempts to get them to do so. Let this interaction go on for about five minutes. Then ask the students to take their regular seats. Ask the following questions.

- What were you feeling when you were doing this exercise?
- What do you think the purpose of this exercise was?
- What is peer pressure?
- Why is it important to know about peer pressure?

Slogans

Have the students develop a list of slogans used by tobacco, alcohol, and OTC drug manufacturers. Discuss what the slogans are attempting to convince the consumer to do. Discuss the irrational appeal often used in this advertising approach. Then have the students come up with counterslogans that attempt to convince the consumer to do the opposite.

Affirmations

Have each student come up to the front of the class and say, "Sometimes I don't feel so good about myself." Then have the student turn his or her back to the class. Have other students then volunteer to affirm one fine quality about that individual. Every student should get three affirmations from the class. These may refer to being a loyal friend, being kind, being a good student, being fair, being friendly, and so on.

19. Sex and Family Life Education

Few controversies in American life have endured so long, or been argued so passionately, as the debate over how to teach children about sex—or in fact whether to teach them at all. It is a subject of labyrinthine complexity, involving as it does such broad areas as religious belief, public and private morality, the law, and control of the school curriculum. The arguments, moreover, are suffused with the personal attitudes people bring to the discussion, attitudes firmly rooted in their own psychosexual lives.—John Tebbel

PROGRAM GOALS

Sex and family life education are among the most controversial areas facing the teachers. Many people see inclusion of these subjects as an attempt to teach sexual technique, encourage premarital coitus, and lower the morals of today's school children. The fact is that an effective family life program seeks to develop an appreciation for self and the opposite sex and the responsibilities of family members.

Before any family life curriculum can be taught, parental approval must be obtained. Most communities will support such a program if the school administration and community really understand what is to be taught. This is a most important first step, which cannot be ignored.

The appreciation for self must start early in life and be built upon each year if children are to feel comfortable with their sexuality through the preadolescent, adolescent, and adult years. As should be emphasized in all aspects of health education, children must recognize that they will have to eventually accept the responsibility of their sexuality. Children must realize that sexuality is more than biological functioning. Sex and family life education should seek to strengthen the bonds of a loving relationship within families.

If society is not willing to promote comprehensive sex and family life education, then that component of a young person's total being will be shortchanged. Personal and social problems such as unwanted pregnancies, sexually transmitted diseases, impotence, sexual nonresponsiveness, and divorce will continue to plague us. A worthwhile educational effort in sex and family life must include social, psychological, moral, and biological components. In this chapter, each of these areas will be examined.

ESTABLISHING GUIDELINES

McCary (1978) recommends that information be provided in a formal sex education class a year or so earlier than students would learn it from their peers. This would allow the children to "hear it accurately and in a wholesome atmosphere."

Teachers must be sensitive to their qualifications and must prepare themselves thoroughly before undertaking sex education. They must always present accurate and factual information; obtain materials for teaching from professional sources; not be embarrassed when teaching sexual material; and present a balanced viewpoint of the controversial issues associated with sex education. For example, abortion, premarital sex, or religious doctrine should be presented in a balanced manner, with one viewpoint receiving no more emphasis than another. In essence, the teacher should seek to "educate, not indoctrinate; teach fact, not fallacies; formulate a code of ethics, not preach strict self-denial; be objective, not subjective; be democratic, not autocratic; and seek knowledge, not emotionally biased constructs" (McCary, 1978).

Gaining Support for Sex Education

Schiller, (1973) lists 11 steps for gaining support for a sex education program. They are as follows:

1. A proposed program must first gain support from the highest level of authority within the school organization. Administrators and parent leaders alike must provide backing.
2. A small committee is then formed to determine the receptiveness of parents and other appropriate individuals. If there is likely to be strong opposition from some individuals, informed professionals should meet with these individuals to answer questions and lessen anxieties.
3. An advisory committee representative of appropriate community components should be formed. This group should be chaired by an influential leader and will function to advise and support professional personnel on overall policy concerning the nature of the program, its philosophy, concepts, and approaches.
4. The advisory committee spearheads parent meetings to describe what sex education is and why it should be taught. At such meetings, it is essential to give attendees a chance to meet in small groups to discuss their feelings.
5. After the meetings, a questionnaire should be distributed to parents to determine their feelings about sex education. They should be asked about content, approaches, and qualifications desired of those running the program.
6. Technical experts should help in developing a curriculum for the sex education program.

7. Educator training needs to be accomplished through in-service programs, workshops, college courses, or other practical means.
8. Educators ought to be volunteers and should be carefully screened as to their attitudes, values, and ability to relate to students, parents, and other involved individuals.
9. The initial program should be small to allow for pilot testing and evaluation. The advisory committee should be met with frequently and consultants should be utilized.
10. If the program is successful, it should be revised and broadened to make it better. This helps keep everyone involved and facilitates program understanding. If not successful, alternate approaches should be considered.
11. Parallel to the basic program should be parent education or education for other significant groups.

Health Highlight: Guidelines for Sex Education

To those groups responsible for developing school and community programs in sex education we suggest the following guidelines:

a. Such education should strive to create understanding and conviction that decisions about sexual behavior must be based on moral and ethical values, as well as on considerations of physical and emotional health, fear, pleasure, practical consequences, or concepts of personality development.

b. Such education must respect the cultural, familial and religious backgrounds and beliefs of individuals and must teach that the sexual development and behavior of each individual cannot take place in a vacuum but are instead related to the other aspects of his life and to his moral, ethical and religious codes.

c. It should point out how sex is distorted and exploited in our society and how this places heavy responsibility upon the individual, the family and institutions to cope in a constructive manner with the problem thus created.

d. It must recognize that in school sex education, insofar as it relates to moral and religious beliefs and values, complements the education conveyed through the family, the church or the synagogue. Sex education in the schools must proceed constructively with understanding, tolerance and acceptance of difference.

e. It must stress the many points of harmony between moral values and beliefs about what is right and wrong that are held in common by the major religions on the one hand and generally accepted legal, social, psychological, medical and other values held in common by service professions and society generally.

f. Where strong difference of opinion exist on what is right and wrong sexual behavior, objective, informed and dignified discussion of both sides of such questions should be encouraged. However, in such cases, neither the sponsors of an educational program nor the teachers should attempt to give definite answers or to represent their personal moral and religious beliefs as the consensus of the major religions or of society generally.

g. Throughout such education human values and human dignity must be stressed as major bases for right and wrong; attitudes that build such respect should be encouraged as right, and those that tear down such respect should be condemned as wrong.

h. Such education should teach that sexuality is a part of the whole person and an aspect of his dignity as a human being.

i. It should teach that people who love each other try not to do anything that will harm each other.

j. It should teach that sexual intercourse within marriage offers the greatest possibility for personal fulfillment and social growth.

k. Finally, such a program of education must be based on sound content and must employ sound methods; it must be conducted by teachers and leaders qualified to do so by training and temperament.

Taken from a statement on sex education by the National Council of Churches, the Synagogue of America, and the United States Catholic Conference.

Teaching Sex and Family Life Education

For effectively teaching sex and family life education, as with any topical area, classroom rapport and a sensitivity to the childrens' needs are necessary. In addition, the teacher must have a strong knowledge base and the ability to communicate this knowledge. Specifically, Johnson and Belzar (1973, pp. 24–36) suggest the following criteria:

1. The teacher must have come to terms with his or her own sexuality and to have admitted not only to its existence but to its full status in the dynamics of his or her total personality functioning.
2. The teacher needs to know the appropriate factual material associated with the subject matter that he or she is to teach.
3. The teacher of sex education needs to be able to use the language of sex easily and naturally, especially in the presence of the young.
4. He or she needs to be familiar with the sequence of psychosexual developmental events throughout life.
5. The teacher needs an acute awareness of the enormous social changes that are in progress and of their implications for changes in our patterns of sexual attitudes, practices, laws, and institutions.

SOCIAL ASPECTS OF SEXUALITY AND FAMILY LIVING

Various cultural, historical, legal, religious, and other institutional factors influence families and the sexuality roles within the family. It is important to remember that many forms of the family can be found. With this in mind, some typical characteristics of the family will be examined.

Types of Families

The family fulfills a most important role in providing stability for the individual and society. The term *family* is used to describe two or more persons living together who are related by blood, marriage, or adoption (Eshleman, 1981). A *nuclear* family might be composed of a husband and wife, a brother and sister, one parent and a child or children, or both parents and one or more children. An *extended* family consists of a number of nuclear family groupings, often with blood ties. Extended family members can include uncles, aunts, grandparents, or cousins.

Since most people marry, they will be part of two different nuclear families, one in which they are born and one they start after selecting a marriage partner. The nuclear family to which we are born is the first and most basic provider of socialization. The extended family also has an influence on our socialization.

Changing Nature of the American Family

American youngsters in past generations generally grew up in one city or town, married someone from the surrounding area, and lived in the immediate locality. Chances were that members of the extended family, such as aunts, uncles, and

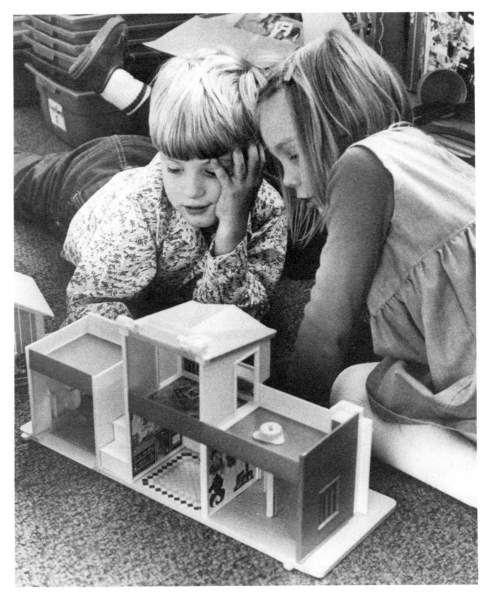

The family serves an important role by providing stability in the individual and society.

grandparents, lived in the area also. In today's society the nuclear family may be intact, but chances are that the extended family is not. For example, parents and grandparents may live in widely separate locations. As a result, grandparents may visit only on holidays or other special occasions. Thus the interaction between these family members is not as frequent as in the past. The mobility of today's society and frequent job changes or transfers have served to separate the nuclear family from the extended family.

The advent, sometimes of necessity, of two-career households has brought about several changes. Families tend to have fewer children and the care of the children may be left to day care centers or other individuals who are not family members. Consequently, children may come in contact with many more individuals during their early years than was the case in previous generations. Divorce may also change children's perspective and the roles and responsibilities they have to handle.

Technology has influenced the family. Easy access to transportation has enabled the family to move throughout the country quite easily. Sometimes this has led to the family members engaging in activities as individuals rather than as a unit. Television and other media have presented a variety of social values to children. In the past, the value system a child initially accepted was a combination of beliefs fostered by the church, family, and school. Now, the child can witness a whole spectrum of values in a relatively short period of time by viewing, listening, or reading.

What a child becomes is socially, morally, and psychologically influenced by all of the above-mentioned factors. Understanding the world is perhaps more difficult than ever before because of these transitions and because of a barrage of mixed signals. No wonder then that many young people are confused about their roles in society and the expectations of society.

The family is changing. However, it seems that people will always need others to whom closeness, sharing, and love are binding elements. Changes in child-rearing and household responsibilities have required family members to make necessary adjustments, but a complete upheaval in the basic family structure seems unlikely.

MATE SELECTION

Although various lifestyles are available to us, more than 90 percent of the American population marry at least once in their lives. About four out of five who divorce marry again. Some form of courtship is usually engaged in before marriage. The sequence is usually courtship, engagement, and then marriage. The length that each phase lasts, including the marriage, depends on the couple. All too often the couple does not take advantage of the courtship and engagement periods to gather useful information about each other. Unfortunately, we drift from a movie script involving romance to the day-to-day reality of marriage. Many people do not know what their partner expects of the marriage or realize that marriage is not one long romantic adventure. As wonderful and exciting as this time of life can be, every effort should be made to keep in mind the realistic aspects of marriage.

Love and Intimacy

From the socialization process we learn that we are supposed to form relationships and "fall in love." Attempting to define love is a most difficult task. Love has been defined as "that condition in which happiness of another person is essential to your own (Heinlein, 1961). This definition of love would be characterized by the popular songs we listen to, the scenario of Romeo and Juliet, and the reason Edward VIII left the throne to marry Mrs. Simpson. Certainly the element of caring must be present.

Without caring, what is thought to be love may be strong desire. We may desire to have sex or gain wealth and status by pretending to be in love. The problem is determining what love really is. Erich Fromm wrote that caring and respect for another is central to love, and that people can achieve a meaningful type of love only after they are secure in their own identity. Fromm (1956) goes on to define mature love as "union under the condition of preserving one's integrity, one's individuality." Fromm suggests that a lover must feel, "I want the loved person to grow and unfold for his own sake and in his own ways, and not for the purpose of serving me."

The English language is limited in that only one word is available to describe a wide variety of feelings and relationships called love. The ancient Greeks had a variety of terms to describe more precisely the different kinds of love. *Eros* referred to passionate or erotic love. *Storge* meant affection such as the feelings parents have for their children, while *philia* indicated the type of love in friendships, and *agape* referred to a kind of love associated with the traditional Christian view of being undemanding, patient, kind, and always supportive. In our society, love has been defined in terms of romantic, rational, and mature love. Romantic love is an intense emotional experience that can totally captivate our existence. Another type of love is rational love, which is based on acceptance of the partner's imperfections as well as affections and is more likely to lead to fulfilling, long-lasting relationships. Mature love is maintained through communication and separateness of the partners. It involves respect, admiration, and the desire to help each other. Mature lovers are best friends who are committed to each other and their relationship.

To help deal with the concept of love, Coutts (1973) has described five levels of love. The first is called sentimentality, which centers on one's own feelings, needs, fears, and insecurities. If we remain at this level, we become insensitive and exploitative in our relationship. The second level is awareness. Sharing and caring develops mutually between the partners, and an intimacy emerges based on facts, not impressions. The third level is involvement, in which the partner sees what is needed and works very hard at offering the support. The fourth level is dedication, in which the partners are willing to make sacrifices of their needs, safety, and comfort. The fifth level of loving is commitment. This is the most powerful of all love relationships. It encompasses intellect, emotions, body, lasting awareness, and involvement. As difficult as love is to define and identify, perhaps it will help to pose several questions to help distinguish between healthy and problematic love (Peele & Brodsky, 1976):

1. Do both lovers have a secure belief in their own value?
2. Are the lovers improved by the relationship?
3. Do the lovers maintain serious interests outside the relationship, including other meaningful personal relationships?
4. Is the relationship integrated into, rather than being set off from, the totality of the lovers' lives?
5. Are the lovers beyond being possessive or jealous of each other's growth and expansion of interest?
6. Are the lovers also friends? Would they seek each other out if they should cease to be primary partners?

As love develops, so does intimacy. Like love, intimacy needs time to develop and goes through several stages. Those stages are (Calderone, 1972):

1. Choice: two people meet; they like each other; and begin to become closer.
2. Mutual: their desire for closeness is mutually shared.
3. Reciprocity: they give to each other and grow by confiding in each other. There is an equal sharing of confidences.
4. Trust: they begin to share at deeper levels, becoming aware that their deepest feelings and thoughts are accepted.
5. Delight: they have unconditional acceptance of one another and delight in the relationship.

To be intimate means to be vulnerable. It means a risk of rejection or suffocation of one's self. However, compatible partners replace those risks with trust and satisfaction. Essentially, individuals must remain responsible for themselves, yet help each other with their goals, problems, and desires. Enjoying, sharing, and caring should be the outcomes of living with someone with whom love and intimacy are shared.

Why People Marry

People marry for both personal and societal reasons. There is no single reason why people marry. Some marry because they do not want to be alone. They want someone to share confidences, and they want to give and receive affection. A happy marriage can offer intimacy, sharing, and support and can stimulate personal growth.

Some people marry for economic reasons. For example, they may wish to pool their incomes or the husband may provide financial security to the wife and children, while the wife runs the home and cares for the children. Most people marry because they enjoy that person on whom they can depend in times of need and with whom they can share both joy and sorrow.

Dating and Courtship

Most people experience some form of dating. The development of an extensive dating system seems to be a modern American innovation. Lacking standards of right and wrong or institutionalized patterns of behavior, most couples have to seek their own modes of behavior. Dating as courtship is influenced by parents, church, and other aspects of our society that have a vested interest in continuing a traditional form of society. It is through dating that we select our mates. The beneficial features of dating are that it aids the process of socialization, personality development, and learning to get along with the opposite sex. Typically, the characteristics that people look for in a marriage partner include dependable character, emotional stability, pleasing disposition, mutual attraction, good health, desire for home and family, and refinement (Kephart, 1977).

Choosing a Partner

We tend to marry someone from more or less the same background as ourselves. We may be attracted to certain types of people but seldom consider how various factors affect the chances of a successful marriage. The following are some of the factors that are involved in selecting a marriage partner:

Love. As difficult as it is to define, most people marry because of the feelings of love they hold for their partner. A desire for sharing experiences and sexual intimacy, as well as a deep concern for the partner, are the ingredients of love. As important as this factor is, love can be maintained only if the couple develops communication, understanding, and a desire to enhance each other's happiness. The nature of love tends to change over the years of marriage and is enhanced by emotions over the years. Certainly, love should not be confused with sexual attraction. Although sexual desire may confirm one's feeling of love for the partner, a couple may have a good sexual relationship without loving each other.

Background. We all bring unique histories to our relationships. Several factors seem to be important considerations in the selection of a potential mate. Included are the considerations of age, race, health, education, intelligence, religion, economic status, family background, and previous marital status.

Age. Research indicates that the younger the age of the couple, the less chance the marriage has of surviving. Between 50 to 67 percent of marriages in which the individuals are below age 20 will end in divorce. The average age of marriage in the United States is now 24 for men and 21 for women. For men, marriage before age 22 decreases the probability of success. In four out of ten marriages, the man is three to nine years older than the woman. Certainly, age differences between couples are not uncommon, but the motives for marrying someone extremely older or younger should be examined. For example, does the older person represent a parental figure or offer immediate economic security?

Race. In many communities, interracial marriages are not well accepted and may present difficult barriers, even though the percentage of such marriages has been increasing steadily. Besides the societal problems an interracial marriage faces, problems that evolve around customs, values, and attitudes must also be faced. These factors are present in any marriage but may be even more pronounced in an interracial marriage and should be discussed when such a marriage is planned.

Health. Factors such as genetics may be important if one or both partners have conditions that could be manifested in offspring. Conditions such as alcoholism or mental health problems are indications of possible problems for a marriage. An important aspect of success in marriage is the mental and physical health of the partners. Warning signs of serious problems in either area should not be ignored.

Education. Although marriages can succeed with a variety of educational levels within a relationship, it is important to assess one's feelings if a wide disparity in educational levels is present. A pronounced difference in this area could lead to feelings of inferiority. However, any differences can be overcome if love, interests, and expectations are similar.

Intelligence. Like education, differences in intelligence should not hinder a relationship if partners are given the freedom to be themselves. The positive aspects should be emphasized. A point of warning is that wide variations in intelligence can lead to a drifting apart of the couple since educational, social, and intellectual interests may become different as the partners develop their individuality.

Religion. One of the most difficult aspects to overcome is the difference in religious affiliation and devoutness of the partner. Although interfaith marriages are quite common, few couples take the time to discuss religious beliefs regarding raising children, sexual behavior, and finances. For some, religion has little meaning, while for others it has the potential to either unify or serve as a powerful wedge in the relationship. This area should be discussed thoroughly between the couple, their parents, and clergy so that the couple clearly understands the issues and obligations surrounding their partner's religious views.

Economic status.   Adequate income is essential to a successful marriage since this factor can represent a major area of contention. A couple should examine their values and determine whether their available income allows for the lifestyle they desire, or if marriage would be better delayed. Job potential should be assessed to determine whether the desired lifestyle requires both partners to work full-time.

Marriage

For most members of society marriage is viewed as the cornerstone of family organization. Reiss (1980, p. 50) defines marriage as "a socially accepted union of individuals in husband and wife roles, with the key function of legitimation of parenthood." Eshleman (1981, p. 82) identifies six criteria that have been found to exist for marriages regardless of social or economic background. They are

1. A heterosexual union, including at least one male and one female
2. The legitimizing or granting of approval to the sexual relationship and the bearing of children without any loss of standing in the community or society
3. A public affair rather than a private, personal matter
4. A highly institutionalized and patterned mating arrangement
5. An assuming of mutual and reciprocal rights and obligations between the spouses
6. A binding relationship that assumes some permanence

Marriage serves many functions for individuals, including establishment of a family, companionship, happiness, love, economic security, a sexual outlet, and children. The greater success in meeting these needs, the greater the likelihood the marriage will remain intact. Since each year more than two million marriages take place in the United States, it seems safe to say that marriages exist to fulfill basic needs associated with the husband-wife relationship. For these individual needs to be met, each partner must be committed to the marriage, develop effective communication, and accept the responsibility to nurture and enhance the marriage.

PARENTHOOD

When children enter a family, the married couple must assume new roles. The wife must become a mother and the husband a father. The exclusiveness of the partners to each other as well as the time demands and interest of the couple must change. Parenthood is a most difficult task, and yet couples are expected to automatically fulfill this role with little or no formal training. Parenthood is a lifetime commitment. Individuals can quit their jobs or divorce their mate, but there is no honorable way to withdraw from the role of father or mother. Many groups are now teaching parenthood education programs that promote parenting skills. These courses attempt to teach ways to facilitate communication between parents and children, improve methods of discipline, and develop appropriate behavior for parents and children.

Advantages and Disadvantages of Parenthood

The obvious advantage of parenthood is the opportunity to love and nurture another human being. The psychological pleasure from being part of a loving family and helping direct its development can bring a couple closer together with the long-term benefit of pride in having done so. Besides the extreme economic cost of having and raising children, parenthood usually requires an adjustment in the career of at least one of the partners. Further, a child will take away from the emotional sharing time of the couple. Much time will be spent in guiding and showing affection to the child. Some personal activities will have to be changed or eliminated, and there is constant need to transport the children to various activities and functions as they become older.

Single Parenthood

Parenthood is difficult when two partners share the nurturing and love that each child requires. It can become even more difficult if only one parent is present. Through death, desertion, or divorce, single-parent situations often arise. Some individuals cope quite successfully with single parenthood, while others struggle with the many roles and situations they face in raising their children.

A single parent may experience various problems. It may be difficult to meet the emotional needs of the child. There are a variety of ways to express love for a child. Telling them they are loved, demonstrating that love, and helping them, all serve to express love; however, the demands of working and maintaining a home may be so overwhelming that this aspect is lacking. It also may be hard for the single parent to provide proper supervision for the child. Making arrangements for the child's care and supervision is difficult and costly and may take a large share of the budget. In addition, since women tend to make less money than men, households headed by women can experience financial difficulties. Finally, the single parent may experience unfulfilled emotional and sexual needs. Unmet emotional needs can develop because of the lack of time to seek or spend in a relationship. Since most single parents wish to hide their sexual involvement, finding a time and place can present problems. Nevertheless, being a single parent does not have to be a disaster. It is important that the single parent have sufficient financial, material, and emotional support to meet the demands of the child and themselves.

Divorce

Death, annulment, and divorce are all ways in which a marriage may be terminated. The most frequent method for dissolving a marriage is through divorce. Divorce is usually viewed as a failure of the family system as well as a great personal crisis. However, it is also a way to end physical abuse and emotional tension associated with a marriage. Divorces can be obtained in most societies and the divorce rates have risen throughout the world. Personal factors given as reasons for divorce include financial problems, physical abuse, mental abuse, drinking, in-law problems, lack of love, adultery, and sexual incompatibility. Kephart (1977, p. 470) lists six social factors that are contributing to the increased divorce rates. They are as follows:

1. *Changing family functions.* Outside sources may now fulfill functions that were once considered primary family responsibilities. These may include medical, religious, and recreational aspects of family life.
2. *Casual marriages.* Hasty and youthful marriages complicated by pregnancy are often unstable.
3. *Jobs for women.* With greater job opportunities available to a large number of women, a great barrier to divorce for many women was removed.
4. *Decline in moral and religious sanctions.* Although not openly so stated by all churches, most have taken a more liberal attitude toward divorce. Also, society does not attach the severe stigma to divorce that it once did.
5. *The philosophy of happiness.* If happiness does not materialize to the degree anticipated, divorce or separation is accepted as a way of dealing with the feeling.
6. *More liberal divorce laws.* The liberalization of divorce laws, including no-fault divorces, has made it easier to terminate a marriage.

The emotional impact of a divorce is most difficult. Anyone who has experienced a divorce will usually describe it as a painful, devastating experience. Problems with finances, personal adjustment, and children create an extremely stressful situation. Perhaps the most stress in a divorce is created for children. Children whose parents are divorcing may develop deep feelings of guilt, fear, and anger. Many times children feel that they must take sides in the conflict, which only serves to enhance their guilt feelings. Because of the emotional conflict between the marriage partners, they may fail to recognize the worry the children feel concerning their own welfare and what is going to happen to them. It is important to remember that despite the family fighting, the children will continue to love both parents. It is extremely important that children have sensitive parents and understanding teachers during and after a divorce. Many children will require counseling but this must usually come from a private source, not the school system.

PSYCHOLOGICAL ASPECTS OF SEXUALITY AND FAMILY LIVING

Individuals have a wide variety of options for displaying their psychological and physiological traits. Also, in today's society there is greater flexibility in sex roles. This section will deal with those psychological aspects of human sexuality and family life that help determine how people feel and react as individuals.

Gender Development

From birth, social expectations largely guide gender development. Parents consciously and unconsciously manipulate their children's gender development from infancy based upon the sole criterion of sex. From dress and toys to behavior, the child learns to accept the parameters of being either a girl or a boy. By age two, children know what sex they are and understand some of their society's expectations for that sex.

By the time children have reached school age, task orientation and emotional responses are based almost solely on what has been learned about gender. Children's activities are tied to traditional social images of adult roles. Boys are focused on achievement and sports, while girls are pointed toward personal beauty or roles of wives and mothers. This is not to say that girls do not participate in sports or aggressive activities, but these activities are not stressed for girls to the extent they are for boys.

Throughout the school years, for the most part the student observes traditional concepts of adult roles. For example, most elementary teachers are female while most administrators are male. Boys typically are encouraged toward achievement, competition, and occupational goals. Girls typically are encouraged toward compliance, dependence, and submissiveness of occupation and position to males.

Gender identification is a most important organizer of expectations and conduct. Society places a great deal of emphasis on socializing and maintaining gender differences. In some cases this process may be beneficial, in others detrimental to the potential of both boys and girls.

Sex Roles

Since the 1960s, there has been a growing realization that both males and females have a right to expand their individual potential and not be held to traditional roles and stereotypes. Traditional sex roles are learned in the same ways as is gender identity. The emphasis in sex roles should be on the humanness of people, not on their respective genders. Through such an emphasis, factors that inhibit the complete development of the individual can be discarded. Sharing household duties, child rearing, and economic responsibilities can all contribute to the personal development of both partners. Males should not always be expected to be aggressive, nor females always passive.

Overcoming traditional sex roles is not easy since they are established early in life and are constantly reinforced throughout the years. Self-evaluation and a sense of adequacy are linked to sex role performances as defined by parents and peers in childhood. Some say that sex roles are a natural part of growing and learning. However, it is important not to use "tradition" to psychologically lock people into traditional sex roles that inhibit their growth as individuals.

Developing Sexuality

All aspects of human sexuality develop over a long period of time, from early childhood through the adult years. The groundwork for sexual values begins to develop in infancy, as children learn trust, initiative, and love. As they grow older, they try to achieve self-confidence in their interactions with parents, adults, and peers. Development of self-confidence is crucial to the development of the child's sexuality. If children grow up feeling at ease with themselves they are more likley to appreciate themselves and members of the opposite sex.

Anything that affects a child's developing identity will eventually affect his or her sexuality as well. If the child learns to be defensive, unforgiving, or mistrusting in daily life, these attitudes will carry over into the sexual component of that individual's personality. Consequently, it is imperative that children learn to give and receive love and have a positive self-image if they are to be at ease with their sexuality later in life.

BIOLOGICAL COMPONENTS OF SEX EDUCATION

While teachers of younger elementary school children will not be called upon to discuss the human reproductive system in as much detail as teachers of older elementary school children, all children are curious about birth in general and how they themselves came to be. As a result, it is essential for all teachers to have a basic knowledge of the reproductive system and how it works.

The Female Reproductive System

The female reproductive system, shown in figure 19.1, is comprised of the external genitalia and the internal organs consisting of the vagina, uterus, fallopian tubes, and ovaries. The external genitalia are the *labia majora* (the outer lips) and the *labia minors*. The *clitoris* is a small structure at the top of the labia major that serves to facilitate sexual stimulation. The *vagina* is an elastic canal extending from just behind the cervix to the opening of the external genitalia. It serves as the organ for sexual intercourse and as the birth canal. The *uterus* is a pear-shaped organ that serves as a cavity where the fetus develops. The uterus has three layers called the *perimetrium*

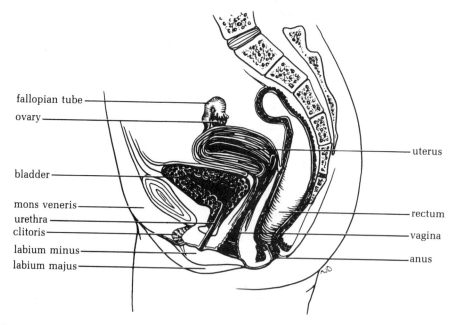

Figure 19.1
Female reproductive system.

(outer layer), the *myometrium* (muscular layer), and *endometrium* (inner layer). It is the endometrium that is sloughed off during menstruation. Two armlike projections called the *fallopian tubes* branch from the uterus. These tubes are three to five inches long and have *fembria* (small fingerlike projections) at the far ends next to the ovaries. Through these tubes the eggs or *ova* pass. If fertilization takes place, it occurs in the upper third of one of the fallopian tubes. Two *ovaries* produce ova and secrete hormones that bring about the development of the female secondary sex characteristics such as the rounding of the female figure, breast development, voice, and pubic hair.

Each ovary contains 200,000 to 400,000 saclike structures called *follicles* that house immature egg cells. At the onset of puberty, due to the release of *FSH* (follicle stimulating hormone) into the bloodstream from the anterior lobe of the pituitary, several follicles are activated in the ovary each month. Only one will evolve into a mature ovum. Simultaneously, estrogen begins being secreted by the follicle. Estro-

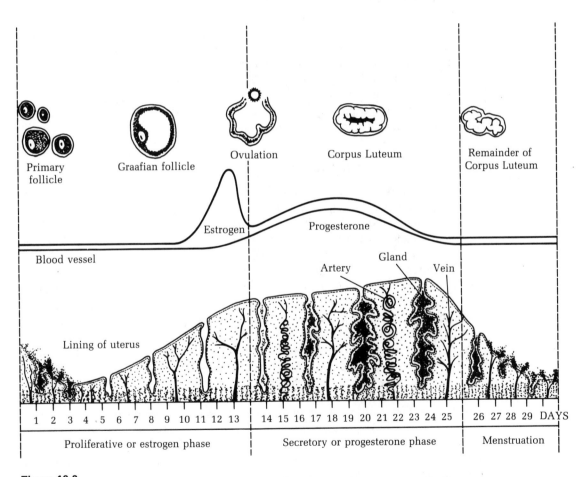

Figure 19.2
The menstrual cycle.

Source: J. J. Burt, L. Meeks, & S. Pottebaum, *Toward a healthy life style through health education in the elementary school.* Belmont, Calif.: Wadsworth, 1980.

gen signals the womb or uterus to prepare for a potential pregnancy by filling its lining with blood and nutrients for nourishment of the embryo.

As the maturing follicle and its ovum move to the surface of the ovary, with the follicle continuing to secrete estrogen, *LH* (luteinizing hormone) is released into the bloodstream from the anterior lobe of the pituitary. The production of LH causes rupture of the follicle and the release of the mature ovum into the fallopian tubes. This process is known as *ovulation* and usually occurs midway into the monthly reproductive cycle of 28 days. This cycle is shown in figure 19.2.

During ovulation, estrogen is at its highest level and causes cessation of additional secretions of FSH. At the same time, LH continues to be secreted and produces closure of the ruptured follicle. The empty follicle, now called the *corpus luteum,* along with the mature ovum begin to produce another hormone in addition to estrogen called *progesterone*. Progesterone further prepares the uterus for implantation of a fertilized egg and continues to maintain the uterus during pregnancy. Simultaneously, the levels of estrogen begin to decrease.

If the mature ovum is not fertilized within 24 to 48 hours after ovulation, it disintegrates, thus diminishing the amount of estrogen and progesterone in the bloodstream. Around the twenty-fourth day of the cycle, the corpus luteum also stops secreting progesterone and estrogen. As a result, several days later the uterus expels its blood-rich lining through the vagina. This process is referred to as *menstruation*. Following menstruation, the reproductive cycle begins again in preparation for possible fertilization and pregnancy. Menstruation begins with puberty. The onset of menstruation at this time is called *menarche*.

The Male Reproductive System

The male reproductive system, shown in figure 19.3, is not cyclical and thus not as hormonally or endocrinologically complex as that of the female. The major male sexual endocrine glands are the two *testes,* or testicles, which are contained and protected in a saclike structure called the *scrotum*. At puberty, the testes begin producing mature *sperm,* the male reproductive cells. Attached to the top of each testis is the *epididymis*. This structure consists of tightly coiled tubes through which the sperm pass to the *vas deferens*. The two vas deferens serve as storage areas for the mature sperm and are the means by which sperm move to the *urethra*. The two vas deferens eventually form into one structure called the *ejaculatory duct*. This tube connects with the urethra. The urethra is a tube that runs the length of the penis. The *penis* is the male organ for sexual intercourse and consists of spongy material called *erectile tissue*. The head of the penis is called the *glans penis*. This area contains many nerve endings and is very sensitive to sexual stimulation.

The *seminal vesicles, prostate gland,* and the two *Cowper's glands* manufacture substances important to the sperm and ejaculation. The seminal vesicles produce a simple sugar, fructose, that adds volume to the ejaculatory fluid, called *semen,* and activates the movement of the sperm. The prostate gland provides a highly alkaline milky fluid that helps to neutralize the highly acid vagina, which facilitates the movement of sperm through that organ. The pea-sized Cowper's glands also produce an alkaline fluid that lubricates and neutralizes the urethra, which is highly acid. The Cowper's glands secrete this substance prior to ejaculation. The combined

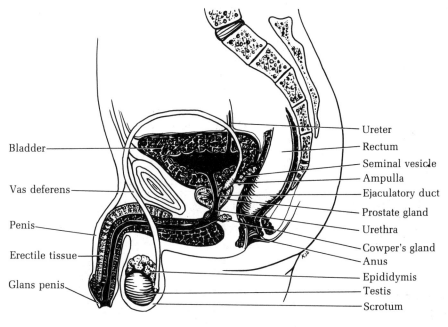

Figure 19.3
The male reproductive system.

fluid produced by the seminal vesicles, prostate, and Cowper's glands, along with the sperm it contains, is semen.

It should be noted that the testes manufacture mature sperm on a consistent basis from puberty through old age. Upon release of *ICSH* (interstitial cell-stimulating hormone) into the bloodstream from the anterior lobe of the pituitary, the testes also secrete *testosterone*. Although it plays many diverse roles, testosterone is needed to trigger the male adolescent growth spurt, which is accompanied by the development of secondary sex characteristics.

CONCEPTION AND PREGNANCY

Conception occurs when a single sperm fertilizes an egg to produce a *zygote*. Conception usually occurs in the upper third of the Fallopian tube and must take place in the first or second day following ovulation. When a sperm enters an egg, the membrane thickens to prevent further penetration by sperm.

Indications of Pregnancy

The first indication that the woman may be pregnant may be the missing of a menstrual period. The woman may develop morning sickness, or nausea. The term morning sickness is not altogether appropriate since the nausea can occur at any time of the day. The breasts may increase in size, and the nipples may enlarge and become darker. The woman may also need to urinate more frequently. One of the most common methods for determining pregnancy is a laboratory test based on the presence in the urine of a hormone called human chorionic gonadotropin. This hormone becomes detectable about 10 days after the missed menstrual period. The hormone is produced by the developing placenta (uterine lining). Home pregnancy tests are available as over-the-counter products, but these should be used only as a preliminary diagnosis since one study found that 20 percent of all women who used the tests obtained false negative results. Consequently, a physician should confirm whether the woman is actually pregnant.

The Embryonic Period

Immediately after conception, the zygote begins to divide to form other cells. It travels down the Fallopian tube and within ten days attaches to the uterine wall. From the time it attaches to the wall until the eighth week, it is called an *embryo*. The embryo divides into three layers of cells from which the various body organs and systems develop. The innermost layer, the *endoderm*, becomes the digestive and respiratory systems; the next layer, the *mesoderm*, forms the skeletal, muscular, circulatory, and reproductive systems; and the *ectoderm*, or outermost layer, becomes the nervous system and skin. The head develops first, with the lower body developing last. After eight weeks, the embryo is called the *fetus*.

The *amnion* is a thin protective membrane that is filled with a fluid called the *amniotic fluid*. This fluid serves as insulation and protection for the embryo against shocks and blows to the mother's abdomen. The fluid also allows for changes in position as growth and movement occur. The *umbilical cord* connects the placenta and the embryo.

The placenta is the organ through which the embryo receives nutrients, vitamins, antibodies, and other substances such as drugs, alcohol, and diseases. The fetus also gives off waste products such as nitrogen compounds and carbon dioxide, which, are carried through the umbilical cord to be diffused through the placenta and given off in the mother's urine and through her lungs. This is accomplished even though there is no mixing of the embryo's and mother's blood. The placenta is expelled shortly following the birth of the child and is referred to as the *afterbirth*.

Trimester Development

From the moment that conception occurs, the woman's body begins to change. Through pregnancy a weight gain of 17 to 24 pounds is normal and looked on as desirable since this helps ensure adequate development of the fetus. The average fetus weighs approximately 7 pounds at birth. Table 19.1 lists the development of the fetus through each trimester.

Multiple Births

Several factors contribute to multiple births. Heredity, age of the mother, and social factors seem significant (McCary, 1982). Multiple births occur more often in certain families than in others. Women in their thirties are more likely to have multiple births than are women in their twenties. Blacks have more twins than whites. Whites have more than Orientals.

Table 19.1
Development During Pregnancy

First Trimester Development

A small mass of cells is implanted in the uterus.
Development into a fetus begins.
Major organ systems are present and recognizable.
During the fourth to eighth weeks, the eyes, ears, arms, hands, fingers, legs, feet, and toes develop.
By the seventh week, the liver, lungs, pancreas, kidneys, and intestines have formed.
By the end of the first trimester, the fetus weighs two-thirds of an ounce and is about 4 inches in length.
From this time on, development consists of enlargement and differentiation of the existing structures.

Second Trimester Development

By the end of the fourteenth week, movement can be detected.
By the eighteenth week, a fetal heartbeat can be detected.
By the twentieth week, the fetus will open its eyes.
Around the twenty-fourth week, the fetus is sensitive to light and can hear sounds. It will also have periods of sleep and wakefulness.

Third Trimester Development

Fat deposits form under the skin.
During seventh month, the fetus turns in the uterus to a head down position.
By the end of the eighth month, the fetus weighs an average of 5 pounds 4 ounces.
At birth, the infant weighs approximately 7.5 pounds and is 20 inches long.

Identical twins develop from a single fertilized ovum that divides to form two individuals. Such twins are always the same sex and look very much alike. *Fraternal twins* develop from two different ova. The ova are fertilized at about the same time. However, fraternal twins may not be of the same sex and look no more alike than any other sibling born to the parents.

Triplets usually involve two fertilized ova, one of which separates and then develops into twins. *Quadruplets* usually involve two fertilized ova that then divide and develop into two pairs of identical twins.

CHILDBIRTH

The process of birth occurs in three stages and is referred to as labor. This process begins when the amniotic sac that has protected the fetus ruptures and the amniotic fluid flows from the vagina. Labor pains occur at regular intervals, usually fifteen to twenty minutes apart, with the cervix dilating to three to four inches to permit the emergence of the fetus through the vagina. This first stage of labor may last twelve to sixteen hours (or even longer) for the first birth but usually is shorter in subsequent births.

The second stage begins when the cervix has fully dilated and the baby's head enters the vagina. It ends with the birth of the baby. Contractions are quite severe and last from a minute to a minute and a half, with a two-to-three-minute interval between contractions. The contractions serve to move the baby down the birth canal.

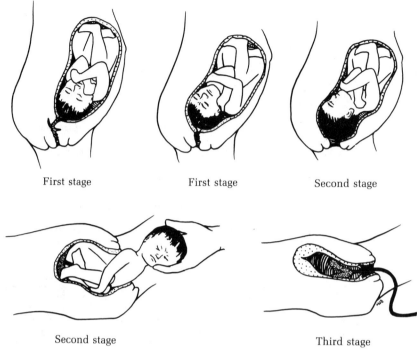

First stage   First stage   Second stage

Second stage   Third stage

Figure 19.4
Stages of birth.

Just before the head of the child appears, it rotates to the side to pass the pelvic bone. The neck and shoulders emerge and the rest of the body follows rather quickly. The physician cuts the umbilical cord and checks to ensure that the baby is breathing. This stage lasts from fifty to sixty minutes for the first delivery but may be as short as twenty minutes in subsequent births.

The third and final stage lasts only a few minutes and consists of the delivery of the placenta. The placenta separates from the wall of the uterus and is expelled as afterbirth. It is examined to determine that all of the organ has been delivered.

Occasionally complications do arise during labor. For example, some conditions may require a *cesarean section.* When this procedure is used, an incision is made through the abdominal wall. Another incision is made in the uterus and the baby is removed. The reason for a cesarean section is usually a contracted pelvis, in which the baby is unable to pass into the vagina. Other reasons are that the baby is in a *breech* (buttock or leg presenting first) position, the placenta has prematurely separated from the uterus causing a loss of oxygen, a vaginal infection is present, or the mother is incapacitated because of injury or trauma. To help identify potential complications, a fetal monitor may be used during the birth process.

Methods of Delivery

Several methods are commonly used to help reduce the pain associated with labor. A general anesthetic is sometimes used to induce a light sleep in which the mother is partly awake. The problem with any type of general anesthesia, however, is that it also enters the baby's bloodstream and can cause sluggish respiration in the infant. A complaint against local anesthetics is that they are often used unnecessarily, therefore increasing the potential for harm to the woman and the infant. Anesthetics may also dull the experience and excitement of birth. Another procedure used is a surgical incision in the vagina called an *episiotomy.* This is done to prevent undue stretching or tearing of the vagina.

For many couples today, it is essential that the father be present and that the mother be totally aware. A method known as prepared childbirth is an outgrowth of this desire. Introduced into the United States by Fernand Lamaze, it is known as the Lamaze technique. This technique requires pretraining sessions to learn relaxation and controlled breathing. This type of childbirth is not an endurance test since a mild painkiller may be given, but the use of a general anesthetic is avoided unless the mother so chooses during labor. The husband is taught how to help his wife relax through birth. A major advantage of the Lamaze method is that both the man and the woman learn what happens to the woman's body during birth and what to expect during delivery. Prepared childbirth may be done either at the hospital or in a special childbirth center where a midwife usually assists in the labor process.

Frederick LeBoyer, another French physician, has developed a procedure that attempts to provide a nonviolent birth for the baby. This approach advocates placing the baby in warm water immediately after birth and surrounding the baby with dim lighting and very little noise. LeBoyer believes this type of environment makes birth gentler for the baby. He also advocates not cutting the umbilical cord immediately and allowing breathing to begin gradually (LeBoyer, 1966).

In addition to alternative methods of birth, some women are choosing to have their children in birth centers or in their own homes. The alternative birth center may be associated with a hospital and typically emphasizes the needs and desires of the mother. The birthing room may consist of a double bed and be decorated more like a bedroom than a hospital room. This serves to provide a homelike situation but still has any medical equipment readily available that might be needed. Other women prefer to have their babies in their homes. However, it may be difficult to find a physician who is willing to deliver in a home. Some states do allow midwives to deliver babies in the home setting, but there is still the major drawback of not having emergency medical equipment if needed. The advantages are that it costs less, places control in the parents' hands, and allows the woman to avoid procedures she finds unnecessary or objectionable.

Breast-Feeding

At one time in the United States, few women breast fed their children. However, a group called the La Leche League has been a leader in educating American women to the advantages of breast-feeding.

Breast-feeding seems to be an important means of bonding between the mother and child by ensuring close contact and by providing a sense of security for the baby. Additional advantages are that the mother's milk is easier on the baby's digestive system, has more iron, viramins, minerals, contains more antibodies that provide immunity against allergy and disease, is always the right temperature, and is free from bacteria. In addition, sexual interest returns more rapidly for breast-feeding women than for non–breast-feeding women.

Any woman who does not enjoy or is unhappy with breast-feeding should discontinue it since it can disrupt the mother-child relationship. Other disadvantages of breast-feeding are that any substances the mother ingests (such as alcohol, nicotine, drugs) can have a negative effect on the baby; some women find that their breasts drip milk, which can become a nuisance for them; the baby may not drink enough milk and as a result the breast will become swollen and tender; the nipples may become sore; it may be difficult for the mother to know if the baby is consuming enough; and the father may feel he is not part of the process because he cannot feed the baby. Finally, some women feel that breast-feeding prevents them from resuming their regular activities or returning to work.

Genetics

The human body is made up of trillions of cells that provide for various specialized functions. Each cell contains a nucleus. This nucleus contains *genes* that provide the hereditary information in smaller rod-shaped bodies called *chromosomes*. Twenty-two pairs of autosomal chromosomes account for individual facial features, hair color, height, body build, and myriad of other characteristics. Gender is determined by the twenty-third, or sex-determining, chromosomal pair. One member of the pair is called an X chromosome. The other can be either an X or Y chromosome. If two Xs pair, a female develops. An XY pairing produces a male offspring.

Mitosis is ordinary cell division. This process results in two new cells that each contain the full complement of 46 chromosomes. *Meiosis* is the cell division by which sperm and ovum are formed. These cells are called *gametes* and contain only 23 chromosomes. When a male gamete (sperm) unites with a female gamete (ovum), the 23 pairs unite to determine gender. The ovum always contains the X chromosome, while the sperm can have either an X or a Y chromosome. If a sperm with a Y chromosome fertilizes the egg, the baby will be a male, XY. If an X sperm fertilizes the egg, the baby will be a female, XX. For a more complete discussion of genetic defects, see chapter 3.

Contraception

For many people the problem is not how to conceive but how to prevent conception. Contraception, or the prevention of pregnancy, can be accomplished in various ways. It can be accomplished by preventing ovulation, fertilization, or implantation. Some of the common methods employed are coitus interruptus, rhythm, fertility awareness, condoms, vaginal spermicides, diaphragms, cervical caps, hormonal contraceptives, intrauterine devices (IUDs), vaginal sponges, and sterilization. The last should be considered a permanent procedure for prevention of pregnancy.

Abortion

Abortion is the removal of an embryo or fetus from the uterus. However, if the body rejects the embryo or fetus, it is called a spontaneous abortion or miscarriage. Most miscarriages occur in the second or third month of pregnancy. About 33 percent of all fertilized eggs abort before the next menstrual period. An additional 25 percent of all pregnancies miscarry between the time of fertilization and labor (McCary, 1982). Some of the causes for miscarriage include diseases such as syphilis, genital herpes, and diabetes; poor uterine environment; a defective fetus; or malformations of the female reproductive organs.

Probably no issue has been more controversial than that of artificially induced abortions. Many consider it to be an act of murder. Others just as strongly believe that abortion is a matter of choice for the individuals involved. In 1973 the U.S. Supreme Court ruled that every woman was entitled to an abortion if she so desired. Since the legislation of abortion, more than one million have been performed each year.

The abortion issue, however, is far from settled. Many states have circumvented the 1973 ruling by establishing laws that make abortions more difficult to obtain. The U.S. Congress has placed restrictions on government-paid abortions by prohibiting Medicaid funds from being used to pay for the procedure except when the mother's life is in danger.

PROBLEMS OF ABUSE AND VIOLENCE

Spouse Abuse

Spouse abuse occurs in all social and economic classes. Usually it is the wife who is the recipient of the abuse, but there are some cases in which the husband is physically abused by the wife. Only a small percentage of abuse cases are ever reported. The typical wife abuser seems to be a man who is angry, resentful, and suspicious, yet extremely dependent on his wife's support and nurturance. To the outside world, he may appear to be a self-assured, independent individual. Unfortunately, he harbors deep feelings of insecurity and is unable to vent his anger on what he views as a threatening world. Abusive husbands see themselves outclassed and unable to assume the "ideal" that has been presented to them during their upbringing.

Perhaps the most mystifying question is why wives remain in such a deplorable situation. Many women feel that they are somehow to blame and actually deserve what they receive. Others have a very real fear of having to deal with the husband if they should call the police—what happens to her after the police leave or the husband is released—from jail. Finally, many women are reluctant to leave because they have nowhere to go and no way to support themselves or their children.

There is good evidence to suggest that if a husband and wife seek professional help together, violence in the home often can be eliminated. Unfortunately, abusive husbands rarely are willing to seek therapy as a solution. If a husband refuses to seek outside help, a wife should not remain in the household and expose herself to additional abuse.

Child Abuse

Child abuse is a particularly difficult problem to combat because the abuse usually occurs in the home and because there is often a public reluctance to intervene and report what is thought to be a family matter. The National Center of Child Abuse and

Health Highlight: Information for Teachers

1. Child sexual abuse (molestation) involves the misuse of power by an adult or older child to engage a younger child in sexual activities to gratify the adult's needs.
2. Both touching and nontouching offenses are included in the category of sexual abuse. Examples of nontouching behaviors include showing children pornography or having children pose for pornographic pictures. Touching offenses include fondling and penetration.
3. While the actual behavior involved in child sexual abuse varies, the following characteristics are common to most cases.
   A. It usually starts at an early age before children are aware of the inappropriate nature of the activity.
   B. The adult takes advantage of the child's need for approval, trust, and lack of knowledge.
   C. The behavior is surrounded with secrecy.
   D. The adult uses authority to threaten, bribe, or trick the child into complying.
   E. The child feels responsible for the abuse.
4. The child's reaction to the situation is dependent upon his or her perception of the offense and the reactions of those important to him or her, rather than the legally defined severity of the offense.
5. Current information suggests that at least one in four girls and one in seven boys are physically molested by the age of 18. In 80 to 90 percent of the reported cases, the perpetrator (offender) is someone who is known to the child; in over 50 percent of the cases, the offender is a family member.
6. Most often, the perpetrator is someone the child knows well. The child may be emotionally tied to the individual and may even love him or her. Therefore, it should be emphasized that abuse can happen with someone we know or love; do not overemphasize danger from strangers.
7. Some children are aware of the inappropriateness of abusive behavior but are still unable to terminate it. Others are unable to recognize or respond appropriately to abusive or potentially abusive situations.
8. The educator should be sensitive to the manner in which material is presented and to the reactions of the students. Disclosure is often vague or indirect.
9. *Talking About Touching* by Harms and James and the *Personal Safety Curriculum* by Crisci are excellent cirricula that contain lesson plans, resources, and activities for grades K-6. A list of audiovisual and written materials is provided after each section of the instructional sequence and in the annotated bibliography.
10. Define the subject according to the child's age. For young ones, explain that, while most adults are good and care, some do not make good decisions about touching children. They may try to touch children on private parts of the body for no good reason. A broader range of offenses and behaviors can be included when defining molestation to older children. Use examples of touching and nontouching behaviors to make sure they understand the entire concept.
11. It is equally important for children to understand the characteristics of healthy interpersonal and familial relationships. Indicate that most adults do care and want to help children. Use examples of positive interpersonal relationships as well as negative ones in teaching the material.
12. Lessons for younger children need to stress developing the self-confidence and self-esteem needed to resist the attention and gifts often "earned" through participating in the abuse. Older children should begin to recognize characteristics of cooperative and exploitative relationships and relate these to their daily activities.
13. Touches can be categorized according to one's personal reaction to the touch. Good touches make one feel warm, secure, happy; bad touches make one feel angry, hurt or ashamed. Those touches that confuse are often sexual touches, or touches that are delivered in a contradictory manner that perplexes the child. Refer to resource materials for additional information about the Touch Continuum.
14. Lessons should include opportunities to role play and use the skills taught. For examples of assertiveness and decision-making activities, refer to resource materials.

Neglect estimates that one million children are maltreated by their parents each year. Of these children, as many as 100,000 to 200,000 are physically abused; 60,000 to 100,000 are sexually abused; and the remainder are neglected. Each year, more than 2,000 children die in circumstances of abuse or neglect.

Aside from the obvious physical effects, a child's psychological development can be seriously handicapped by abusive treatment. Many abused children are emotional cripples for the rest of their lives. A child who is abused in the home is one who loses the chance to be a child. Unable to understand why they are being punished, these children come to believe that they deserve such treatment because they are "bad." They see the world as cold and hostile and have little faith in themselves or in their ability to succeed in life. They learn that using force is an acceptable way to deal with others and, most tragically, often become child abusers themselves.

Most parents become abusive either because of their failure to understand the needs of their children or in response to overwhelming stress. They typically do not have the self-confidence, ingenuity, and ability to cope with crisis within the family. For them, any crisis presents a greater danger than for someone with better coping skills. Even a minor occurrence may be enough to lead to loss of self-control and an abusive attack on the innocent child. There is hope for re-education if the matter can be brought to the attention of the proper authorities.

Every state has laws that make it mandatory for teachers to report suspected child abuse. Teachers should keep in mind that a child's development into a healthy, happy adult may depend on receiving love and concern. Not every bruise should be considered abuse, but if a pattern of injury is observed, teachers should express concern to the proper authorities.

Rape

Rape is the act of being forced to have sexual intercourse against one's will. It is a crime of violence and is often not sexual in nature or motivation. Forcible rape is distinguished from statutory rape, which is intercourse with a partner below the age of consent, even if force is not involved. In her book *Against Our Will,* Susan Brownmiller asserted that rape is essentially an act of aggression, control, and degradation aimed at proving male superiority (Brownmiller, 1975). The profile of the typical rapist is a man of 20 to 24 years old, from a low-income, culturally deprived background. The rapist is typically of dull to normal intelligence. The family backgrounds of rapists are typically unstable, and the rapist often expresses feelings of inadequacy and low self-esteem. A history of teenage offenses is common.

In an attempt to deal with the various personalities that commit rape, a classification system has been developed (Cohen, 1977). The four types of rapists are: the aggressive-aim rapist, the sexual-aim rapist, the sex-aggression-fusion rapist, and the impulse rapist. The aggressive-aim rapist is motivated by a desire to hurt his victim. The emotional state during the rape is one of anger. The attacker's victim is typically a stranger. Hurting the victim, not sex, is the intent. For the sexual-aim rapist the motivation is clearly sexual. He uses a minimal amount of violence and aggression and is highly sexually aroused. The act is usually committed outdoors, and the victim can escape quite easily if she resists this type of attacker. The sex-aggression-fusion rapist seems to be sexually excited by violence. Rapist-murderers are an extreme version of this type. Needless to say, this type of rapist is the most dangerous. Fortunately, he is also the rarest. The impulse rapist has neither a sexual nor an aggressive motive. Rape is committed on impulse. He sees an opportunity and seizes it and is not bound by normal societal restraints against rape. The motivation is that the rape is satisfying to him.

Group or gang rapes have been estimated to constitute 70 percent of all rapes. These types of rape occur most often when group members seek esteem by challenging their peers to join in an assault. Responsibility for the assault shifts from the individual to the group. The attacks are usually planned in advance, with the attackers between the ages of 15 and 19.

Many myths are associated with rape. Among these myths are the patently absurd notions that women secretly want to be raped; some women deserve to be raped; rape keeps women in line; nice women do not get raped; or rape is provoked by the woman. Nothing in the research substantiates these claims even partially. They may serve to ease the rapist's guilt feelings, but the fact remains that he has committed a heinous act of aggression and violence against an innocent victim.

The victim of rape may react in one of two ways. The expressive reaction may include hysteria, crying, guilt, and fear. This type of reaction may first appear as a very controlled reaction followed at some later time by a severe emotional reaction. The second type of reaction is referred to as the silent reaction. In this case, the victim may tell no one of the attack because she feels responsible for the rape or feels she could have prevented it. Unfortunately, this reaction may also be motivated by the fact that many men reject their wives or girlfriends after a rape. Regardless of the type of reaction, victims of rape suffer from a wide variety of conditions, including rectal bleeding and pain, irritation of the genitals, headache, nervousness, sleeplessness, fear, nausea, a sense of humiliation, and a desire for revenge.

Counseling is extremely important in helping the victim work through her feelings. Many cities have rape crisis centers designed to help the victim with the physical and emotional problems. Many centers also help the victim with the police and court procedures. Self-defense instruction is important for women in avoiding rape. It is imperative that proper training be taken before self-defense measures are taken, since even greater physical harm can occur to the victim if the self-defense techniques are not done properly. Others suggest that we need to change the way we socialize males and females. The stereotype of females being weak and passive while the male is aggressive seems to be one root cause. In societies in which males are taught to be nurturing rather than aggressive, rape is virtually unheard of (Mead, 1935).

Incest

Sexual intercourse between two persons who are too closely related by blood or affinity to be legally married is considered incest. When the act occurs against the will of a party involved, it is coercive. Most incest goes unreported; thus, it is difficult to know its exact occurrence. Father-daughter incest was once thought to be the most common. Researchers now feel that brother-sister incest is the most common (Renshaw, 1983).

Taboos aganst incest are found in virtually every society. Genetically, the factor of inbreeding can cause serious consequences. A study done in Japan compared marriages between cousins with nonrelated marriages. It was found that the children of the blood-related marriages were significantly lower in school performance, physical skills, and certain measures of health than were the offspring of the nonrelated marriages. In addition, incest may cause conflict within the family, guilt, and resentment that may last a lifetime for the individuals involved. Finally, incest is not bound by family education or economic level. The evidence indicates that families from all walks of life can be affected.

IMPLICATIONS FOR SEX AND FAMILY LIFE EDUCATION

In the early elementary years, children have a natural curiosity about the human body, emotions, babies, and the differences between boys and girls. Family relationships and responsibilities should be explored since children need to gain insight about their contributions to family functioning. Special concern should be shown for single-parent families and the sensitive feelings that may be involved when discussing family life. The concepts of love, concern, and caring for family and others should be introduced in the early elementary years. Another important concept is the issue of child abuse. This issue should be discussed and children should realize that no one has the right to violate their personhood.

In the upper elementary years, children may begin to experience a rapid growth spurt. A greater curiosity about their own bodies develops as well as a greater interest in the opposite sex. Students usually feel the need to improve their social skills with the opposite sex, yet are very self-conscious when dealing with the opposite sex. The physical changes some of the students are experiencing in late elementary school should be addressed. The responsibilities and privileges of adolescents should be discussed. Interpersonal skills that help the students deal with the emotions of adolescence should be emphasized.

SUMMARY

No area in health education is more controversial than that of sex and family life education. The goal of sex and family life education is to develop an appreciation of self and others and to aid children in assuming the responsibilities of being members of society. This process must start early in the life of children and be built upon each year if they are to develop a healthy appreciation of their own sexuality.

The biological aspects of sex education are an important component of a total sex and family life education program. Children should be taught the names of the parts of the reproductive systems and should understand the basic facts concerning fertilization, pregnancy, and birth. An understanding of menarche and puberty should be achieved in the later elementary school years.

Dating, mate selection, marriage, and parenthood are all aspects of an individual's total sexuality. Each fulfills basic needs of the individual or society and serves to maintain a highly institutionalized social pattern. The increase in premarital intercourse and in the incidence of divorce are often viewed as a failure of our family system. The American family is in transition and is subject to greater stress. However, the family as the basic unit of society continues to thrive.

All aspects of sexuality develop over a long period of time. It is extremely important that a positive self-image be developed if children are to grow to adulthood with

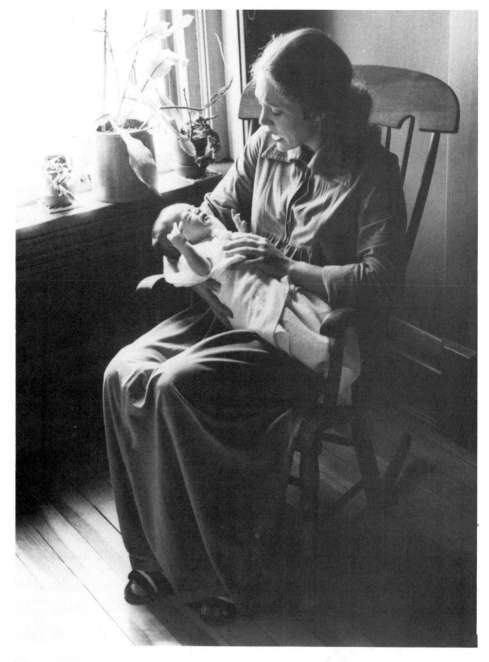

What a child becomes socially, morally, and psychologically is determined by many different factors.

the ability to respect others and give and receive love. Involved in this process is the development of the roles children must assume in their lives. These roles should not be so rigid that they inhibit the right of each individual to develop to optimum potential.

DISCUSSION QUESTIONS

1. Discuss why parents might be opposed to family life education.
2. Discuss the steps recommended for establishing an effective sex and family life education program.
3. What qualifications should a teacher have for teaching sex and family life education?
4. What are secondary sex characteristics?
5. Discuss the female reproductive cycle.
6. Discuss the development that occurs at each trimester during pregnancy.
7. According to Eshleman, marriage serves many functions. Discuss some of these functions.
8. Discuss how sex roles are learned and some of the possible shortcomings of inflexible sex roles.
9. Concerning sexual adjustment, why is it imperative that a child have a positive self-image?
10. How do children learn their sexuality?
11. Discuss child abuse.

REFERENCES

1. Bossard, J. "Residential propinquity as a factor in marriage selection." *American Journal of Sociology,* September, 1932.
2. Brownmiller, S. *Against our will.* New York: Simon and Schuster, 1975.
3. Calderone, M. "Love, sex, intimacy and aging as a life style." In *Sex, love, intimacy— Whose life styles?* New York: Siecus, 1972.
4. Cohen, M. et al. "The psychology of rapists." *Seminars in Psychiatry,* July, 1977.
5. Coutts, R. *Love and intimacy: A psychological approach.* San Ramon, Calif.: Consensus Publishers, 1973.
6. Eshleman, J. *The family: An introduction.* Boston: Allyn & Bacon, 1981.
7. Fromm, Eric. *The Art of loving.* New York: Harper & Row, 1956.
8. Heinlein, R. *Stranger in a strange land.* New York: Putnam, 1961.
9. Hyde, J. *Understanding human sexuality,* second edition. New York: McGraw-Hill, 1982.
10. Johnson, W., & Belzar, E. *Human sexual behavior and sex education.* Philadelphia: Lea & Febiger, 1973.
11. Kephart, W. *The family, society and the individual.* Boston: Houghton Mifflin, 1977.
12. Kinsey, A. *Sexual behavior in the human female.* Philadelphia: W. B. Saunders, 1948.
13. LeBoyer, Frederick. *Birth without violence.* New York: Alfred A. Knopf, 1966.
14. McCary, J. *Human sexuality.* New York: Van Nostrand, 1978.
15. McCary, J., & McCary, S. *McCary's human sexuality,* fourth edition. Belmont, Calif.: Wadsworth Publishing, 1982.

16. Mead, M. *Sex and temperament in three primitive societies.* New York: William Morrow, 1935.

17. Monahan, T., "Are interracial marriage really less stable?" *Social Forces, 48* June, 1970.

18. Peele, S., & Brodsky, A. *Love and addiction.* New York: New American Library, 1976.

19. Reiss, L. *Family systems in America.* New York: Holt, Rinehart, & Winston, 1980.

20. Renshaw, D. *Incest—Understanding and treatment.* Boston: Little, Brown, 1983.

21. Schiller, P. *Creative approach to sex education and counseling.* New York: Association Press, 1973.

22. U.S. Bureau of Census. *Statistical abstract of the United States.* Washington, D.C.: U.S. Government Printing Office, 1979.

23. Woodward, K. L. "Saving the family." *Newsweek,* May 15, 1978.

20. Techniques for Teaching Sex and Family Life Education

What is included in a sex education program in any setting depends upon who makes the final decision. Various groups decide on their own programs based on criteria that are thought to be sound in their particular situations. Individuals may debate the exact placement of content as well as the appropriateness of specific learning activities.—Clint E. Bruess and Jenold S. Greenberg, Sex Education: Theory and Practice.

BUILDING SELF-ESTEEM AND RESPONSIBLE DECISION-MAKING

Traditionally, the area of sex and family life education has always been the primary responsibility of the family. The church and other social institutions also played a significant role. For a complex variety of reasons, these sources are no longer always completely adequate. For children, the result is often confusion, misinformation, guilt, self-doubt, anxiety, and unhealthy adjustment. However, the schools, by supplementing—not replacing—traditional sources, can lessen this possibility by providing well-designed and tested sex and family life education programs that can provide beneficial results for all concerned—children, parents, and society in general.

In your classroom, you can offer an open, nonthreatening atmosphere where reliable and accurate information can be presented about sex and family matters. But sex and family life education is more than just factual information. An effective program must be based on the development of self-esteem and responsible decision making. If children learn to feel good about themselves, they are less likely to need to exploit others and less likely to be open to exploitation in sexual and family functioning. Sex and family life education strives to teach equality and respect between the sexes and an appreciation for self and others.

The suggestions in this chapter will help you work toward these goals. Included as activities in a community-supported program, these learning opportunities will assist your students in obtaining factual knowledge, developing their value systems, and growing psychologically as individuals.

Concepts to be Taught

- There are many different types of families; not all families consist of a husband, wife, and children living together.

- Each member of a family is important and each has certain privileges and responsibilities.

- Interpersonal skills are necessary for strengthening individual and family life.

- Friends help one another feel good about themselves and provide support.

- Positive self-image is necessary if we are to be at ease with ourselves.

- Understanding of self and others is a foundation for successful adulthood.

- Children have rights and no one should be mistreated, taken advantage of, or abused by another person or adult.

- Heredity and environment influence growth and development.

- Physical, social, and emotional growth occur over a long period of time; such growth differs in each individual.

- All living things can reproduce.

- Wholesome attitudes toward sexuality constitute a basic factor for happiness throughout life.

- Sexual values and sexual responsibilities are often individual decisions.

Cycle Plan for Teaching Topics

Topic	K	1	2	3	4	5	6
				Grade Level			
Types of Families	*	**	**	***	**	***	**
Roles of Family Members	**	*	**	**	***	***	***
Family Problems	*	*	**	***	**	**	***
Physical Growth and Development	**	**	**	***	***	***	***
Child Abuse	**	*	**	**	**	**	***
The Opposite Sex	*	*	*	**	**	***	***
Sexual Feelings	*	*	*	*	**	***	***
Genetics and Heredity	*	*	**	*	**	***	***
Reproduction	*	*	*	**	**	**	***

Key: *** = major emphasis, ** = emphasis, * = touched upon or reviewed.

VALUE-BASED ACTIVITIES

Rights and Responsibilities

Have the class prepare parallel column lists of their rights and responsibilities as family members. Under the "Rights" column, they may list such things as being provided with food and shelter, having free time to play or watch television, being allowed to express their opinions on certain family matters, and spending their allowances as they wish. Under the "Responsibilities" column, students may list such things as keeping their rooms clean, taking out the trash, helping with housework, caring for a younger sibling, being honest in family matters, and accepting parental decisions. After the lists have been prepared, discuss the significance of the items listed. Ask questions such as the following:

- Do you think that your rights and responsibilities are equally balanced?

- How have your rights and responsibilities changed as you have gotten older?

- Do boys in a family have certain rights and responsibilities that girls do not have? Do girls have certain rights and responsibilities that boys do not have?

- How much say-so should children have about their rights and responsibilities?

- If you made all the rules in your home, what changes might you consider? Why?

- What do your rights and responsibilities suggest to you about your own level of maturity?

- How would you feel if you had no responsibilities?

Attitude Inventory

Prepare individual sheets like the one shown here and ask the students to offer their opinion about each statement. Follow with a general class discussion.

Agree	Disagree	Not sure	
——	——	——	1. Each child is an important member of his or her family.
——	——	——	2. Families do a lot of fun things together.
——	——	——	3. Mothers should hug and kiss their children more than fathers.
——	——	——	4. Children who have no brothers or sisters are unhappy.
——	——	——	5. Mothers and fathers should not hug and kiss each other in front of their children.
——	——	——	6. The more I learn about myself, the better I like myself.
——	——	——	7. Children who don't help with the housework should not get an allowance.
——	——	——	8. The best way to learn about sex is to ask friends.
——	——	——	9. I'd be too embarrassed to ask my parents about sex.
——	——	——	10. Sometimes I dread becoming a teenager.
——	——	——	11. I have trouble telling friends how I really feel.
——	——	——	12. My friends often pressure me to do things I don't want to do.

Agree	Disagree	Not sure	
____	____	____	13. When a friend does something wrong, I usually tell the person how I feel.
____	____	____	14. Children should be allowed to set some of the family rules.
____	____	____	15. Adults are free to do what they want most of the time.

Getting to Know Me

Prepare sheets or cards with the following statements or categories on them. Pass out a sheet to each student to complete. Then collect and shuffle all the responses. Either as a class or small-group activity, see if students can identify each other by the responses. Have the students consider what this suggests about the unique individuality of each person.

Something that I do well: _____ .
Music that I like: _____ .
Three words that describe me: _____ .
If I could have a dream come true, it would be: _____ .
What I like to do in my spare time: _____ .
I'm looking forward to: _____ .
One thing I like about myself: _____ .
Who am I? _____ .

The Perfect Friend

Ask the students to make a list of five qualities they would like in a perfect friend. Have them describe each of these qualities in a sentence, such as "My perfect friend gives me good advice when I am not feeling happy" or "My perfect friend accepts me for who I am." Ask students to share their ideas in class and prepare a master list on the chalkboard. Then ask the class how they can each be their own "perfect friend." Have them cross out "my perfect friend" in their sentences and substitute the word "I." Discuss how each of us can be more of a "perfect friend" instead of sometimes being "your own worst enemy."

Decision Stories

Present decision stories such as the following, using the procedures outlined in chapter 5. The content of the stories that you present should be appropriate for the developmental levels of your students. The examples here range from stories suitable for the early elementary grades to the upper grades but are not identified as to grade level since appropriateness must be determined in the social context of your own community.

Am I Stuck with Me?

Kevin is overweight and not very good at sports. In fact, he is often chosen last in team sports and games, which bothers him a lot although he tries to make a joke of it. In fact, he makes a great many jokes because he wants the other kids to like him. And they do. They think Kevin is a lot of fun. But Kevin doesn't just want to be the class clown. He wants the other kids in class to respect him for what he is. He would like the girls in class to think more highly of him, too.

Focus Questions: What might Kevin do to feel better about himself? Are there some changes he can make? Are there some things that he should not change? Why or why not?

The Crush

Jackie couldn't seem to stop thinking about the boy who lived down the street. He was a lot older than she was and he thought that she was "just a kid." Jackie went out of her way to be around him. She hoped that he would invite her out on a date, even though she wasn't really old enough to start dating. Then, one day Jackie saw him with another girl—one closer to his own age. She felt terrible. How could he do this to her?

Focus Question: What should Jackie do next?

John's World

John's parents were divorced last year. John is living with his mother, but he sees his father regularly. One weekend, while John is staying with his father, he finds out that his father is going to get married again. "John," his father says. "This is Janet. I know that you're going to like each other." But John doesn't like his father's woman friend. He is still feeling bad about the divorce. Now this! Will this woman become his stepmother? What will happen to his real mother? What kind of a family will this be? John is confused, very angry, and deeply unhappy.

Focus Question: Why does John feel the way he does?

Stories or Facts?

One day after school, some of the girls are talking about how babies are made. Susan is listening with interest. Some of the things she hears are new to her. She has learned a little bit about sex education from her parents and in school. But she is still not sure about all the details. Now she is more confused than ever. She wishes that she knew which of these things were really true.

Focus Questions: What can Susan do to get accurate information? Whom should she try to talk with? Should she rely on her friends for information?

Fooling Around

Bob and his friend George are spending the afternoon together in George's home. It is raining so they have to stay inside. George's parents are not at home. The two boys start to talk about sex. Then George suggests that the two of them "fool around" together and play with each other's bodies. Afterwards, Bob feels that maybe he did something wrong. He feels guilty and frightened. The next day, he feels even worse about what happened. He is afraid to tell his parents what happened.

Focus Question: What should Bob do?

The Party

Tina's friend Marie is having a party and has invited her. At the party, Tina knows only a few of the other guests. Everyone seems to be having a good time. There is music, and the boys and girls are dancing. Later, Tina notices that some of the couples are kissing and making out. A boy named Carl comes over to her. "Would you like to dance with me?" he asks. She is not sure. She doesn't really know Carl. What if he tries something? What could she do? She feels flattered that Carl is paying her attention, but she is also unsure of herself in situations like this.

Focus Questions: What should Tina do? Why does she feel uncomfortable? What decisions does Tina have to make now and in the future?

DRAMATIZATION

The Answer is *No*

Have the students divide into pairs of their own choosing. Explain that one student will play the part of a parent, while the other will play the part of that parent's son or daughter. Then set up the situation. The child tells the parent that he or she wishes to go to a party. Both boys and girls will be present at the function. Have the student acting the part of son or daughter ask permission and then explain all the details about the party: who will be there, where it will be, and so on. After listening, the student acting as parent refuses permission. The son or daughter continues to argue for permission, but it is still refused. Let several pairs of students act out the situation in front of the class, but do not require anyone who does not wish to participate to have to do so. Discuss how the different pairs of students handle the same situation. Then, without having told the class that you will do so, have selected pairs of students switch roles and repeat the activity. Use discretion in choosing which pairs of students to use for this second part of the activity. Follow with a general discussion. What differences did the class note in individual roles when these roles were reversed? What insights can they gain from this activity?

How Would You Handle It?

Divide the class into pairs, this time making sure that close friends are not paired. Explain that there will be no role switching in this activity. Then have each pair act out situations such as the following:

- Asking for and getting a date

- Asking for and being refused a date

- Introducing a friend to one's parents (a third child should play the part of the friend)

- Telling a divorced parent that you don't care for the person the parent is dating

- Introducing yourself to a member of the opposite sex to whom you feel attracted

- Being polite to someone you don't care for; handling rejection upon being socially rebuffed

Understanding Others

Explain that not everyone is alike; some people are bossy and others are shy, for example. Then assign different roles to various children, such as Noisy Ned, Bossy Betty, Shy Sam, Iceberg Irene, Chatterbox Chester, Silent Sylvia, Blustery Ben, Whirlwind Wanda, Studious Stu, Laughing Larry, Somber Sarah, and Flighty Frank. Make sure that the children assigned to each role do not have the characteristics of the role they are to play. Have each child act out the part for a few minutes. Then ask the children to discuss how they might deal with these different personality types. Ask individual students to note what they find appealing about the characteristics of each personality type. Ask the same students why others might be put off by these characteristics. Discuss the value of variety among individuals, noting that not every person will be universally liked by every other person, but that each individual has qualities that are worthwhile.

Superkid

Have the students divide up into pairs. One student will play the part of Superkid, the other will be his or her press agent. Have the pairs decide just what qualities each Superkid will have. These qualities might include the ability to fly, to speak any language, to sing or play a musical instrument so well that the person is a superstar, to be a great athlete, and so on. First, have the student playing the part of press agent introduce the Superkid and describe his or her abilities in the most glowing terms. Then, have the Superkid acknowledge his or her popular acclaim, but note to the class that life is not perfect even for a Superkid. The student should then explain why being a Superkid isn't as completely wonderful as the press agent has said. If the person is described as an athlete, for example, he or she might explain the anxieties about getting injured on the field, the pressure of competition, and so forth. The object of the activity is to make the students realize that no one is perfect and that the grass isn't always as green on the other side of the fence as it may seem at first glance. Conclude by emphasizing that in some ways each of us is "super" but that life is not without anxieties for anyone.

DISCUSSION AND REPORT TECHNIQUES

Me and My Self-Confidence

Discuss characteristics that can cause people to feel self-conscious, such as being overweight or underweight, being very short or very tall, having a large nose, or having skin problems. Note that some of these characteristics are either temporary or ones that can be changed, while permanent or difficult-to-change characteristics can actually become an asset. Discuss famous individuals noted for unique or unusual physical features. These might include Barbra Streisand and her nose, Wilt Chamberlain and his height, or Paul Williams and his shortness. You should emphasize that each of these individuals relied on developed talent rather than inherited physical characteristics to achieve success. Note that self-confidence is often the key to success.

Opportunities for All

In years past, many occupations were considered as appropriate only for males or females. Today, this social attitude is changing, as are our conceptions of sex roles and sex stereotyping in general. After discussing this point with the class, have them divide up into small groups to talk about and research individual instances of this phenomenon. Suggest that some groups look into changing occupational opportunities while others look at changing social or familial roles. For example, many police officers in cities and towns throughout the nation are now women, where formerly only men worked in law enforcement. Some men now stay home and care for the children, often while working at a skilled profession at home such as a computer programmer. Ask each group to compile a report on how changes in their area of research have resulted in greater opportunity for both men and women. Also have each group discuss the social ramifications of the changing roles in our society.

Information Please

Prepare a worksheet, as indicated here, giving possible sources of information on sex and family life. Have each student rank order the list from the source most likely to provide accurate information to the least likely source. Then discuss the different rank orderings in class. Be sure to point out that even what might be considered the most informed source may not be able to supply information on a particular question without research. Also note that it is unlikely that any one source will have all the answers on every sex-related subject, although some sources are likely to be more reliable than others. Avoid disparaging any valid source of information but suggest that some are probably more useful than others. If appropriate, you might also note that sometimes more than one source should be consulted for more complete information.

Possible sources of sex and family life information:

_____ Movies and television
_____ Health teacher
_____ Minister, priest, or rabbi
_____ Friends
_____ Parents
_____ Books from the city library
_____ Physician (doctor)
_____ Newspaper columns
_____ Magazines
_____ Textbooks used in school

Legal Rights

Unfortunately, many children in this country are sexually abused. Such abuse may come from other family members or from trusted adults or friends. Often, children are completely unaware of their legal and moral rights in such instances. After becoming informed yourself on legal recourses, present an objective lecture on the subject to your class. It is very important that you preface your discussion by emphasizing that the child has no reason to feel guilty or ashamed for being a victim of sexual exploitation of any kind. Suggest sources that children can turn to for help if such exploitation is occurring. A good first choice is the school psychologist or physician.

Families Are Different

Invite adults of your acquaintance to come to class to discuss different types of families in which they grew up. Have individuals from a wide variety of familial backgrounds, including traditional American nuclear families, extended family situations, single-parent families, and so forth. This is not an easy activity to do, but it can be a most valuable one. Your guests should not gloss over any difficulties they had growing up in their particular situation, but children should not get the impression that singular events are typical of any situation. The intent of the activity is to help children realize that today there may be no "typical" family structure but that any family structure can provide a loving and healthy environment for personal growth.

Individual Reports

As appropriate for the developmental level of your particular students, assign individual report topics on aspects of physical and emotional growth. Have the students use your health textbook and other approved informational sources to research particular areas, such as the growth spurt that occurs in adolescence, puberty, menarche, first encounters with the opposite sex in social situations, and dating behavior in the early teen years. On a separate sheet of paper, have students list questions that they did not find answers for during their research. Consult with each student on an individual basis to assist in finding appropriate solutions to these questions. In doing this activity, rely on the advisory committee to your sex and family life education program for appropriate responses to individual student questions or dilemmas.

Why Not?

After discussion and approval of this activity by all members of the family life advisory committee, invite various representatives of sex education groups in your community to lecture to the class on the ramifications of certain sexual decisions that each individual must make, such as the decision to have intercourse outside of marriage. Make it clear before the activity that you as the teacher are not advocating any behavior that goes against general community norms.

EXPERIMENTS AND DEMONSTRATIONS

Guppies

After discussing the concept that all living things can reproduce, let students observe the birth process in live-bearing fish. Obtain some young female guppies and young male guppies. Raise them in separate aquariums. Point out to the class the physical differences between the females and the males. Note that the female guppy is larger and somewhat drab in coloration in contrast to the smaller, brightly colored male. Explain that in many animal species there are obvious differences between the male and female, as there are with human beings. When the fish are mature, place one or more males in the tank with the females. In a few weeks, one or more of the females will become pregnant. This will soon be obvious. With luck, birth may take place while class is in session. Have the children observe the birth process. Discuss similarities in the live birth of guppies and the live birth of other animals, such as common species of mammals. Also point out differences. For example, many fish and all birds are egg layers. As soon as the female guppies give birth, separate the adults from the young, as guppies are cannibalistic.

Baby Animals

If appropriate, you may wish to breed white mice or other rodents in the classroom. After the female has given birth, have the children observe the offspring. Ask questions about how the young are like the adults and how they are different. Observe the care that the mother gives to the young. Ask why such maternal care is vital to the survival of the offspring. Relate this demonstration to the nurturing process that occurs among different species of animals. Do some animals have families that are in any way like human families? Discuss similarities and differences.

Genetics

If you decide to breed mice or other animals in the classroom, you can also use the project to demonstrate inherited traits by using a male and a female with different physical characteristics, such as fur coloration. Use a male and female with different colorations. Then observe how many of the offspring have inherited coloration traits similar to those of the male or those of the female. For upper elementary school children, discuss dominant and recessive traits. Ask the children to offer other examples of such traits that they have observed in the offspring of pet cats or dogs.

Inherited Traits

The human genetic code contains information about thousands of inherited traits. These include hair, eye, and skin color, shape of ears and nose, and general physique. Emphasize to your class that even individual rates of growth are to a large extent genetically controlled, which explains why some children are early bloomers while others are late bloomers. To demonstrate that some genetic traits are less obvious than others, ask the class to roll their tongues. Some children will be able to roll their tongues, while others will be unable to do so. This ability is a genetic trait.

PUZZLES AND GAMES

Reproduction Systems Crossword Puzzle

Prepare crossword puzzle sheets as shown in figure 20.1. This activity will help children build necessary vocabulary.

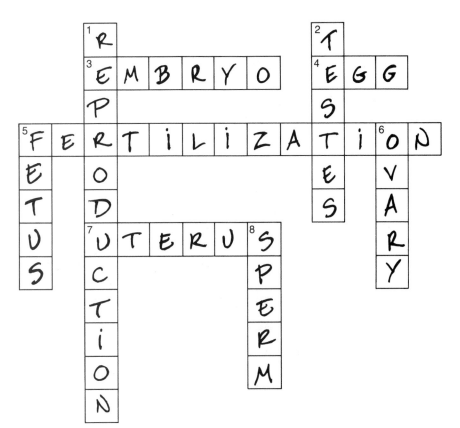

Down

1. the act of producing or recreating

2. the part of the male reproductive system where sperm are developed

5. the name given to the unborn child from about 2½ months till birth

6. the part of the female reproductive system where eggs are stored

8. the male sex cell

Across

3. the name given to the unborn child during the first stages of development

4. the female sex cell

5. the union of egg and sperm

7. the muscular organ of the female reproductive system that holds the baby before birth

Figure 20.1
Crossword puzzle.

FETUS   EMBRYO   SPERM   FALLOPIAN TUBE   EGG   TESTES

OVARY   FERTILIZATION   REPRODUCTION   UTERUS

U	U	H	F	K	F	E	T	U	S	I	X	W
Z	T	D	Y	F	L	M	N	B	I	E	F	C
G	S	E	T	L	Y	B	O	V	H	A	E	X
E	Q	P	R	K	I	R	I	R	J	W	R	B
B	N	M	R	U	Q	Y	T	J	X	L	T	Y
U	P	E	O	N	S	O	C	K	J	F	I	A
T	E	S	T	E	S	P	U	D	W	E	L	T
N	M	N	M	B	O	G	D	U	S	G	I	Z
A	V	J	T	I	H	G	O	E	D	G	Z	U
I	C	R	C	O	W	K	R	D	C	P	A	G
P	Q	O	U	N	A	E	P	G	V	F	T	V
O	V	A	R	Y	P	T	E	M	Y	K	I	H
L	O	M	B	B	H	P	R	A	R	D	O	Q
L	R	Y	S	Z	T	X	Z	N	O	E	N	W
A	M	Z	A	J	I	C	U	Q	T	X	P	L
F	A	S	B	L	S	E	V	U	F	R	Q	S

Figure 20.2
Student activity sheet for Word Hunt.

Word Hunt

Duplicate sheets as shown in figure 20.2 and have the students find each of the words.

Find each of the words listed here. Circle each word. The words may read in any direction—up, down, across, or diagonally.

Scrambled Sentences

Have the students unscramble each of these sentences about the human reproductive systems.

1. Canal acts birth as the vagina a. (The vagina acts as a birth canal.)
2. Ova the hormones and ovaries produce. (The ovaries produce ova and hormones.)
3. Tubes occurs in fertilization the fallopian. (Fertilization occurs in the fallopian tubes.)
4. Begins females in at menstruation puberty. (Menstruation begins in females at puberty.)
5. In the fetus uterus the develops. (The fetus develops in the uterus.)

6. Are cells the male sperm reproductive called. (The male reproductive cells are called sperm.)
7. Testes produced in the cells sperm are. (Sperm cells are produced in the testes.)
8. Fluids other and semen of made is up sperm. (Semen is made up of sperm and other fluids.)
9. Puberty begins at sperm produced to be. (Sperm begins to be produced at puberty.)
10. At testosterone the triggers spurt male puberty growth. (Testosterone triggers the male growth spurt at puberty.)

Matching Parts and Functions

Draw a large diagram of the female reproductive system on the chalkboard. Draw leader lines from each of the parts and allow room for labeling. Prepare a similar diagram for the male reproductive system. Divide the class into two teams. Point to a part on either diagram and ask the first player to identify it. If the student knows the answer, he or she should come to the board and label the part. If the student does not know the correct answer, the first player from Team B gets a chance. Score one point for each correct answer. After a part has been correctly labeled, ask the next player to explain one function of that part. If the student knows the correct answer, he or she should come to the board and write the function next to the name of the part.

True or False?

Divide the class into two teams and ask each player to decide whether a statement that you make is true or false. Score one point for each correct answer. Then write each of the *true statements only* on the chalkboard. Review the true statements at the end of the game. Sample statements might include the following:

- Girls should not swim during menstruation (false).
- A wet dream is a sign that a boy is reaching puberty (true).
- Fertilization leading to pregnancy occurs when a sperm unites with an egg (true).
- The beginning of menstruation means that a girl can now become pregnant (true).

BULLETIN BOARDS

Many Kinds of Families

Prepare a bulletin board display showing some of the many different kinds of families. Use pictures from magazines to make the display. Family types should include one-parent families, families with no children, families with many children, extended families, and so forth.

Expanding Roles

After discussing sex roles, have the children find pictures in old magazines that show males and females in nontraditional roles. These should include both occupational and social roles. For example, look for illustrations showing girls and women engaging in activities that were only associated with males in the past. Also look for examples of boys and men engaging in expanded roles. Prepare a large bulletin board display or a collage.

Growth and Change

Trace frontal silhouettes of a male and a female at different stages of growth. Provide four silhouettes for each, showing physical changes from childhood to young adulthood. Under each, write in information about typical aspects of development at that age. Give height and weight ranges, description of physical changes such as rounding of the body in females and muscular development of the upper body in males, and so forth. Emphasize to the class that the display shows average changes but that changes in individuals can vary widely because of hereditary factors.

OTHER IDEAS

Growing Up

Have each student trace his or her hand on a sheet of paper. Ask the students to take their tracings home and have one or both parents trace their hands over the child's tracing. The next day, discuss how the body parts grow and why parents are larger than children. Tie this activity into a general discussion of growth and development.

Family Activities Collage

Have each student search through magazines to find pictures of family activities. These activities can include watching television together, going on trips or outings, working around the house, talking with one another, and so forth. Explain to the students that the pictures they choose need not exactly mirror their own families as long as the illustrations represent an activity. Thus a picture of a television set by itself can represent watching television together, an airplane can represent a trip to relatives in another part of the country, and so on. Have each student prepare a colorful collage and then explain to the class the meaning of each component.

My Family Tree

Have each student prepare a family tree using the format shown in figure 20.3. Younger children may need the assistance of their parents to fill in the names of earlier forebears. After the diagrams are completed, discuss each family tree. Ask children what physical features they have in common with siblings, parents, grandparents, and so on.

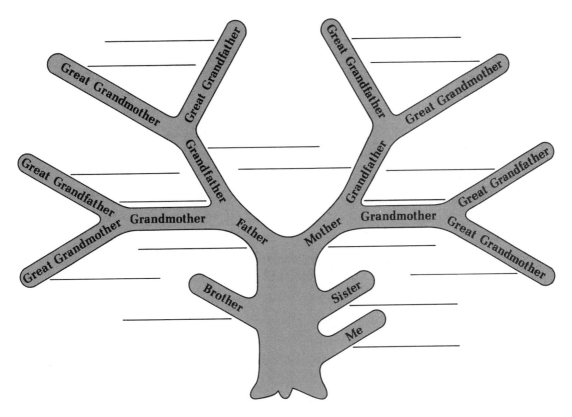

Figure 20.3
Family tree format.

Why Are They Like That

Certain aspects of the behavior of boys is often a puzzle to girls, and vice versa. Have each student write one question about some aspect of the "typical" behavior of the opposite sex that is puzzling or perhaps annoying. The questions should be unsigned. Collect all the questions and read those out loud that seem most germane to a discussion of behavior among boys and girls at your class's grade level. Have volunteers attempt to explain the point of view of the opposite sex that might shed light on a particular aspect of behavior. For example, girls may be more interested in boys at a certain age than boys are interested in girls. Maturational differences explain this fact. As a result, girls may be attracted to older boys, giving boys their own age the feeling that they are not seen as sexual peers. Act as moderator in the discussion and provide factual information as necessary.

Advice Column

With your assistance and supervision, have the class put together a newspaper advice column. First, have each student write a letter to the column asking for some advice about a sex or family life matter. Students may ask for simple factual information, such as "What is masturbation?" or for advice on handling a personal problem, such as "How can I ask someone for a date?" Collect all the letters, which should be unsigned or signed with something like "Puzzled" or "Wondering," and group them into categories. Restate a typical example for each category, writing this paraphrase on the chalkboard. Then have each student write an answer for the "column." Again using your discretion, collate the different suggestions offered and discuss them with the class. Properly handled, this activity can offer you important insights into the sexual development of students in your class. As "managing editor" of the advice column, however, you must make sure that topics covered stay within guidelines set up for your school's sex and family life education program.

21. Aging

The way our nation deals with aging and with its elderly citizens should be a subject of interest not only to the elderly themselves but to us all.—From the 1981 White House Conference on Aging

THE NORMALCY OF AGING

Aging is a normal developmental process, not a pathological phenomenon, as it is often viewed. When we speak of aging, we must avoid the misconception that the process affects only those over 65; each of us is aging every day. We generally consider the changes taking place in the body as "growth" until postadolescence, and "aging" after that. Most people in our society view growth as positive and aging as negative. But, in fact, it is all one process. Aging is a continuous experience that begins at birth and ends at death.

Exactly how we age is not clearly understood. Many theories have been advanced, but some aspects of the aging process are still mysteries. In any case, the number of elderly in the United States has risen sharply in the past two decades, and this trend will continue. Because of advances in medical technology, improved health care delivery, reduced infant mortality, and control of diseases, more people are living longer. In this chapter, we will examine the ramifications of this fact and consider the ways in which aging is viewed in our society.

THE SIGNIFICANCE OF AGING EDUCATION

Aging education is relatively new compared to other health topics. Few schools include the topic of aging in their curricula, yet the aged are the fastest growing demographic group in our country. The aged possess many skills, but these skills are going to waste. This group could have a tremendous impact on our society through their talents, wisdom, and psychological support for younger age groups.

421

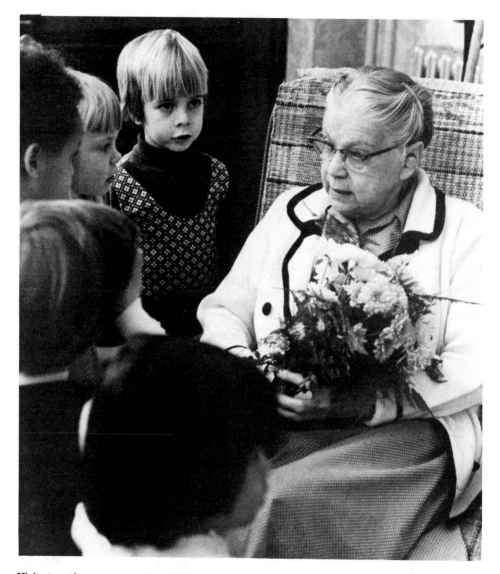

Visits to retirement centers are enjoyed by both students and residents.

People face many changes and challenges in life as they age. The problems of the elderly are problems that affect all of us. Major challenges facing the elderly include income, health, housing, mandatory retirement, and the changing character of American society.

Our society places a great deal of emphasis on youth and productivity; the elderly person's role is considered less significant. Also, because of financial reasons (sharing housing costs) and social factors (desiring to live with or near peers and living nearer service-oriented agencies), some elderly people have opted to move into housing and communities for the aged. This further segregates them from the remainder of society and makes them less visible.

Children today are more likely to lose contact with the older generations than in the past (DiMarco, Eckman and Wolford, 1984). Some children see older persons daily, but do not mingle or socialize with them. This lack of contact with the elderly, coupled with misleading stories they read and hear, often leads to fears and misconceptions. Children need to be taught about the elderly and aging early in their lives. They need to see that they themselves will one day be old. They also need to understand that the elderly were once children like themselves.

If the schools fail to include aging education, the myths and stereotypes about aging will continue to abound. The goal of health education is to teach all aspects of growth and development through the life cycle, including the latter stages. Through the study of aging, elementary school children will become more aware of issues facing their parents and grandparents today. It will also prepare them for their own aging. Effective aging education can lead to more satisfactory living for today's elderly by promoting understanding and empathy among those who will one day also be old. A major objective of aging education is to promote and enhance the quality of life in all the years that a person lives.

DEMOGRAPHIC ASPECTS OF THE ELDERLY

The 1980 U. S. Census counted over 25 million persons 65 or over. This is approximately 11 percent of the population. In comparison, only 3.1 million persons were 65 or older (4 percent of the total population) in 1900. The older population should increase in percentage even more in the next generations because a lower birth rate is keeping the numbers of younger people down and because improved medical technology is allowing more older people to live much longer. Also, those persons born during the postwar baby boom of the 1940s will be elderly by the turn of the century. For these reasons, the number of citizens over 65 is expected to double by the year 2050, and they will comprise 22 percent of the population (Eustis, Greenberg, and Patten, 1984, 2).

A child born in 1900 could be expected to live an average of about 47 years. A child born in 1981 can be expected to live 71 or more years. This increased lifespan is due primarily to improved public health measures—especially in sanitation—and a reduction in infant mortality. The life expectancy of a baby boy born in the United States now is approximately 70.8 years; for a baby girl, it is approximately 77.3 years. Blacks and other minorities have somewhat shorter life expectancies, partly because of generally lower socioeconomic status.

A popular myth is that most elderly are in nursing homes or other homes for the aged. In fact, only 5 percent of older people in this country live in such institutions. The majority, 70 percent, live with a spouse or other family, and the remaining 25 percent live with nonrelatives in homes or apartments. More elderly are now living in cities than was the case for the previous generation of elderly Americans. This is partially due to the availability of government housing in cities and to the fact that many cities have expanded to incorporate what formerly were suburbs where the aged person's house is located. Black elderly are more heavily concentrated in cities than are white elderly (Haynes, Feinleib, Ross, & Stallones, 1980). Half of the elderly are concentrated in a very few states: California, Illinois, New York, Ohio, Pennsylvania, Texas, and Florida. Florida has the highest percentage of elderly in a state population—over 17 percent (Burdman, 1986). Many social statistics regarding the elderly are dismal. For example, 14 percent of older people live below the poverty level. This is due to a variety of reasons, the chief among them being mandatory retirement, low income levels during the working years leading to lower retirement incomes, poor planning for retirement income, and lack of opportunity to work, either for social or physical reasons. Only 3 percent of the elderly are involved in the labor force. Again, some have been forced to retire, while many are women who have never been in the labor force, and some are physically incapable of working. Only one-half of today's elderly completed an elementary school education and only 8 percent graduated from college.

FACTORS RELATED TO AGING

Aging is a complex function, influenced by physiological, psychological, and sociological factors. Wantz and Gay (1981) classify the factors that cause aging into two categories: intrinsic components and extrinsic components.

Intrinsic Components

The intrinsic, or internal, components of aging are based on biological and physical factors, over which we have little or no control. These intrinsic components of aging include sex, race, intelligence, personality, and genetics.

Sex. Women have a longer life expectancy than men. This is primarily due to the fact that men are more susceptible to disease at every stage of life, especially chronic diseases. Also, men are more prone to stress than women.

Race. Whites have a higher life expectancy than nonwhites. This difference can be partly attributed to the fact that some nonwhites, especially black males, are more prone to hypertension than whites. Also, the general differences in education, economic levels, living conditions, nutrition, and health care between whites and nonwhites are factors.

Intelligence. College graduates have a greater life expectancy than nongraduates. Assuming that college graduates are generally more intelligent than nongraduates, the premise is that more intelligent individuals often make wiser decisions regarding factors that can increase their life spans.

Personality. Individuals who are very nervous will probably not live as long as those who are more relaxed. Also, some personality types may be more prone to taking risks or may pursue a more physically taxing lifestyle.

Genetics. The genetic code in our bodies provides a blueprint that may dictate how long we will live. Also, genetic diseases affect the number and quality of our years.

Extrinsic Components

The extrinsic components are environmentally related. Most people have some degree of control over these factors, which include employment and income, education, and social attitudes toward aging.

Employment and income. The more money an individual has, the better diet and lifestyle the person usually enjoys. Also, people with higher incomes generally have less financial stress.

Education. The more education an individual has, the better job the person might get. Better educated individuals are also more likely to be aware of the importance of a good diet, proper exercise, and the dangers of tobacco and alcohol misuse.

Social attitudes. Many of the elderly in our country today feel "old" because they are behaving in the way they are expected to by the younger generation. Our society often treats the aged as sickly and unproductive. If people accept these social expectations of behavior, their lifestyles will certainly be affected as they age.

THE AGING PROCESS

Before the specific changes associated with the aging process are discussed, it should be emphasized that the changes occur to different people at different times. Most of these changes are gradual, and adjustments can often be made to offset them. Further, many of the changes can be retarded through proper exercise and other preventive health maintenance.

Biological Aspects of Aging

The following physical changes occur to the body with the passage of time.

1. The skin becomes less elastic, turns dry and wrinkled, and exhibits age spots.
2. The hair becomes thinner in men and women. It loses its pigmentation and changes color to gray or white.
3. The joints of the skeleton stiffen because of a reduction of lubricating fluid, diminished weight bearing, and postural changes.
4. The rapid voluntary movements in muscles become more difficult.
5. The total mass of muscle fiber is reduced, and there is a loss of muscle power.
6. There is a loss in the total bulk of brain substances, and a decrease in the total number of brain cells. In some individuals, there is a hardening or occluding of the vessels in the brain.
7. The sense of touch is diminished and response to pain lessens.
8. The reflexes are weakened and reaction time lengthens.
9. Short-term memory is reduced.
10. Vision tends toward farsightedness.
11. Hearing sensitivity decreases.
12. The sense of smell is reduced, and the sense of taste appears to decline.
13. The loss of teeth and ill-fitting dentures in some elderly affect normal speech.
14. There is diminished cardiac output and increased blood pressure.
15. Lung capacity decreases and there is a reduction in vital capacity.
16. There is reduced motility of the stomach and reduced peristalsis in the intestines; these changes often result in constipation.
17. The rate of filtration by the kidneys is reduced.

18. Males and females experience menopause that affects the reproductive organs. This is more pronounced and empirically observable in females.
19. There is a decrease in the ability to maintain a constant body temperature. This is due to a reduction of metabolism and sometimes improper nutrition.
20. Older people tend to perspire less.

Health Highlight: Alzheimer's Disease

Alzheimer's disease is a term often used to describe senile dementia. This is an incurable disease in which abnormal changes in the tissue of the brain result. Problems of memory, particularly recent or short-term memory, are common in the early stage of the disease. Mild personality changes also occur early in the illness. Tasks that require abstract thinking or judgment become more difficult. The latter stage of

Alzheimer's is characterized by difficulty in communication, memory, and coordination. There appears to be a hereditary link in the causation of Alzheimer's. To date, there is no cure for the disease.

Source: Pajk, Marilyn, "Alzheimer's Disease: Inpatient Care," *American Journal of Nursing*, 1984, pp. 216–223.

Psychological Aspects of Aging

The psychological changes that accompany the aging process affect some elderly more than others. Many of these are the result of negative attitudes and behavior toward the elderly by younger people. Detrimental psychological aspects of aging include

1. A regression to childhood days
2. A restless, wandering feeling
3. Confusion
4. Combative nature
5. Persistent talk about the wish to die
6. Paranoid delusions
7. Inappropriate dependency
8. Becoming critical and demanding
9. Depression
10. Isolation and alienation
11. A sense of worthlessness
12. A sense of devaluation
13. A loss of self-esteem

Better treatment of and more positive attitudes toward the elderly would do much to limit many of these detrimental changes. In helping individuals cope with changes that do occur, it must be recognized that the elderly face many losses, including peers, jobs, spouse, and physical senses. These problems of adjustment overwhelm some elderly people, while others are able to face the challenges and find satisfaction.

Sociological Aspects of Aging

Sociological aspects of aging in America include

1. A loss of the child-rearing function (the empty-nest syndrome)
2. Loss of spouse
3. Mandatory retirement (or if voluntary, nonetheless a change in role)
4. Problems with transportation
5. Lack of community involvement
6. Lack of knowledge of community resources
7. Inadequate medical services
8. Financial problems
9. A need for leisure activities—proper use of time
10. Loneliness
11. Loss of role identification
12. Victimization through crime or abuse

Again, it should be noted that many of these sociological aspects of aging are the result of the discrimination and inappropriate treatment from younger people. With proper education and attitudinal changes in the general population, many of these detrimental changes could be alleviated among some of the elderly in America. The validity of this premise can be demonstrated by contrasting the role of the elderly in America with that of the elderly in some other cultures, such as that of Japan. In Japan, individuals enjoy higher social status and prestige as they grow older—almost the opposite of what happens in our country.

MAJOR CHALLENGES FACING THE ELDERLY

Chief among the challenges facing the American elderly is the lack of financial resources. As mentioned, many elderly live below poverty level. Lack of sufficient income is the result of inflation that has eroded the savings many elderly acquired dur-

---

Health Highlight

The following is a partial list of the recommendations from the 1981 White House Conference on Aging to "promote and maintain wellness among the elderly of our country."

1. To disseminate information to the elderly stressing the importance of a healthy lifestyle
2. To promote and maintain a sense of well-being among seniors
3. To provide nutrition programs for older Americans
4. To provide financial reimbursement of individuals for expenses paid for preventive care and the maintenance of wellness

5. To develop a national health care policy for health care management for the elderly
6. To establish health assessment centers for older Americans
7. To pay a wage to family members for caring for elderly loved ones, if they desire to keep them at home

Source: Final Report of the 1981 White House Conference on Aging, Volume 3.

ing their working years. Retirement benefits from Social Security are not sufficient to meet all of their needs, yet they are only allowed to make $6,000 additional income before their Social Security benefits are reduced.

Housing continues to be a major issue for the elderly. Nearly two-thirds of the elderly in our country own their own home. But even if the house is paid for, the owners are still responsible for taxes and insurance costs. Also, if the home is older, it has higher maintenance costs. Some elderly have to make a decision between drastic improvements in their present home and moving. They are sometimes limited financially as to where they can move. Some government housing is available based on present income—the less the income, the less the monthly payment. Some elderly share housing to reduce the monthly costs. For many elderly, however, there are few housing options. Other housing alternatives are apartments for the aged, sponsored by private, public, and nonprofit church-related groups. Also, for the aged dependent, boarding homes and nursing homes, providing both intermediate and skilled care are available. One of the recommendations from the 1981 White House Conference on Aging was to pay a salary to family members who care for an elderly loved one in their home.

Maintaining good health is a major challenge of growing old. An individual's health affects every aspect of life—relationships to spouse, family and community, income-producing ability and leisure pursuits (National Council on the Aging, 1979). The health problems that beset the elderly are usually associated with the aging process, in addition to those related to environmental causes, trauma, and heredity. Chronic ailments, such as heart disease, are the most common affliction of the elderly.

Escalating medical and health-related expenditures are a major concern for the older population. Of economic necessity, the health care of many elderly people is crisis-oriented. Since they cannot afford to visit a physician every time they are ill, many do not seek help until they feel it is absolutely necessary. Additionally, there are many areas in which the elderly needlessly spend money on health remedies or could spend their money more wisely for greater health benefits. Federal programs such as Medicare and Medicaid have helped in some ways, but even these programs do not pay enough of the health care bills of some elderly because of the ever increasing costs of health care delivery. Medicare is a health insurance program for those age 65 and over that is designed to help pay for hospital insurance and medical insurance. The hospital insurance helps pay for hospital care and certain follow-up care after the person leaves the hospital. The medical insurance primarily pays for a doctor's services and outpatient hospital services. Medicare pays for about half of the medical expenses incurred, but the remaining amount must come from the elderly person. Medicare has incorporated a prospective payment system based on diagnosis-related groups and implemented a freeze on reimbursement levels for physicians accepting Medicare assignment. These reforms have saved money at the Federal level, but have cost hospitals, physicians, and the elderly more money. Further, the reforms have adversely affected the quality of health care given to elderly persons (Brodsky & Ezell, 1985, 61).

Some of the health problems faced by the elderly are due to improper nutrition. Nutrition is as important for the elderly as it is for other age groups. Because of limited finances, loneliness, various disease states, and a reduction in the senses of smell and taste, many elderly skip meals or do not otherwise eat well. Sometimes, emotional problems, such as depression, keep elderly from eating. Because an elderly person's basal metabolism is reduced, the person's caloric need is also reduced. For this reason, better planning is required to ensure proper nutrition. Less quantity of food is required, but the quality has to remain high. Programs such as Meals on Wheels, which delivers meals to homebound elderly, and the federal government's Food Stamp Program and Nutrition Program for the Elderly (Title VII of the Older Americans Act of 1965) help defray the cost and improve the nutrition of the elderly.

Drug use in older adults may cause greater problems than in younger persons because of slower metabolic rates and more illnesses. It is very common for older persons to be taking many different drugs. Some recommendations to help prevent drug problems among the elderly are for the physician to keep a drug schedule as simple as possible, to keep a daily record of the drugs taken, to keep the physician informed of all medications taken, and to discard old medicines (Avorn, 1984).

Crime affects everyone. However, older people fear crime much more than the general population does. The elderly are weaker and more vulnerable. After being victimized, many elderly persons are too embarrassed or depressed to talk about what happened and do not report the crime. Thus far, no effective means have been identified for protecting the elderly from crime (Atchley, 1980). Some phony mail order schemes seem deliberately designed to trap the elderly. Medical quackery also affects them. Arthritis sufferers, mostly older individuals, spend 300 million dollars yearly on quack remedies. Other types of crime against the elderly range from muggings and theft to financial exploitation and physical abuse by members of their own family.

Transportation is a major challenge for some elderly Americans; many of them do not drive. Others drive, but have not adjusted to today's complicated traffic patterns. Also, those who drive with failing eyesight and hearing are more likely to be involved in accidents. The cost of automobile maintenance and gasoline prohibit some older persons from operating a car. Nondrivers must seek other means of transportation. Taxis can be expensive, and public transportation, while cheaper, is much less convenient; it requires more walking and takes more time. Often it is not designed with the elderly in mind. For these reasons, many elderly are restricted to their homes and apartments except for health care, groceries, and other necessities.

AGEISM

Ageism is a term used to describe the biased values that a culture holds against the elderly (Ray, Raciti, & Ford, 1985). Our society promotes ageism by exalting youth and vigor and emphasizing efficiency, speed, and mobility. We are critical of those considered unproductive. This attitude causes much discrimination and fosters many false beliefs about the elderly. Research studies confirm that young people generally have a negative image of the elderly. Younger individuals tended to downgrade the appearance of old people, felt that the old resented the young, and preferred to avoid personal contact with the elderly (Atchley, 1982).

Intergenerational misunderstandings are reduced when the old and young work, play, study, and socialize together. When the young and old see each other frequently and interact in meaningful ways, they generally express a high regard for each other.

Unfortunately, this does not occur often enough in our country (DiMarco, Eckman, & Wolford, 1984). Younger people are quick to emphasize the problems that occur with aging and the aged. While people do face special problems and challenges as they grow older, the problems are not so widespread as many younger people believe. For example, it is a myth that most elderly are incapacitated. In fact, most older people are able to work and live independently. Only 5 percent of the elderly are institutionalized, and elderly individuals average less than 15 days a year in bed because of ill health (Watson, 1982). Here are some other misconceptions about the elderly (Burdman, 1986):

1. All old people are senile (a term used excessively to explain the behavior and condition of very few elderly.
2. Old people are unproductive.
3. Old people sit around a lot because they have nothing better to do.
4. Old people are not very good at getting things done.
5. Old people are not very bright or alert.
6. Old people are uncooperative and unsociable.
7. Older people should not be allowed to engage in work or activity that requires mental or physical effort.

INTERGENERATIONAL CONTACT

Intergenerational contact programs can be one of the most effective ways for elementary teachers to implement an aging-education program. Such an experiential approach to intergenerational contact has been implemented in programs throughout the country. Notable examples are the Foster Grandparent Program and the Retired Seniors Volunteer Program. Volunteers and paid-aide programs, tutoring projects, free lunches, and guest speaker days have all served as ways to involve the elderly with the schools. Only as children are given the opportunity to understand aging and the aged will many false beliefs be dissolved. The positive attitudes gained from aging education can assist children in realizing their full potential throughout their lives as they themselves age.

AGING IN THE FUTURE

As a result of the increasing numbers of elderly people and greater realization of the complex issues that surround aging, many organizations, public and private, are offering expanded services to the elderly. These services include homemaking services, chore services, health services, personal counseling, mobility and transportation assistance, financial and income tax counseling, and visiting services. Portable meals for the homebound, lunch programs at senior citizens centers, employment services, and information and referral services that tell the elderly about the services available to them in their communities are also becoming more widely available.

The elderly in the year 2000 will be better organized and more of a political and economic force in society. They should be able to do much to improve the quality of

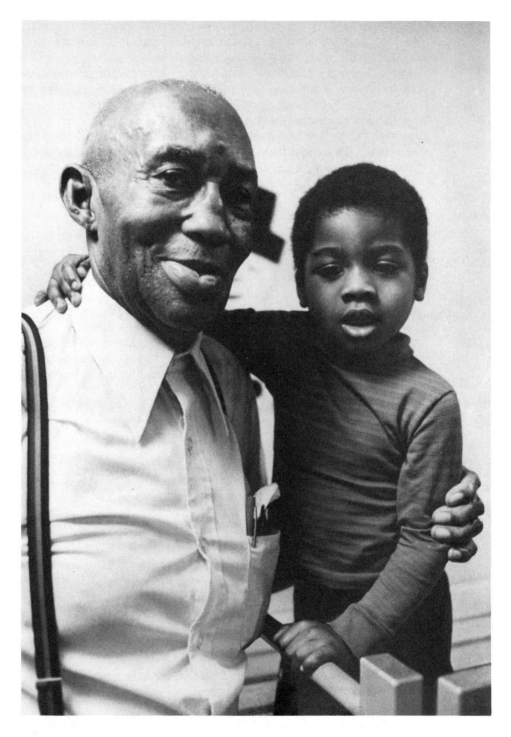

By studying aging, students will be better able to understand and interact with their parents and grandparents.

life for the aged (Waton, 1982). They will be better educated as a group than the elderly of today. Many will have been activists in organizations and movements in their younger years, concerned with such matters as environmental issues and women's rights. They will probably continue to be activists, helping to improve the quality of life for all older individuals. The elderly of the future will most likely have higher incomes, better retirement plans, better living standards, better housing, and better health care programs. The next generation of elderly Americans will be larger in number, comprise a higher percentage of the total population, and be more evenly distributed throughout the nation. Finally, more government and private organizations will probably be created to meet the needs of the elderly. The organizations' programs and services will most likely temper the negative attitudes of younger people toward the elderly.

SUMMARY

Aging is a normal part of the life cycle, not a pathological condition. We are all aging every day. The number of elderly has risen sharply in the past two decades and this trend is likely to continue. The life expectancies for all Americans are increasing. The majority of older Americans still own their own homes, and only 5 percent are institutionalized. Half of the elderly are concentrated in only seven states.

The aging process remains poorly understood for the most part. Many factors, both intrinsic and extrinsic, also affect the aging process for each individual. Many biological, psychological, and sociological changes occur as a person ages. Some of these changes present unavoidable problems for the elderly, but other changes can be successfully adjusted to.

Elderly Americans face many challenges in life. These issues affect all members of society, not just the aged. Among these challenges are income, retirement, housing, health problems, nutrition, crime, and transportation. Some of the problems facing the elderly are the result of discrimination and misconceptions. Stereotypes about the elderly largely result from lack of knowledge and insufficient contact with the elderly. Intergenerational contact programs in schools can be one of the most effective ways to help children understand aging and the elderly, helping to dissolve some of the many myths about aging.

The elderly of the future will generally enjoy a better standard of living. There will probably be many public and private organizations, programs, and services developed to meet their needs as the elderly become a stronger social and political force in the United States.

DISCUSSION QUESTIONS

1. Discuss aging as a normal part of the life cycle.
2. Describe how ageism affects the elderly in our society.
3. Describe the current living arrangements of the American elderly.

4. Compare the intrinsic and extrinsic components of aging.

5. Explain the factors that can help delay or retard the physiological changes that occur in aging.

6. List the reasons why elderly persons have problems with nutrition.

7. Describe Alzheimer's disease.

8. Enumerate suggestions for intergenerational contact programs for school-aged children and the elderly.

9. Describe the new prospective payment system in the Medicare health care delivery system.

10. Discuss the factors that will lead to better quality lives for the elderly in the future.

REFERENCES

Atchley, R. *The social forces in later life,* third edition. Belmont, California: Wadsworth Publishing Company, 1980.

Atchley, R. "Culture and aging: Lifestyles and intergenerational relationships." In Lesnoff-Caravaglia, G. (editor). *Aging and the human condition.* New York: Human Sciences Press, 1982.

Avorn, J. "Drugs and the elderly." *The Harvard Medical School Health Letter, 9,* 8, June, 1984.

Brodsky, D., & Ezell, G. "Impact of availability of health care information on the market behavior of providers and consumers." Unpublished research report submitted to the AARP/Andrus Foundation, Washington, D.C., December 31, 1985.

Burdman, G. *Healthful aging.* Englewood Cliffs, New Jersey: Prentice-Hall, Inc., 1986.

Butler, R., & Lewis, M. *Aging and mental health: Positive psychosocial approaches,* third edition. St. Louis: C. V. Mosby, 1982.

DiMarco, C., Eckman, M., & Wolford, C. "An action-oriented approach to aging education." Presentation at the American School Health Association, National Convention, Pittsburgh, Pennsylvania, October, 1984.

Eustis, N., Greenberg, J., & Patten, S. *Long-term care for older persons: A policy perspective.* Monterey, California: Brooks/Cole Publishing Company, 1984.

Haynes, S., Feinleib, M., Ross, J., & Stallones, L. (editors). *Proceedings of the second conference on the epidemiology of aging.* Bethesda, Md.: U.S. Department of Health and Human Services, July 1980.

National Council on the Aging. *NCOA public policy agenda, 1979–80.* Washington, D.C., 1979.

Pajk, M. "Alzheimer's disease: Inpatient care." *American Journal of Nursing, 84,* 2, February, 1984.

Ray, D., Raciti, M., & Ford, C. "Ageism in psychiatrists." *The Gerontologist, 25,* 5, October, 1985.

Wantz, M., & Gay, J. *The aging process: A health perspective.* Cambridge, Mass.: Winthrop Publishers, 1981.

Watson, W. *Aging and social behavior.* Monterey, California: Wadsworth Health Sciences Division, 1982.

White House Conference on Aging. Final report of the 1981 White House conference on aging. Washington, D.C.: White House Conference on Aging, 1981.

22. Techniques for Teaching About Aging

Aging cannot be excluded in the life continuum, nor in the educational programs which teach this process.—Ruth Engs and Molly Wantz

Our culture typically propagates ageism through inaccurate portrayals of elderly people in television, movies, and literature. The elderly are often characterized as noncontributors to society, and rarely are characterized as energetic, creative, or industrious. These stereotypes are shared by young people in this country, primarily because of a lack of opportunity to learn about aging and the aged, and through a lack of contact with older persons. While American families formerly shared one house with three generations, now the generations are more apt to live apart, sometimes in different communities or even in different parts of the country. Young people often fear older persons and the aging process.

We need to present realistic and accurate information to students about aging and the aged. Through these educational experiences, students can learn that aging is a natural part of the life cycle and that they have much more in common with elderly people than they might suppose. This type of education will allow students to decide for themselves what aging and the elderly are really like. When students are able to understand and develop healthy attitudes toward aging (including their own aging), they will be able to live a higher quality life as they grow older.

Concepts to be Taught

- Aging is a natural part of the total life cycle.
- The body changes as a person ages.
- Exercise and proper diet can retard the aging process to some degree.
- Most elderly people are healthy and alert.
- Responsibilities change as a person ages.
- People use their retirement years for different activities.

- Elderly people make positive contributions to society.

- Grandparents and grandchildren can share activities.

- Older people face many changes and challenges.

- The elderly in America are often discriminated against.

- Many social agencies provide services for the elderly.

Cycle Plan for Teaching Topics

Topic	K	1	2	3	4	5	6
				Grade Level			
We All Age	**	*	**	***	**	***	***
Theories about Aging	*	*	*	**	***	**	**
Life Expectancies	*	*	*	**	**	*	**
Physical Changes in Aging	*	*	**	**	**	***	**
Social Changes in Aging	*	**	**	*	**	***	***
Psychological Changes in Aging	*	*	**	**	***	**	***
The Elderly in Our Society	**	**	**	***	**	***	***
Problems of the Elderly	*	**	**	**	***	***	***
Intergenerational Contact	***	***	***	***	**	**	***
Services for the Elderly	*	*	*	**	**	***	**

Key: *** = major emphasis, ** = emphasis, * = review.

VALUE-BASED ACTIVITIES

Rank Ordering

Prepare a list of positive qualities often associated with aging. After discussing these qualities, have students individually rank order each, using the format shown here. Follow with a discussion of why some students feel certain qualities are more desirable than others. Note the importance of individual preferences.

> Number each of the following from 1 to 5. Use 1 to show that quality or condition about becoming older that appeals to you most, 2 for the second most appealing quality or condition, and so on.
>
> _____ Retirement
> _____ Wisdom
> _____ Grandchildren
> _____ Leisure time
> _____ Satisfaction

Sentence Completion

Instruct students to complete each sentence by writing down their immediate reaction to the statement. Point out that statements should be honest, even if some are negative. After the exercise, discuss the responses on a volunteer basis. Note varying points of view and discuss possible reasons for these opinions.

1. Aging is _____ .
2. Growing old is _____ .
3. When I grow old, I _____ .
4. My grandparents _____ .
5. Retirement from full-time work is _____ .
6. I think that old people are _____ .

Attitude Scales

Use a Likert scale format to have students determine their attitudes toward different aspects and issues concerned with aging. Employ statements such as the following.

	Strongly Agree	Agree	Not Sure	Disagree	Strongly Disagree
1. Retirement is the worst part about growing old.	___	___	___	___	___
2. Grandparents are fun to be around.	___	___	___	___	___
3. Growing old makes a person wiser.	___	___	___	___	___
4. Growing old is a normal part of life.	___	___	___	___	___
5. Old people are not very bright.	___	___	___	___	___

Decision Stories

Use the procedures outlined in chapter 5 for presenting decision stories such as the following.

The Old Woman Next Door

Jill and her parents have just moved into a new house. An old woman lives in the house next door. Her name is Mrs. Larsen. One summer day, Jill and some friends are playing in the back yard. They are making a lot of noise and having a good time. Mrs. Larsen comes out. She looks upset. "Do you have to make so much noise?" she says to Jill. Then she goes back inside. Jill gets angry. What right does her neighbor have to tell her and her friends what to do?

Focus Questions: What should Jill do? Why might Mrs. Larsen have asked the children to make less noise? Can Jill and Mrs. Larsen be good neighbors?

A New Member of the Family

Susan's grandfather lives by himself since his wife died a few years ago. Now Susan's parents tell her that Grandfather is coming to live with them. He has been sick and cannot live by himself anymore. Susan doesn't really know her grandfather very well because he has been living in another city some distance away. She is not sure how the new arrangement will work out.

Focus Question: How can Susan help her grandfather feel like a part of the family?

What's So Funny?

Larry is walking home from school with a couple of his friends. At a street crossing, they see an old man. He is having trouble getting across the street. The traffic light has changed and he is trying to walk as fast as he can, but he still has a way to go. "Why don't you get some roller skates?" one of Larry's friends yells. He laughs, and so does Larry's other friend.

Focus Question: What should Larry do?

Going for a Visit

Martha's grandparents live in a retirement village in another state. Her family is going to fly there for a visit next month. But Martha doesn't want to go. She visited her grandparents a few years before, when she was younger. She remembers that there was nothing for her to do at her grandparent's home. There were no other kids around. And her grandparents made such a fuss over her. They were nice, but they treated her like a baby. Martha didn't like that and she wished her grandparents would realize that she was growing up now.

Focus Question: What should Martha do?

DRAMATIZATION

Now I am Old

Have two volunteers role play situations where two elderly retirees are planning the day's activities. One situation could include two retirees who are very active, and another where the two retirees are inactive. Follow up the activity by asking the students with which of the characters they most identified.

Facing Retirement

Ask each student to think about a job or career he or she might like to have. Students should then find out more about the chosen area. What is appealing about this occupational role? What are some of the problems that a person doing this job faces. Then have each student act out the job in the front of the class or explain what is involved. Now, the student should explain that the time for retirement has come. What feelings does the person have about retiring? What problems will the person no longer have to deal with? What new problems will come with retirement?

Doing Things Together

Assign students to work in pairs. Do not pair close friends. Let one student act the part of a grandparent and let the other act the part of the grandchild. Each pair should then act out some activity that the grandparent and grandchild could do together. Activities might include doing some household chore, having lunch in a restaurant together, going to the park, or working on a homework assignment. Have the students note in their skits that grandparents and grandchildren often have different views on things. Suggest the following bits of dialogue to illustrate. In a restaurant, the grandparent might say, "A bowl of soup is all I want." The child might say, "I want a double cheeseburger and a chocolate malt." Helping with a homework assignment, the grandparent might say, "How can you learn mathematics if a hand calculator does all the work?" The child might say, "Why make things harder than they have to be? Anyway, I still have to know the concepts before I can use a calculator." The skits should emphasize appreciation for different points of view and the idea that older people and younger people can each learn from the other.

Gray Power

Divide the class into groups of five or six. Have them pretend that they are all elderly people facing a common problem. Assign a different problem to each group. Problems might include lack of low-cost housing, victimization by street criminals, need for better medical services, desire for more social opportunities in the community, and transportation problems. Explain that the members of each group are activists who have come together to talk about finding solutions to the problem. Then have the groups act out what they might do, what tactics they might develop, and so on.

A Visit to the Doctor

Have students role play the parts described below and answer the discussion questions afterwards.

Mrs. Johnson (72 years old, widowed)

You have not been sleeping well the last two weeks. Finally you can't take it any longer. You know you have very little savings in reserve for doctor's fees or medications but you have to do something. Since you have no personal transportation you decide to take the bus. Unfortunately, your regular doctor is located across town so you decide to go to a doctor whose office is nearby. You become more and more anxious during your bus ride. You feel weak and worry not only about having enough money but also about the new doctor and what he may be like. As you walk into the waiting room the nurse takes your name and tells you to have a seat as it will be a one to one-and-a-half-hour wait due to an emergency case. The waiting room is crowded with people waiting to see the doctor. Many are becoming impatient and start harrassing the nurse about the long wait. This upsets you even more and you begin to wonder if the doctor has the time or skill to really help you. At last, the nurse shows you to the examination room. The doctor comes in and after a brief examination, decided to prescribe sleeping medication.

Dr. Brown

Your day started off routinely enough but soon it turned into a real bear! An emergency call from one of your regular patients came in at about 10:00 A.M. and even though the emergency room staff could handle it you felt obliged to respond. You knew you had a full day's schedule but they would have to wait. When you got back to your office you were a full two hours behind schedule. Then you remembered you promised your family you would take them out to eat and a movie. You consider calling home and cancelling the night out but that would be the third straight time that you broke your promise in the last two weeks. You decide to rush through your patients and try to hold to your promise.

Things are getting hectic in the waiting room and the nurses are complaining about the overload. You're getting hungry because you decided to skip lunch to save time. It's getting to the end of the day and your next appointment is with Mrs. Johnson. You have five appointments after her and time is getting tight. You don't know anything about her medical history or what medication she's been on. You walk into the examination room. You check BP, heart rate and respiration and decide to prescribe sleeping medication.

Questions

1. How should Mrs. Johnson prepare for the visit? What should she bring with her?
2. What information should be shared during the visit? What should be asked and what should be volunteered?
3. What can be done to ensure that Mrs. Johnson will follow her doctor's instructions concerning the prescription to induce sleep?
4. What questions might be asked of her pharmacist?
5. What information should be reported to the doctor once the medications are being taken?

DISCUSSION AND REPORT TECHNIQUES

Panel Discussion

Divide the class into small groups and have each group research a problem area for elderly Americans. These areas should include health problems, financial problems, problems due to stereotypes and misconceptions, forced retirement, crime, and loneliness. After research is complete, have each group present a panel discussion of their findings. Group members should be prepared to answer questions from the class about the problem area that they have researched.

Aging Questions

Read the following statements to the students to stimulate discussion about attitudes and opinions about the elderly.

1. Grandparents should live with their children and grandchildren in the same house instead of living in a nursing home.
2. City bus services should offer free rides to the elderly.
3. Health care should be free or very inexpensive for the elderly.
4. Labels on products should be larger so the elderly can read them easily.
5. Retirement should be mandatory at age 60.

Services for the Elderly

Ask a member of a local service bureau to come to class and explain the different services provided to elderly people in your community. Or, find out about such services yourself and present a lecture to the class.

What is Old?

Note to the class that the concept of "oldness" is changing as people live longer. Compare life expectancies today with those 20, 50, 100, and 200 years ago. Point out that at one time a person of 45 was considered to be old. Today, this age is considered to be prime of life. Discuss how changes in technology and society have altered our concept of "oldness." As an extension, note that individuals are considered "old" for a particular activity at different stages of life. For example, an Olympic swimmer is "old" at 17 or 18. A professional football player is "old" at 30. But a race car driver may not be considered old even at age 40 or 45.

Elderly Role Models

Have students discuss elderly persons with whom they have come in contact or about whom they have heard that they would most like to be like when they get older. Conversely, have them discuss an elderly person they would not like to be like when they get older. Have them discuss the differences between the two role models.

EXPERIMENTS AND DEMONSTRATIONS

Last Year's Clothing

Have students bring in articles of clothing that they wore a year before and try them on. Use this activity as a springboard for a discussion of growth and aging. Note that the process is a continuum and a normal part of the life cycle.

Aging in Animals

Bring to class two small animals. Rabbits, mice, or guinea pigs will be suitable. One of the animals should be of advanced age, while the other should be young. Have the class observe the two animals and note differences in physical condition and behavior. Use this activity to lead into a general discussion of aging in animals. Supplement the discussion with visual aids, such as photos of young and older animals in their natural habitats.

Aging in Plants

As a year-long project or seasonal project, have the children observe the changes that take place in plants. Observation of annuals, such as many flowers, will permit a view of an entire life cycle, from budding stage, through flowering, to withering. Long-term growth can be observed and compared in different trees.

Aging in Humans

Bring in photographs of some well-known person taken over a period of many years. Have the students note the aging process in the person's features from year to year.

PUZZLES AND GAMES

Scrambled Sentences

Have the students unscramble these sentences to form correct statements about aging and the elderly.

1. Homes most own own people older their. (Most older people own their own homes.)
2. Life aging a part natural is of. (Aging is a natural part of life.)
3. People health most good in elderly are. (Most elderly people are in good health.)
4. Very senile few are old people. (Very few old people are senile.)
5. As occur ages changes the body. (Changes occur as the body ages.)
6. Little everyone day a ages each. (Everyone ages a little each day.)
7. Happy age of life old time be can a. (Old age can be a happy time of life.)
8. Community people the to elderly are important. (Elderly people are important to the community.)
9. Have sometimes people older physical problems. (Older people sometimes have physical problems.)
10. Process is gradual a aging. (Aging is a gradual process.)

Scavenger Hunt

Have each student bring to school some small object that can be described as "old." Objects can include clothing, books, photographs, tools, toys, and household items. Have each student describe the object brought in. What makes it old? How did the object change as it got older? Is it still useful? Compare the objects with people as they age. Note to the class that some objects get more useful or valuable as they become older. For example, discuss how certain cheeses or wines must age. Also talk about antiques. Is an antique valuable simply because it is old? Or does the antique possess qualities that become more valuable with age?

Games People Should Play*

Do you really understand what it feels like to be old or chronically ill? Try these simulations and see how your attitudes change.

Arthritis/Stiff Joints

In order to simulate stiff knees, get two elastic bandages (3 or 4 inches wide), wrap one firmly, but not too tightly, around each knee, and try walking. First move around the room; then climb some steps. Place these same elastic bandages around your elbows and try to put on a coat, or eat or drink something. To feel what it's like to have arthritis of the hands and wrists, put on a pair of bulky gloves and try to button your shirt or blouse.

---

*Sehnert, Keith W. "Put Yourself in Their Place." *Family Health*, April, 1976. pp. 28-40, 53

Stroke or Paralysis

If you are right handed, take a pencil in your left hand (vice versa for you southpaws) and try to write your name. Would the teacher give you an A in penmanship? Simulate the speech problems that follow a stroke by placing a ping pong ball or a small rubber ball (please wash it first) in your mouth. Now recite the Pledge of Allegiance. Call a friend on the telephone and chat for a few minutes. Did he recognize your voice? Hold a yardstick against the outside of one leg and secure it with pieces of heavy rope at six-inch distances. Walk around the room, then try going up and down stairs. Feel awkward?

Hearing Loss

Place a cotton ball in each exterior ear canal, then don a pair of earmuffs. (If you have stereo headphones, use them since they're more soundproof.) Then call someone in from the next room and strike up a conversation with her. How many times did you have to ask her to repeat something? Did you find yourself lipreading? Turn the TV set down to its lowest level, sit at the opposite end of the room and listen to the evening news or the local talk show. Hard work, isn't it?

Visual Problems

Take a pair of swim goggles or old glasses and cover them with wrinkled cellophane or Saran wrap. Read the newspaper for a few minutes or watch TV. It won't be long before your eyes feel strained. Again, watch TV. But this time turn it slightly out of focus. See how long you can watch before you become irritated.

Loss of Smell

Take a sheet of tissue paper, tear it in half, and gently push one piece into each nostril. Or simply clamp your nose between your thumb and index finger of your left hand. Then grab an apple or your favorite snack and eat it while still holding your nose. Not very tasty, is it?

Loss of Touch

Cover your fingers with rubber cement. Let it dry and then try to thread a needle. Not so easy, is it? This time cover your hand with a sandwich bag or sandwich wrap. Again try threading that needle and see how long it takes.

BULLETIN BOARDS

Famous Older Americans

Have students create a bulletin board display about famous older Americans, including individuals who became best known when they were already elderly, such as Harlan Sanders (Kentucky Fried Chicken) or Ronald Reagan. Discuss the contributions made by each person featured.

How We Grow and Age

Prepare a bulletin board display composed of pictures from magazines showing individuals at different times of life, from early childhood, through maturity, to old age.

Pictures chosen should emphasize the fact that individuals can have active, fulfilling lives regardless of age.

Advantages and Disadvantages of Growing Older

Have students prepare a two-column display listing some of the advantages and disadvantages of becoming elderly. To bring the point home that every stage of life has advantages and disadvantages, also have students prepare similar displays for childhood, adolescence, and young adulthood.

Person of the Week

Each week, prepare a display highlighting some elderly person in your community. Have the children do most of the research. Individuals featured should be ordinary citizens, including grandparents of the students, retired people connected with the school, and so on. Feature the individual's photograph and a short biography. The poster should also show the person's current interests and involvement with the community or with a student's family. Note to the class the diversity of lifestyles featured individuals have.

Older People in My Life

Have each student make a drawing showing interaction with some older person, either a family member or a nonrelative. Drawings should be based on actual experi-

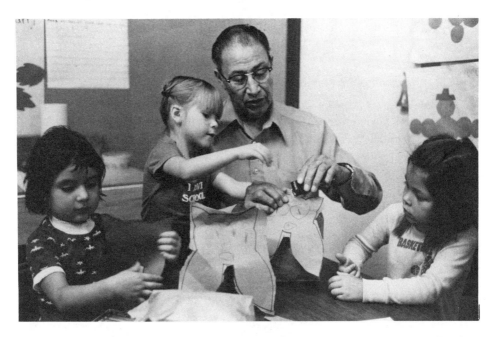

Contact with the elderly, as well as classroom discussion, will prevent students from forming misconceptions about aging.

ences. Display the completed pictures around the classroom and have each student describe the scene portrayed in his or her drawing.

OTHER IDEAS

How Would You Feel?

To make your class more aware of the discrimination that older people often suffer, divide the class into small groups. Assign one student in each group the part of an elderly person. Then have each group carry on some activity, such as working out plans for a class picnic. The student playing the part of the elderly person should attempt to take part by offering suggestions. However, the group should ignore the person or not treat the person as an equal. Let the interaction continue for five or ten minutes. Then ask the student who played the part of an elderly person to tell about how it felt.

Pictures of Me Through the Life Cycle

Have students draw pictures of what they perceive they would look like at 35, 55, and 75. Have them react to what changes they have shown in the three pictures, and how they differ from the way they look now.

Field Trip

Arrange to have your class visit a local senior neighborhood center and take part in the activities that go on there. Encourage interaction between the center members and the children, perhaps by arranging some group activity.

Intergenerational Contact Programs

One of the best ways to dispel myths about aging is to encourage social contact between young and old persons. Voluntary grandparents are useful in this activity. You could also encourage your students to be adoptive grandchildren of elderly pesons in a nearby nursing home.

What Was It Like Then?

Present living American heritage to your students. Search out very old Americans to report on past lifestyles, historic moments for your community and country. Another suggestion is to find a veteran of World War I and/or the Depression and have that person report on his activities during the war or depression, and how society was different then.

23. Consumer Health

*The goal of health education is the health-educated consumer who . . . wisely selects and uses health care resources, products, and services. . .—*The Governing Council of the American Public Health Association

A NATION OF CONSUMERS

We are all consumers. A consumer is anyone who selects and uses products to fulfill personal needs and desires. Consumer products range from the clothes we wear to the foods we eat to the over-the-counter drugs we buy for self-medication. Consumer services include those provided by physicians, dentists, and other medical professionals. In this chapter, we shall examine the area of consumer health—the selection and use of health-related products and services. At first, this may seem only a small percentage of consumer goods and services, but in fact many more are health-related than may be supposed. For example, buying a car may not seem to be a health-related matter, but it is, at least in part. One car might be safer to operate than another. Also, money spent unwisely on such a major purchase may result in a person having to cut corners on more directly health-related consumer expenditures.

This chapter cannot discuss all aspects of consumer health—only the more directly health-related issues. In addition to products and services, we will look at consumer psychology and how various forces attempt to manipulate consumer attitudes and behavior. In addition, we will discuss consumer rights, consumer-oriented legislation and government agencies, and the role of the teacher in consumer health education.

ADVERTISING AND CONSUMER BEHAVIOR

Everyone, including beginning elementary school children, has consumer needs and desires. From childhood, we are barraged with advertising that attempts to foster these needs and desires so that one blurs into the other. A need becomes a desire and a desire is perceived as a need. Our economic system is built on supply and demand and producers do all that they can to nurture a growing demand.

This manipulation of consumer psychology and behavior begins in early childhood, often by means of Saturday morning televisons commercials aimed specifically at young childrren. Typical products promoted are toys, candy, and breakfast cereals. Although the target audience of children may be unsophisticated, the methods used to advertise the products are quite sophisticated indeed. By law, advertising of any kind may not be false or misleading, and the rules are particularly strict for advertising aimed at children. However, the advertising agencies do an excellent job of stimulating desire and creating a belief about need, as any parent of a young child can attest.

Businesses spend over $60 billion a year on advertising; more money is spent on advertising health products than any other category of items. Approximately 5 percent to 35 percent of the gross sales of drugs and health aids is spent on advertising (Cornacchia & Barrett, 1985). A great deal of psychological research goes into advertising so that the target group—children, homemakers, adult males, or older adults—can be effectively reached and manipulated. The entire point of this endeavor is to get consumers to buy a particular product. Advertising does not seek to inform, but to persuade.

There are dozens of different brands of products to choose from. In many ways, the American consumer is fortunate to have so great a choice. Competition for the consumer dollar also stimulates the development of better and more efficient products and services. Consider the level of quality that would be available if only one brand of each type of product or service were offered. By providing us with so much choice, however, our economic system also makes it more difficult to make correct and informed decisions about purchases. Many of the products on the market are virtually indistinguishable from one another as far as quality and effectiveness are concerned. Price may be the only difference, and even that may not be much of a factor. For example, all brands of aspirin are basically the same in quality and effectiveness, regardless of advertising claims to the contrary.

Keep in mind that the purpose of advertising is not to inform but to persuade. As a result, most advertising contains little informational content. Even that which appears to be informational is carefully selected so that the product being advertised will appear to be uniquely better in some way. Certainly, no manufacturer could be expected to state, "Our product is no different than those of our competitors, but please buy ours anyway."

ADVERTISING APPROACHES

Young children might be expected to be taken in by misleading claims of superiority in advertising, but would a rational, experienced adult be? Yes. Advertising is a sophisticated kind of manipulation. Advertising experts understand that, despite the lack of information conveyed about the actual merits of a product, consumers can be convinced that one particular brand should be sought out from among the dozens of very similar products on the market. The reason for this is that advertising does not attempt to appeal to the rational aspects of human psychology but instead to the irrational aspects. By making a particular product sound more appealing—for any reason—an advertiser can increase the market share of the product. This can be done in a variety of ways, almost all of them noninformational in nature. Here are typical approaches used to create appeal.

Costs

Two advertising approaches are related to the cost of the product. If the cost of the item is less than the competition, the "cost effectiveness" of the item will be emphasized. However, if the product costs more than the competition, the quality of the product will be stressed as being more important than the initial cost involved in the purchase.

Repetition

Consider the number of times you have seen a television commercial only to see it repeated five minutes later. A mistake by the broadcaster? A waste of money by the advertiser? Not at all. Advertising experts understand the impact of repetition, even if such repetition may annoy or puzzle the consumer. They know that constant repetition of the same message for a product has an impact upon the consumer. Even when the consumer attempts to ignore or block out the commercial, as is usually the case, the message gets through to some degree. A catch phrase, a jingle, or a visual image is remembered. When it comes time for the consumer to make a choice in a store, that memory can be the deciding factor. More often than not, consumers will choose a product they have heard about over one they have not heard about, even when the message essentially provides no useful consumer information.

Testimonials/Authority Figures

Some commercials or advertisements attempt to persuade consumers by offering testimonials from famous individuals. Most informed adults, and even many children, realize that the person who gives the testimonial is being well paid and may not even be a regular user of the product. But there is an appeal of reflected glory; by using this product, you will have something in common with a famous movie star or athlete. Testimonials by "plain folk," often supposedly done on "hidden camera," attempt to persuade consumers that people just like themselves have found the product effective. Note that while the camera may be "hidden," no claim is ever made that the person offering the testimonial does not know that he or she is making a commercial. Such individuals, who may or may not be professional actors, are paid for their services.

Comedy Appeal

Some advertisers use comedy to promote acceptance of their product. Since there is nothing funny about most health problems, this approach is of limited use, but it has been applied to analgesic and antacid products quite successfully.

Bandwagon Appeal

This widely used approach attempts to convince the consumer that "everyone" uses the product. Typical phrases employed are "the nation's leading," "used by millions," "preferred by most for more than 20 years," and so on. The implication is that if the product is so widely used, it must be good and effective. Left unsaid is that advertising alone may have created the widespread use of the product, regardless of effectiveness or need.

Scientific Appeal

This is the "hospital tested" or "many doctors recommend the ingredients in . . ." approach. That a product was tested in a hospital means nothing. The product may have been tested and found to be no better or worse than similar products. That many doctors recommend the ingredients in a product does not mean they endorse a particular product containing those ingredients. The scientific appeal may also involve an actor recommending the product in a scientific-looking set with laboratory equipment or medical books in the background. The actor may also be wearing a white laboratory coat to heighten the effect.

Snob Appeal/Superiority

This can either be one of the most blatant or the most subtle of approaches. Testimonials are sometimes based on snob appeal by attempting to get the consumer to identify with the famous person endorsing the product. Snob appeal can also be fostered by insinuating that the consumer being addressed is much smarter than most people and that the facts presented in the commercial or advertisement will be the sole deciding factor in that person's decision to buy or not buy the product. "People who know, use . . ." is the basic message used to manipulate the consumer with this ploy.

Fear Approach

This method of manipulation is a favorite with insurance companies. "One out of every ten Americans will spend some time in a hospital this year. Will you be one of them?" The statistics used may be technically accurate but still misleading. In any case, the consumer must ask—but often does not—if this insurance company will provide the best coverage for dollars spent.

Other Common Advertising Approaches

Many advertisers combine the approaches mentioned above with visual and/or emotional imagery. Whether in a magazine ad or television commercial, the visual aspects of the advertisement are just as important as the written or spoken message. If the visual message of the commercial is pleasant, the reader or viewer will more likely associate positive thoughts with the product.

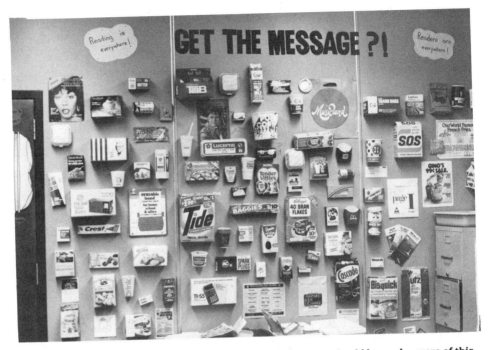

Packages and advertisements can be powerful stimuli. Students should be made aware of this.

Advertisers also use subliminal messages to appeal to the emotions or subconscious mind. One ad for an alcoholic beverage had "sex" written in several places on the picture of a drink, and pictures of food have been displayed for an instant during films at drive-in theaters (Corry, 1983). What consumers, including children, must learn to recognize is that there is a great deal of puffery in almost any commercial or advertisement, regardless of the approach used to convey the message. Often, there is little difference in effectiveness between one health product and another and price is not a big factor either. We are all manipulated by advertising, and even if a person actually feels better about using one product over another, usually there is no difference in health consequences whether Brand X or Brand Y is selected. What is important to consumer health is for individuals to develop an understanding of how advertising seeks to manipulate them, so that, when more serious health problems arise, the consumer will not be deceived by advertising claims and fail to seek out proper treatment. The limited effectiveness of all OTC drugs and self-medication must be recognized.

OTHER INFLUENCES ON PRODUCT AND SERVICE CHOICES

Consumer decisions are influenced not only by advertising but also by an individual's level of education, family beliefs, religion, socioeconomic status, community, and personal goals. A host of other factors may be involvled, including one's physical and emotional needs, motives, and personality (Corry, 1983). Individuals may model their buying patterns and selections on those of family members, friends, or peers. The more status or importance that the person being modeled has, the greater the influence that person has.

With all these influences, it might seem that a person can hardly be blamed for sometimes making poor choices about consumer health products and services. But this denies self-responsibility. Not everything can be blamed on advertising or outside influences. People often make harmful health decisions quite independently of either. They may use advertising claims to shore up these decisions, for example, by relying on OTC products in an attempt to cure ill health when they actually know that they should be seeking more effective medical treatment. Such individuals are only too willing to create a false sense of security or relief by accepting advertising claims uncritically or by enlarging on such claims themselves in order to find easy answers where no such answers exist. In the final analysis, consumers can make informed choices if they desire to do so. By accepting self-responsibility, consumers can then seek out information on products and services, analyze each on its own merits, and make wise decisions accordingly.

CONSUMER MYTHS AND MISCONCEPTIONS

Some consumer health myths might be classified as folk beliefs. Although not based on any scientific facts, many of these myths are widely believed. Here are some common consumer health myths (Cornacchia & Barrett, 1985, p. 5):

- Extra doses of vitamins give more pep and energy.
- Arthritis and cancer are partly caused by the lack of vitamins and minerals.
- Substantial weight loss can occur through perspiring.
- A daily bowel movement is necessary for good health.
- Most things that advertisements say about health and medicines are true.
- Wearing brass or copper jewelry can help arthritic and rheumatic conditions.

In some instances, belief in certain of these myths can lead to unwise consumer health decisions. For example, belief in the need to take supplementary vitamins can cause a person to spend money unnecessarily on all sorts of vitamin and tonic products, when, in fact, most people get all the vitamins their bodies need from a normal, balanced diet. Similarly, a belief that "organic" or "natural" foods are somehow better than regular produce available in stores can lead to wasteful spending on overpriced specialty products. Some consumer health myths are believed because the person is desperate for relief. Sufferers of arthritis, which is an incurable condition at present, may wear a copper bracelet in the hope that perhaps the myth about the curative properties of copper really has some truth to it. They may also spend money on mud baths or other worthless forms of supposed therapy. As some of these treatments do provide relaxation, leading to a feeling of temporary relief, they are not entirely without value, but consumers who place their faith in them are deluding themselves as to long-term benefits.

Consumer misconceptions also lead to wasteful spending, and occasionally to actual harm to health. Perhaps the most common misconception is that producers manufacture only products that are needed—if a product is on the market, it must be fulfilling a need. In fact, many products are marketed to create a need that does not actually exist. A few years ago, for example, some manufacturers began marketing vaginal deodorant sprays. With regular bathing and other sanitary measures, there is no need whatsoever for such a product, but millions of dollars worth were sold. Many mouthwashes, tonics, and other nostrums also provide few health benefits. However, most consumers believe that any product that continues to be sold must be meeting a real need. Constant advertising reinforces this misconception. Shipley and Plonsky (1980) note that even the better educated are often ignorant about consumer health information and hold many misconceptions. For example, when college students were surveyed concerning their knowledge of health care, only 49 percent responded correctly to a series of questions on the subject. Of this same group, 42 percent believed that health articles printed in popular magazines were always checked for scientific accuracy before publication. The greatest number of misconceptions occurred in the areas of health insurance, terminology, legislation, and nutrition.

Clearly, consumers must become better informed if they are to make wise consumer health decisions. They must recognize the negative impact that myths and misconceptions can have on personal health. They must also become more aware of how advertising seeks to manipulate consumer behavior and learn to reject appeals to the irrational in favor of facts and accurate information. Obtaining factual information about health products and services is not always easy. By law, advertisers must tell the truth about their products, prove the claims they make, be specific about any guarantee or warranty, and avoid making misleading statements. Additionally, the Advertising Code subscribed to by most business advertisers puts forth similar guidelines. However, most products are still made to sound more effective than they really are. It is the ultimate responsibility of the consumer to see through this puffery and make wise decisions accordingly.

QUACKERY

There are many models of medical treatment. Some of them are valid and time-tested; some are new and working to gain acceptance. Others, however, do not seek scientific validation and, in fact, avoid scientific inquiry. The first category is comprised of conventional medicine practiced by physicians who are licensed and certified in their field. The second category includes such approaches to health care as biofeedback and holistic health, which may be of value in treating certain health conditions. The third category is quackery—the use of worthless approaches that often promise miracle results.

Quacks usually try very hard to appear scientific. Their offices may closely resemble conventional physicians' offices, even to the framed degrees (but often from diploma mills) on the walls. They may dress as physicians, in white laboratory coats or with stethoscopes around their necks, employ scientific-looking gadgets, and use scientific-sounding mumbo jumbo to explain their supposed treatments. But it is all a sham, and a quack will always find an excuse for not permitting the form of quackery to be subject to independent scientific scrutiny. Although some quacks may sincerely believe in the efficacy of their treatments, most are simply out to victimize the consumer to make money.

Quackery flourishes in the United States for a variety of reasons. The primary reason is ignorance. Many Americans do not know the difference between legitimate and illegitimate medical practitioners. Anyone who claims to be a doctor or a healer is taken at face value. Another reason quackery exists is that quacks often promise cures or relief that legitimate medical practitioners cannot offer. For those suffering from incurable diseases, the false hope that quacks hold out may seem irresistable. As nothing else can help them, they turn to quacks in desperation. People also sometimes consult quacks because they hope to get around the high cost of legitimate medical attention; the quack promises a quick and inexpensive cure. In other instances, people turn to quacks because they wish to avoid surgery or other involved legitimate medical treatment. And, of course, many people actually believe the flimflam claims made by quacks.

Quackery can involve deception in several areas, such as medicine, drugs, healing devices, and diets. Some of the warning signs of quacks include (Hamrick, Anspaugh & Ezell, 1986, p. 69):

1. Offers of a guaranteed, quick cure for an illness with a "miracle" drug or treatment
2. Uses of fear strategies to convince the patient of his need for the cure
3. Claims of victimization by other physicians or the American Medical Association
4. Underrating traditional medical practice
5. No use of surgery
6. Use of devices, gadgets, and secret formulas to convince patients that their illness is cured.

If quacks cannot effect cures, why do so many people continue to have faith in them? In some instances, quacks do seem to provide relief or cures. In these cases, the patient may be a hypochondriac with no actual physical problem to begin with. If the person believes that help is being provided, the "problem" disappears. In cases where an actual problem does exist, the natural healing powers of the body may be responsible for a cure attributed to a quack. Finally, temporary relief or remission may be mistaken for a cure.

HEALTH CARE

The American health care delivery system is in critical condition. Rising medical care costs are a very significant factor contributing to the overall rate of inflation in this country. The reasons for increasing health care costs include present reimbursement practices, increasing technology, and rising physicians' fees and other health care salaries. The poor and the elderly are the ones who suffer most from the present health care delivery system. Government programs such as Medicare and Medicaid help somewhat, but for many individuals the portion of the bills not paid by these

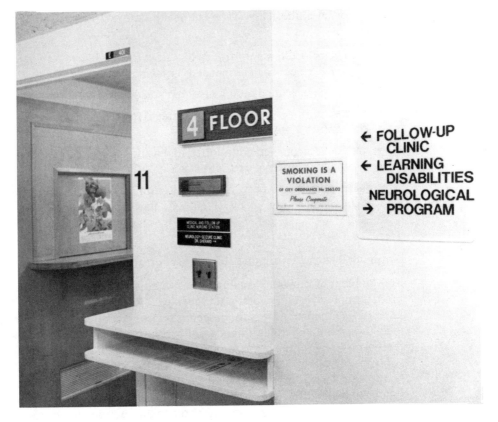

It's difficult to find our way in today's health care maze.

programs is still financially overwhelming. In fact, most people over 65 are paying more of their income for health care now than they did before Medicare went into effect in 1966 (Hamilton, 1982). The Department of Health and Human Services is attempting to reduce costs under the Medicare plan by setting fees for hospital treatments according to diagnostic related groups, or DRGs. A fee is set by DHHS for a specific surgery, and if the hospital charge is more than the set amount, the hospital must absorb the difference in cost (Olsen, Redican & Baffi, 1986).

ALTERNATE FORMS OF HEALTH CARE

Some methods of health care differ from the methods used in traditional medicine. Some of these methods have no therapeutic benefit and can be financially and physically costly since they delay the patient from seeing a legitimate health care provider. Other alternative forms of health care have not yet been accepted as traditional medicine, but, as they are used more frequently, they may gain more acceptance.

Among these alternative forms of health care are (Price, Galli & Slenker, 1985, pp. 502–14):

- hypnosis—a temporary trance-like state in which a variety of conditions may appear in response to verbal or other stimuli

- transcendental meditation—reaching a deeper level of pure consciousness

- acupuncture—a procedure that corrects the blockages of pathways of energy flow; sometimes used in anesthesia

- herbal medicine—includes dried herbs and roots which are brewed and taken internally or externally to cure disease

- naturopathy—the prevention and treatment of disease by using biomedical, psychological, and physical methods that assist the healing processes in the body

National Health Insurance

The problem of providing adequate health care to all Americans has been recognized for many years. Several attempts have been made in Congress to establish a national health insurance plan. In theory, under a national health insurance plan the federal government would finance the cost of medical coverage for families below the poverty level while other families would have deductions from their income to support the system. Various plans have been introduced to provide equal access to health care for all citizens. The advocates of national health care insurance state that such a system would promote cost control by requiring health care institutions to provide care within their annual budgets and put doctors on salary. In general, physicians are opposed to this approach. Other opponents protest that national health insurance would impose too much government control and intervention in health care. Another criticism is that this system of health care would foster an impersonal, assembly-line approach to providing treatment since doctors on salary would no longer be competing for business and thus would have less incentive to provide personalized care. A final criticism is that national health insurance would simply cost too much, with most of the burden falling on middle-income families.

Health Maintenance Organizations

As the debate about national health insurance continues, other attempts to provide better, more economical health care have been made. One promising approach is the health maintenance organization (HMO). These private health care centers provide prepaid group programs that offer a full range of medical services. Good HMOs emphasize preventive medicine. They try to keep their patients well rather than using the crisis-oriented approach of most physicians. The philosophy behind the HMO approach is that it is cheaper to keep people well than to treat them after they become ill. Many HMOs have suffered from poor financial management, however, and this approach to health care still needs refinement. Also, many physicians oppose HMOs because they do not include fee-for-service payments.

Medical Insurance

As fees for medical and health care services continue to climb, it is more important than ever to have adequate medical insurance. Today, most workers are covered by a group plan at their place of employment. Typically, such plans pay 80 percent of medical costs, with the individual responsible for the remaining 20 percent. Premiums for this coverage are paid for by employer contributions and employee pay deductions. Most of these plans provide good coverage, but one problem is that the insurance coverage ceases if the employee leaves the company.

A variation of the third-party reimbursement method of medical insurance as described in the previous paragraph includes the use of preferred providers (PPOs). Under the PPO system, a plan is provided by an employer to minimize insurance claim-filing and costs. The employer contracts with an insurance company and specific health care providers. The employee agrees to use only the health care professionals and institutions under contract. The employer and employee pay lower insurance premiums, the insurance companies save on paperwork and claim filing, and physicians increase their patient load.

Many individuals pay for their own medical insurance. Self-employed people, of course, have no other choice. Taking out personal and family medical insurance has certain advantages. The type and amount of coverage can be tailored to individual needs. However, the more extensive the coverage desired, the most expensive the premiums will be. Nonetheless, every individual should try to have some sort of medical insurance.

SELECTING A HEALTH CARE PROFESSIONAL

Just as everyone should have medical insurance, everyone should have a personal physician. If a medical emergency arises, a person can seek help immediately from a trusted health care professional who knows the patient's history. Just as importantly, by having a personal physician or other health care professional, a person can better maintain good health by means of regular checkups or consultations with the provider about health concerns. You should select a health care professional thoughtfully. Here are some suggestions (Hamrick, Anspaugh & Ezell, 1986, pp. 39–40, 53):

1. Choose your physician while you are in good health. If you wait until a medical crisis arises, you will have to rely on whomever you can find. Having a physician you trust and feel comfortable with before a crisis will lessen anxiety.
2. To locate physicians who are accepting new patients, telephone the local county medical society. The number can be found in the yellow pages. If you are not sure what kind of physician you need, such as a specialist or a general practitioner, the medical society can also offer some initial advice. Generally, you will be given the names of two or three physicians you can call. A local hospital can also be a good source of information about physicians who are accepting new patients.

3. Select a board-certified family practitioner for a family physician, a pediatrician for children, and a gynecologist for females.
4. Check the credentials of physicians you are considering. Don't be afraid to ask questions about how the person is keeping current in the field.
5. Get details about office hours, emergency care, whether house calls will be made, and so forth. Also try to determine how long a patient usually has to wait before seeing the doctor.
6. Determine the fee schedule for checkups and different types of treatment. Doctors often base their fees on recommended prices recorded in a fee schedule book produced by the American Medical Association. The fees are recommended ranges, not fixed prices, and a physician may charge on the high or low end. Keep in mind that the most expensive physician is not necessarily the best.
7. Choose a physician who is able to ommunicate with you in terms you can understand. You have a right to know what is going on during any treatment and the doctor has an obligation to keep you informed. Regardless of their medical skills, however, some physicians are better communicators than others.
8. Choose a physician you feel comfortable with. The doctor's age, sex, and personal manner may all be factors that make you more comfortable or less comfortable. Set up an appointment to talk with the professional to see whether he or she is willing to communicate openly and honestly.
9. Choose a physician you can have confidence in. Even if the person is highly qualified and well thought of in the profession, you may be put off by some personal quality.
10. Don't be afraid to change physicians if you are not satisfied with the way you are being treated. Find a doctor with whom you feel comfortable.

CONSUMER RIGHTS AND PROTECTION

One of the basic premises of this book is that individuals should be responsible for their own health behavior. This is certainly true for consumer health. With so much competition for every dollar we spend, and with so much available to buy, consumers need to guard against wasteful spending on products and services of dubious value. For the most part, consumers do not protect themselves properly through informed consumer health behavior. Fortunately, government agencies and private organizations have stepped in to establish consumer rights and offer some protection.

On March 15, 1962, President Kennedy sent to Congress his Special Message on Protecting the Consumer Interest (Cornacchia & Barrett, 1985). The message stated that additional legislation and administration action were required to assist consumers in the exercise of their rights. Kennedy outlined these rights.

1. Right to safety—to be protected against the marketing of goods that are hazardous to health or life
2. Right to be informed—to be protected against fraudulent, deceitful, or misleading information or advertising

3. Right to choose—to be assured that consumer interests will receive full and sympathetic consideration in the formulation of government policy on consumer matters

In 1970 and 1971, Mary Gardiner Jones of the Federal Trade Commission and Ralph Nader further extended the definitions of consumer rights to include these rights.

1. Right to expect quality of design, workmanship, and ingredients in products and services
2. Right to be charged fair prices
3. Right to receive courteous and respectful treatment from firms
4. Right to expect consumer products and services whose use by the consuming public are consistent with the values of a humane society
5. Right to redress of legitimate grievances related to purchased products and services

These consumer rights, of course, are meaningless unless they are backed up with the power of legislation. Over the years, hundreds of federal, state, and local laws have been passed to ensure the rights of consumers and to protect consumers from fraudulent or harmful products and services.

Consumer Protection Agencies

Many federal agencies work to protect the consumer. One of the most active of these agencies is the Food and Drug Administration (FDA). Responsibilities of the FDA include periodic inspection of foods, drugs, devices, and cosmetics. The agency demands proof of the safety and effectiveness of any new drug before it is marketed and has the power to recall possibly unsafe drugs or other substances from the market. The FDA also enforces the law against illegal sales of prescription drugs, investigates therapeutic devices for safety and truthfulness of labeling claims, and checks importation of foods, drugs, devices, and cosmetics to ensure that they comply with U.S. laws.

Another government agency, the Federal Trade Commission (FTC), is responsible for eliminating unfair or deceptive practices in commerce that curtail competition. In other words, this agency prevents the free enterprise system from being suppressed by a company creating a monopoly on a product or service, or by fraudulent trade techniques. The FTC has the authority to stop the dissemination of advertisement of foods, drugs, devices, or cosmetics when it is in the best interest of the consumer. Also, if a label on a product is misleading, the FTC can order the withdrawal of that product from the shelves.

The Consumer Product Safety Commission, established by the Federal government in1973, protects the public against unreasonable risks of injury from products. This commission oversees the enforcement of the Flammable Fabrics Act, the Federal Hazardous Substances Act, and the Poison Prevention Packaging Act. Under these acts, the Consumer Product Safety Commission is responsible for regulating the manufacture for sale of all highly flammable wearing apparel and fabrics. This is especially helpful for the consumer since the majority of fabrics used in today's clothing will burn quite easily. The commission can ban from sale toys and other articles intended for use by children that present electrical, mechanical, or thermal hazards. In addition, the commission supervises the labeling and packaging of poisonous substances to prevent accidental poisoning by children. Manufacturers are forbidden to package poisonous substances in bright colors or with cartoon figures that would attract children to them. Also, drugs and other medicines must be available in child-restraint containers that cannot be opened by most children under five years of age.

In January 1964, President Johnson established the President's Committee on Consumer Interests. This Committee was replaced by the Office of Consumer Affairs in 1971. The main purpose of this office is to act as a consumer voice in the presidential administration. This organization also coordinates all governmental activities in the field of consumerism, conducts investigations on consumer problems, handles consumer complaints, facilitates communication on consumer affairs between the government, business, and the consumer, and helps disseminate helpful information to the consumer.

Various department-level organizations within the Federal government also aid the consumer. The Department of Commerce encourages industry to avoid packaging proliferation that can lead to consumer confusion in shopping. This department can request mandatory packaging standards. The organization also provides statistics on population, gross national product, corporate profits, personal income, retail sales, balance of payments, manufacturing, and housing—all of which aid the government and consumer to understand the present status of the nation's economy. The Department of Labor provides the Consumer Price Index, the measure of changes in the nation's economy and currency. This agency also surveys employment trends and studies prices of various commodities. The Department of Agriculture (USDA) inspects meat and food animals prior to slaughter to prevent any diseased meat from reaching the stores. The USDA establishes grades of meat to help the consumer in identifying the different levels of quality. The United States Postal Service investigates any incidence of mail fraud and regulates attempts to sell worthless or harmful merchandise or medicines through the mails.

PRIVATE AGENCIES

Many private agencies also assist the consumer by providing accurate, unbiased information about products or by attempting to eliminate fraud and deception by businesses. For example, Consumer's Union publishes *Consumer Reports,* a magazine that provides impartial information about products. This publication informs the consumer about best buys and the most reliable products. *Consumer Reports* also helps the consumer by interpreting advertising on many products.

Better Busissness Bureaus are private, nonprofit, business-supported groups that assist the consumer in mediating misunderstandings between customers and businesses. These groups provide information about a company, help resolve complaints against companies, foster ethical advertising and selling practices, alert consumers to bad business practices, and provide the media with informational materials on consumer subjects. Better Busissness Bureaus have no legal powers. They can arbitrate between consumer and business. When illegal practices are discovered and a business refuses to cooperate, the matter is turned over to the appropriate law enforcement agency. These bureaus are one of the more important sources of help to which consumers may turn when they need assistance, especially in regard to health products and devices (Cornacchia & Bararett, 1985).

Many cities have Chambers of Commerce that are supported by businesses in that community. These organizations publish a business-consumer relations code of ethics. Their work is quite similar to a Better Business Bureau in that they act as liaisons between the consumer and business. They also protect the consumer by attempting to eliminate fraudulent business practices.

Even with all of these government and private agencies working to protect the consumer, it remains the individual's responsibility to be informed about products and services. To increase the probability of satisfaction when purchasing a product, follow these recommendations (Olsen, Redican & Baffi, 1986, pp. 564–5):

1. Keep all sales slips and canceled checks.
2. Take all complaints to the place where you made the purchase.
3. If not satisfied, write to the president of the company and send a copy of the letter to some other high-ranking officer in the company. Be sure to keep a copy of this letter for your own files.
4. If you get no response, send copies of the letter to the Better Business Bureau or other helpful agencies.

Health Highlight: Recognizing Fraudulent Advertising

Bogus remedies are big business in the United States. In fact, $4 to 5 billion a year are spent on cancer remedies of no proven value, $2 billion on worthless cures for arthritis, and $10 billion on diet products and gimmicks. Government controls have not eliminated advertising of quack remedies, partially because the legislation still has loopholes. Each consumer should assume the responsibility to recognize fraudulent advertising by the following signs.

1. It uses words like "miracle," "cure," or "break-through."
2. It does not identify the ingredients.
3. It claims to have support from experts who are not named or fully identified.
4. It offers the substance only through the mail or door-to-door.
5. It makes claims of effectiveness for a variety of conditions.
6. It declares the product is all "natural."
7. It emphasizes opposition or disapproval by the medical profession.
8. It includes testimonials from people who were "cured."

Source: "Quackery: A Brief Manual," *The Harvard Medical School Health Letter*, Volume IX, Number 12, October, 1984, pp. 1–2.

TEACHING CONSUMER HEALTH EDUCATION

With rising prices and a tight economy, support has grown for consumer health education that teaches consumers to learn to make wise decisions about buying and using products and services, especially in health-related areas (Corry & Galli, 1985). Even if you teach at the beginning elementary level, your students are already consumers. As such, they need to become knowledgeable about consumer rights and consumer responsibilities. They have rights as outlined earlier in the chapter, but rights are balanced with responsibilities. These responsibilities include seeking out accurate information about products and services, being skeptical of advertising claims, recognizing the differences between needs and desires, and making wise consumer choices.

The most effective way that all consumers, regardless of age, can protect themselves in the area of consumer health is through preventive health care. By learning about proper nutrition, exercise, and rest, students can avoid the need for many consumer health products such as vitamin supplements, tonics, and diet products. Understanding the dangers of substance abuse will also assist children in avoiding the use of potentially hazardous drugs, whether prescription or over-the-counter products.

The importance of critical thinking cannot be overemphasized when it comes to teaching consumer health education. Children should recognize early that just because a product is advertised on television or in a newspaper does not mean that the product is worthwhile or useful. They should learn to see how wants can be fostered artifically. In addition, they should learn not to accept advertising claims or promises without thinking. Help your students recognize that much of what is said in a commercial is meaningless. For example, a product may be touted as "new" or "improved." Is "new" necessarily better? "Improved" in what way? If a product is advertised as being "25 percent more effective," students should ask, "More effective than what?" Generally, no answer to this question can be found.

Your job is not to teach students what to buy, but rather how to buy. Students should be encouraged to get the facts, comparison shop, consider the consequences of all purchases, and to budget their money. By learning the importance of wise consumer behavior early, children can incorporate the concepts you teach into their own value system. Finally, you should teach children about their rights as consumers and what recourse they have if they are victimized in the marketplace. All consumers have legal rights. Exercising these rights can help put an end to shoddy and deceitful business practice.

SUMMARY

A consumer is anyone who selects and uses goods and services. Consumer health education is concerned with those products that directly or indirectly affect personal health. Overall health can be positively or negatively affected by consumer decisions about products and services.

Consumers become aware of the existence of available products primarily through advertising. Although there are laws and regulations concerning the content of advertisements, the goal of advertising is not to inform but to persuade. Advertising seeks to manipulate consumer psychology and behavior by confusing wants with needs and by fostering desires. An advertisement for a product may be misleading without being legally deceitful. Most health care products try to give the impression that they are more effective than they actually are. Even when consumers understand this on a rational plane, they may still be persuaded to buy a product because of irrational appeal or because of simple and constant repetition of the advertisement.

Quackery is widespread in the United States despite legal measures designed to prevent it. Many consumers turn to quacks for relief either because they are desperate or gullible. Money spent on quacks is money wasted. More importantly, resorting to a quack can prevent a person from getting proper medical attention. The high cost of health care delivery is a problem today. Various plans have been put forward for national insurance schemes, but there has been effective opposition from many different interest groups. Health maintenance organizations can provide some of the benefits of national health insurance, but only limited numbers of people currently are members of such groups. Private and company medical insurance plans, including preferred provider plans, are important safeguards against the financial burdens caused by serious illness.

A health care professional should be selected with care. Consumers should seek out quality professionals whom they can trust to deliver good care at fair prices.

Many government and private agencies have been establahed to protect the consumer. These agencies evaluate the quality and effectiveness of health-related products and also police business practices. However, it is still the primary responsibility of each consumer to become knowledgeable enough to make wise consumer decisions. Helping students learn to become informed consumers is part of the teacher's job in teaching consumer health education.

DISCUSSION QUESTIONS

1. How does advertising manipulate consumer psychology and behavior?
2. Discuss the most typical advertising approaches.
3. Describe the influences, other than advertising, that affect consumer behavior.
4. List and discuss some common health-related consumer myths.
5. What is the teacher's role in combatting consumer misconceptions?
6. Discuss the role of the Better Business Bureau in protecting consumers' rights.
7. Discuss the reasons that quackery prospers in America today.
8. Describe the potential impact of PPOs and DRGs on health care costs.
9. Discuss acupuncture as an alternative form of health care delivery.
10. List the major recommendations to follow when selecting a health care professional.

REFERENCES

Cornacchia, H. & Barrett, S. *Consumer health: A guide to intelligent decisions.* St. Louis: Times Mirror/Mosby College Publishing, 1985.

Corry, J. *Consumer health: Facts, skills and decisions.* Belmont, California: Wadsworth Publishing Company, 1983.

Corry, J. & Galli, N. "The role of the school in consumer health education." *Journal of School Health, 55,* 4, April, 1985.

Hamilton, P. *Health care consumerism.* St. Louis: C. V. Mosby, 1982.

Hamrick, M., Anspaugh, D., & Ezell, G. *Health.* Columbus: Merrill, 1986.

Olsen, L., Redican, K., & Baffi, C. *Health today,* second edition. New York: Macmillan Publishing Company, 1986.

Price, J., Galli, N., & Slenker, S. *Consumer health: Contemporary issues and choices.* Dubuque, Iowa: Wm. C. Brown Publishers, 1985.

"Quackery: A brief manual." *The Harvard Medical School Health Letter,* IX, 12, October, 1984.

Shipley, R. & Plonski, C. *Consumer health: Protecting your health and money.* New York: Harper and Row, 1980.

24. Techniques for Teaching Consumer Health

One human frailty is to believe what we are told by others. However positive and noble this characteristic might be, many have suffered throughout history from their own gullibility. The modern consumer is no exception to this truism. Caveat emptor (buyer beware) is still a relevant warning in the area of consumer health.—Warren E. Schaller and Charles R. Carroll, *Health, Quackery, and the Consumer*

ESTABLISHING CONSUMER BEHAVIOR PATTERNS

The patterns established in childhood of appraising, selecting, and using consumer products and services can influence an individual's physical, psychological, and social well-being for a lifetime. To choose wisely requires accumulating knowledge and formulating attitudes about different kinds of products and services. Children must learn that products and services differ in quality, worth, and intrinsic value. They must also recognize how advertising and social forces influence ideas about needs and desires. Above all, they must understand that the responsibility for making wise consumer decisions ultimately is a personal one.

Consumer health pertains to products and services that either directly or indirectly relate to personal health. Broadly speaking, almost any product or service purchased can in some way be health-related. For example, choice of foods has a bearing on nutrition. Choice of clothing relates not only to physical needs but also to psychological expression of personality. Choice of discretionary purchases, ranging from toys to jewelry to stereo equipment, affects income available for necessities. Most directly health-related products and services include OTC drugs, cosmetics, and medical and dental treatment.

In this chapter, both the rights and the responsibilities of the consumer will be emphasized. A variety of suggestions for learning activities will assist you in helping students establish responsible consumer behavior patterns.

Concepts to be Taught

- Health products and services should be used only when needed.
- It is important to obtain accurate information concerning health care products and services.
- Not all products and services are worthwhile or necessary.
- Advertising seeks to persuade rather than to inform.
- Many advertising claims are inflated or misleading.
- One's family, friends, and peers influence choice of products and services.
- Labels on all health care products should be read carefully and the directions should be followed closely.
- The existence of widespread quackery in health products and services must be recognized.
- There are many ways to spot quack products and services.
- Quack products and services are useless or dangerous.
- Medical attention should be obtained only from qualified and recognized professionals.
- Many government and private agencies work to protect the consumer.
- Federal, state, and local laws enforce the rights of the consumer.
- The best way to make wise consumer decisions is to become informed about the facts concerning products and services.
- Making wise consumer decisions is ultimately a personal responsibility.

Cycle Plan for Teaching Topics

Topic	Grade Level						
	K	1	2	3	4	5	6
Health Care Products	*	*	**	***	**	**	***
Health Care Services	*	*	*	**	*	***	**
Advertising	*	*	*	**	**	**	***
Behavior	*	*	**	*	***	**	***
Quackery	*	*	*	*	**	***	***
Obtaining Medical Services	*	*	*	*	**	**	**
Consumer Protection	*	*	*	*	**	***	**
Consumer Responsibilities	*	*	**	***	**	***	***

Key: *** = major emphasis, ** = emphasis, * = review.

VALUE-BASED ACTIVITIES

Assessing Attitudes

Duplicate statements such as those shown here and have the students assess their own attitudes about each one. By doing so, the children will become more aware of why they make certain consumer choices.

	Agree	Disagree	Not sure
1. Most television commercials give accurate information about the product advertised	____	____	____
2. If my friends have a certain product, I usually want to buy that product, too.	____	____	____
3. I only buy products that I need.	____	____	____
4. Advertisements must tell the truth.	____	____	____
5. Only products and services that are useful are sold.	____	____	____
6. I sometimes buy things that I don't need.	____	____	____
7. There is not much point to saving money.	____	____	____
8. Sometimes I buy things without knowing very much about how good they are.	____	____	____
9. Health care products are always safe to use.	____	____	____
10. The products I buy for myself can affect my health.	____	____	____

Why Do I Buy?

Have each student think of a product that he or she buys from time to time. It can be any sort of product, not necessarily a health-related one. Then write the following reasons on the chalkboard for why a person might buy a product. Have each student determine which three of these reasons most likely influences the purchase of the product being considered. Explain that the students may provide other reasons if they wish. After the exercise, have each student discuss the reasons selected for product purchase. Ask the students to consider how these reasons relate to their values.

1. Advertising has convinced me that this is the best product of its kind.
2. My friends all use this product, so I use it, too.
3. This is the cheapest product of its kind.
4. This is the only product of its kind available for me to buy.
5. I like the packaging.
6. My family has told me that this is a good product.
7. I think this product has the highest quality.
8. I have tried other brands, and I like this one better.
9. I don't really know why I buy this particular product, but I do.
10. I like other people to know that I use this brand of product.

Budget Diary

Have each student keep a notebook diary of all purchases made for a week or longer. Every purchase made should be recorded in the diary, along with the reasons for that purchase. Money spent on food, snacks, toys, video games, school supplies, transportation, books and magazines, pet supplies, hobbies, and health care products should all be recorded. Explain to the class that the amount of money each student spends is not as relevant as *how* the money was spent. After the diaries have been completed for the assigned time period, have each student analyze his or her purchases and answer these questions:

1. What items did you buy that brought you a great amount of pleasure?
2. What items did you buy that disappointed you?

3. Do you think that you spent any money unwisely? Why?
4. Does this diary suggest ways that you could budget your spending money better? How?
5. What does this diary tell you about your consumer habits? Are there patterns in the way you spend your money?

Answers to these questions should be written out so that students can clarify their thoughts better and come to personal conclusions about their patterns of consumer behavior. On a volunteer basis, have students explain to the class what they learned from this activity. Follow with a general discussion.

I'm a Wise Consumer Because . . .

Ask each student to complete the statement, "I'm a wise consumer because . . ." in 25 words or less. Each written answer should be based on actual behavior or attitudes. Discuss each student's response in a general class discussion. Ask students to explain what values their statements are based upon.

Decision Stories

Follow the procedures outlined in Chapter 5 for presenting decision stories such as these.

Broken promises

Ricardo saw a model car advertised on television. It looked like a fun toy. He saved up his money and bought the model. But when he opened the package, the car didn't look as well made as it did on television. He started playing with it and the car broke. He was angry and disappointed. He felt like throwing the car away, but it had cost a lot of money.

Focus Question: Was it Ricardo's fault that the car broke?

Vitamins for Vera?

In her health class, Vera has been learning about the importance of vitamins for good health and growth. She wonders if she is getting enough vitamins because sometimes she feels tired and worn out. One day, Vera's mother asks her to go to the grocery store to buy some milk. While at the store, Vera sees a shelf with many different kinds of vitamin pills on it. She has some money of her own with her. Maybe she should buy some vitamins. Then she might feel in better health.

Focus Question: What should Vera do?

Munch or Lunch

Mike likes to play video games. He spends a lot of his money playing Munchman, his favorite video game. He is getting better and better at it, but playing Munchman often leaves him without any money for other things. His parents give him lunch money every day. Up to now, he hasn't spent this money on anything except lunch. But maybe he could cut a few corners. Maybe he could buy less for lunch and use the rest of the money to play video games.

Focus Question: What should Mike do?

Music, Music, Music

Marsha likes music. She spends a lot of her money buying records and tapes. One day, Marsha sees an advertisement for a tape club in a magazine. For only $10, she can buy any three of her favorite albums on tape through the mail. Marsha sends off a money order, and in a few weeks her three selections arrive. She is very pleased. The tapes are great, and for $10 they are a real bargain. However, the next month three more tapes arrive in the mail. But Marsha didn't order them. Still, there is a bill along with the tapes. The bill is for $25.

Focus Questions: Does Marsha have to pay for the new tapes? How can she find out about her consumer rights in this matter?

Shampoo of the Stars

Valerie's friends have been telling her about a new shampoo called Hairdoyoudo. They say that it makes their hair feel soft and pretty. Valerie has also seen the product advertised on television. A famous young model says that she uses it. The model has beautiful hair. Valerie would like to use Hairdoyoudo, too. But her mother buys another brand of shampoo. It costs much less than Hairdoyoudo and seems to work fine. Valerie asks her mother to buy Hairdoyoudo, but she refuses. She says it is overpriced. Valerie is very put out. She wants her hair to look as nice as her friends' hair. But how can that be if she has to use another shampoo?

Focus Question: What should Valerie do?

Spots and Shaun

Shaun has acne. He is very embarrassed about his spots and blemishes. One day he sees an advertisement for a new acne medication in a magazine. The advertisement promises a "miracle cure." It says that the product will cure acne in 30 days. The product has a money-back guarantee, but it can only be purchased by mail. The advertisement also says that the product has a secret ingredient that no other product has. It sounds like just what Shaun has been looking for, even if the product does cost $12.95 a tube.

Focus Question: Should Shaun send off for the product?

DRAMATIZATION

Now for This Commercial Message

Ask the students to work together in pairs or small groups to reinact commercials they have seen on television for health care products or services. Let each group decide on the commercial they wish to reenact. Draw up a master list so there will not be too much duplication. Then have the students who are working together study the commercial of their choice closely at home. Let them get together and rehearse their reinactment. Each student should play a different role. For example, one student can be the person recommending the product and another student can be the person trying out the product, as in many aspirin commercials. When the students are ready, have each commercial reinacted in front of the class. After the reinactment, the students who played the roles should explain what might have been misleading or overpromising about what they said or did.

Dr. I. M. Quack

Let each student come up with a quack product or service and try to convince the class that this product or service is actually of value. Encourage imagination. For example, one student might try to convince the class that magnetic energy can cure arthritis. Another might claim to have invented a product that will cure the common cold. The class should listen to each presentation without interruption, but then point out the fallacies of each presentation.

Finding a Doctor

After discussing the procedures that can be used for locating a qualified physician, have students role play the techniques. For instance, let one student play the part of a representative from the county medical society who can recommend physicians who are accepting new patients. Another student can call on the telephone to ask for the names of such physicians. Or, one student can play the part of a doctor while the other plays the part of a prospective client. The latter should ask questions about availability of services, fees, qualifications of the doctor, and so forth.

Complaints

Have small groups of students role play how they would act when complaining about a defective or ineffective product or service. One student should act the part of the disgruntled consumer, another the part of the seller, and a third the part of a consumer advocate or representative of a local Better Business Bureau or other consumer-oriented group.

DISCUSSION AND REPORT TECHNIQUES

Presentation by Professionals

Invite members of local consumer-oriented organizations to class to discuss consumer rights. Guest speakers might include a member of the local board of health, a representative of a consumer action group, or a government official who deals with consumer affairs.

Information or Puffery?

Have each student closely watch and analyze a different commercial on television. Because advertising techniques are similar for most products, the commercials chosen do not have to be directly health-related, although many should be. Ask students to determine how much actual useful information is conveyed in the commercial and how much of what is said is mere puffery. Let each student present his or her findings and explain how the commercial attempts to appeal to consumers and manipulate their behavior and attitudes.

Is That So?

Ask each student to find a commercial or advertisement that appears to be quite truthful and informative. Have the students discuss the commercials or advertisements and explain their reasons for believing the claims made. Then ask the rest of the class to offer their own opinions. You may need to point out subtle approaches used in the commercial or advertisement to suggest greater informational content than is actually the case.

Labels Are Important

With the cooperation of parents, have each student analyze the information given on the package of a health product or OTC drug. Students should prepare individual reports about what they find. Follow with a general discussion about the importance of reading and understanding labels before using any OTC drug or health product. Note to the class any warnings or advisory information given on products discussed.

Where Can I Go for Help?

Have students research legitimate health care services available in the community and write reports on their findings. Community health resources include private physicians, dentists, therapists, hospitals, clinics, health maintenance organizations, telephone referral services, and so on.

Panel Presentation on Consumer Agencies

Divide the class into small groups and have each research an assigned consumer protection agency, such as the Food and Drug Administration, the Federal Trade Commission, Better Business Bureaus, and so forth. Each group should present a short panel presentation. Be sure that all members of every group participate in the presentations.

History of Consumer Protection

Assign students to report on past consumer health abuses and how measures have been taken to prevent such abuse today. This is a good library research project.

What's the Pitch?

Have students watch and analyze a television commercial of their choice and then prepare a written report explaining what advertising technique is employed in the commercial, such as snob appeal, fear approach, humor, testimonials, or the scientific approach. Students should note the actual amount of useful information contained in the commercial and decide to what extent the commercial plays on irrational considerations.

EXPERIMENTS AND DEMONSTRATIONS

Is There Any Difference?

Many products are indistinguishable once removed from their packaging. To demonstrate this, bring in some different brand of cola soft drinks. Pour small amounts of three or four different brands into paper cups and have the students do taste comparisons. Let them try to guess which cup contains a particular brand. Discuss the results of the taste testing.

Which Is Better?

Ask students to recommend a particular health-related product such as a shampoo or soap. Then have students trade the products they now use with someone using another brand of shampoo or soap. Let each volunteer student in this experiment use the alternate product for a week or two and then report on the results. Did the alternate shampoo or soap do just as effective a job or were differences noted? Were any differences a matter of individual preference? Are different products perhaps more or less effective for different individuals? Be sure to note that differences or lack of differences in OTC products may not hold true for prescription medications.

Slogans

To demonstrate how advertising tries to manipulate consumers into remembering a particular product so that the product will be chosen from among the many competing brands when it comes time to purchase, prepare a list of advertising slogans and have the class try to guess which product each slogan promotes. Students should note that the slogan used to reinforce the memory of a product often has little informational content, if any at all.

PUZZLES AND GAMES

Consumer Riddles

Let your students solve these riddles about consumerism. Then discuss each one.

1. I am a fraud, but I sound like a duck. What am I? (a quack)
2. An inflated advertising claim is a huff and a _____. (puff)
3. My initials are BBB. I can help you if you have a consumer problem. What am I? (Better Business Bureau)

Scrambled Words

Have students unscramble each of these words that relate to consumerism.

1. mocmlaceri (commercial)
2. qyuracek (quackery)
3. singiadevrt (advertising)
4. elagl githrs (legal rights)
5. aeetngura (guarantee)

START	Buy mouthwash—$2.00	Consult a quack—$100.00	Spend allowance on video games—$10.00	Go to HMO. Save money and get back $35.00 to spend
	Buy unneeded vitamin pills—$8.00	Buy defective product and waste $50.00	Have everything you need—no buying today	Buy most expensive shampoo—$7.00
	Waste money on junk food—$4.00	Buy a new shirt that shrinks—waste $15.00	Find a cheaper and better brand of toothpaste—save $2.00 (get $2.00 back)	Buy a worthless acne cure—waste $6.00
	Do comparison shopping. Save $12.00 (get $12.00 back)	Resist silly commercial for cold remedy—no money spent	Buy a new coat that you like on sale—$25.00	Buy a present for a family member—$15.00
	Go fishing—no cost	Buy a toy that breaks—$11.00 wasted	Visit the dentist for a checkup—$30.00, but $100 saved if dental problem avoided	Buy a book that you want—$7.00
	Dental problem that you could have prevented—$100.00	Buy a new brand of soap—save $1.00 ($1.00 back)	Buy a new bicycle—$120.00 but get $20.00 back because of sale price	END (Continue until END.)

Figure 24.1
Shopping game board.

Consumer Health Tic-Tac-Toe

This game can be played either by two players or by the whole class divided into two halves. Have each side or player come up with a health-related question for one of the tic-tac-toe squares. The opposing side or player elects to try to answer a question for a particular square. The opposing side or player, however, should not know what the question is for that square. If an incorrect answer is given, no mark on the tic-tac-toe board is to be made for that square. Each side plays in turn until there is a winner.

Shopping Game

Prepare a game board as shown in figure 24.1. The game can be played by from two to six players. Each player is given $200 in play money at the start. Participants roll dice in turn to determine the number of moves. The winner is the player with the most money at the end of the game. Play can continue until only one player has any money left. Let each player decide to what extent he or she "won" or "lost" by the consumer decisions the game dictated. Follow with a discussion of options in buying products and services.

BULLETIN BOARDS

Which Would You Buy?

Prepare, or have your students help you prepare, a bulletin board display of different brands of a particular health-related product, such as a shampoo, soap, analgesic, or food product. Make a collage of pictures from magazines of the different products under the heading "Which Would You Buy?" Then have students discuss the merits and differences among the various products.

Believe It or Not

Have students prepare mock advertisements for popular products such as breakfast cereals, toys, and games. Each advertisement should try to sound as appealing as possible. Display the finished products. Then have students discuss the advertising approaches used to promote each product. How believable are the claims made? How much (if any) information is given about each product? Are any of the advertising claims false or misleading?

Needs and Wants

Ask students to prepare bulletin board displays of various products that they consider either needs or wants. Point out that there is nothing wrong with buying a product that is wanted but not needed as long as an individual can afford to pay for it without having to do without any necessity. Discuss this point with the class and elicit different viewpoints about needs and wants.

Don't be Taken In

Ask students to find advertisements that they believe are deceptive or misleading. Have each student display an example and explain to the class what he or she thinks is deceptive about the advertisement.

Rights and Responsibilities

Prepare a bulletin board display illustrating the rights and responsibilities of consumers. Have the students draw pictures to illustrate each right and each responsibility.

Agencies that Help Consumers

Divide the class into groups and have each research a particular government or private agency that works to help the consumer. Each group should prepare a bulletin board display that illustrates and explains the functions of one particular agency.

Not All Doctors Are the Same

Divide the class into small groups and have each research the work of a particular kind of medical doctor. Include general practitioners, gynecologists, pediatricians, dermatologists, psychiatrists, and so on. Let each group prepare a bulletin board display explaining the services offered by each kind of medical doctor.

OTHER IDEAS

Listen Carefully

Tape some representative radio or television commercials, using either audio or video tape. Then play them back for the class. First, play the commercial in its entirety, asking the children to listen or watch for any misleading presentation. Then play the commercial again, this time stopping the tape to discuss statements made, such as "Now, more improved than ever," or "America's number one choice." Note that many statements and claims that seem to say something are actually rather meaningless. Singing commercials are among the least informative. There is an old adage on Madison Avenue that states, "If you don't have anything to say, sing it."

Consumer Reports

Older elementary school children can learn about how products and services are evaluated objectively by reading copies of *Consumer Reports* magazine. Get back issues from the public library and discuss the products tested in the articles. Note that this magazine does not carry any advertising. Ask the students why they think the magazine has this policy.

Comparison Shopping

Have the students develop a list of five or six health care products such as toothpaste, deodorant, soap, eye drops, dental floss, and antiseptic cream. Let each student comparison shop for these items and report on which stores in the community sell each brand of product for the best price. This can be done either by visiting stores or by checking prices in newspaper advertisements. You may wish to have the students comparison shop for specific brands that they normally use or you may suggest that the students look for the cheapest and most expensive brand of each type of product. Compare the results in a class discussion.

Packaging

Some of the appeal of a product results from the way it is packaged. Have the students bring in empty packages from various health care products. Discuss the visual appeal of each one. Then have the students design packages of their own for the products. First, they should try to design a package they think would be very appealing to consumers. Then they should try to design a package that would not appeal to consumers. This activity can teach children how packaging design also serves to manipulate consumer behavior.

25. Environmental Health

The chemicals to which life is asked to make its adjustment are no longer merely the calcium and silica and copper and all the rest of the minerals washed out of the rocks and carried in rivers to the sea; they are synthetic creations of man's inventive mind, brewed in his laboratories, and having no counterparts in nature.

To adjust to these chemicals would require time on the scale that is nature's; it would require not merely the years of a man's life but the life of generations . . . almost five hundred [chemicals] annually find their way into actual use in the United States alone. The figure is staggering and its implications are not easily grasped—500 new chemicals to which the bodies of men and animals are required somehow to adapt each year, chemicals totally outside the limits of biologic experience.
—Rachel Carson, *Silent Spring*

HUMAN IMPACT UPON THE ENVIRONMENT

Maintaining personal health is largely an individual responsibility. Yet none of us lives in a vacuum. We are all subject to the influences of our environment. Thus a person may attempt to exercise the most positive of personal health behavior and still be subjected to health hazards in the form of contaminated drinking water, polluted air, and urban-caused stress factors, such as noise and overcrowded living conditions. Clearly, our environment has an impact on health.

Human beings are the dominant species on earth because of our power to control, manipulate, and alter our surroundings. To a large extent, we have learned to use the natural resources of the planet for our own benefit. But in doing so, we have also created a host of environmental problems. For a long time, many of these problems went unrecognized. However, with the growth of technology and industry the problems became more and more obvious. Even then, many preferred to ignore what was happening to our environment, putting it down to "the price of progress." In any case, there seemed to be no way of correcting many of the problems.

Today, more and more people are becoming aware of the negative impact human activity has had upon the environment. Many of the negative changes that have occurred did not have to happen. Certainly, most do not have to keep getting worse. We can no longer plead ignorance about how our activities affect the world in which we live. We also are increasingly recognizing our responsibility toward protecting the environment and preserving our natural resources for future generations.

Ecology is the study of interactions in the environment. From this study, three basic natural laws have been determined:

1. Every system within nature is connected to every other system.
2. Once created, matter is never destroyed but is recycled in one way or another.
3. Natural resources are finite and nature's capacity to absorb the byproducts of human technology is limited.

The implications of these three laws, separately and together, have great bearing on the health of all people and the state of the environment. At first, it may seem that these principles are beyond control of the individual, but this is not so. Each of us has a responsibility both to understand the laws of ecology and to realize that as individuals what we do affects the operation of these laws. This is the most important single concept in the teaching of environmental health education.

Children must become aware that they are part of the overall ecosystem of our planet and as intelligent members of that ecosystem have both rights and responsibilities concerning the environment. This is a vital concept that must be stressed.

The basic teaching plan for environmental health involves three main areas: ecosystems and ecology, pollution of the ecosphere, and preservation of the ecosphere. Each of these areas will be discussed in this chapter.

ECOSYSTEMS AND ECOLOGY

Each living thing, whether plant or animal, is part of an immediate ecosystem, or habitat in which the living and nonliving components interact and interrelate. For example, all the organisms in a particular field or pond form an ecosystem. By interacting in a balanced fashion with all other parts of the ecosystem, a given species within that ecosystem can generally continue to thrive while perpetuating its population. This interelationship and interdependence with other animals and plants in the environment produces a web of common sharing of most natural resources, including air, water, territorial space, sunlight, and soil minerals. An example of an ecosystem is shown in figure 25.1. Nonliving natural resources are usually referred to as the physical environment comprising the given ecosystem, while living organisms are referred to as the biotic environment of the ecosystem (Dasman, 1972).

Both environmental components of an ecosystem influence the other. When the physical environment is altered significantly, the biotic environment will be altered significantly, and vice versa. As a result, ecosystems are governed and operate through an interwoven natural organization of cycles between groups within the system so that balance and stabilization of the community are sustained. Yet, balance and stability are dynamic processes, ever changing to adapt to the alterations in these cycles as they themselves are changed by the varying interactions between

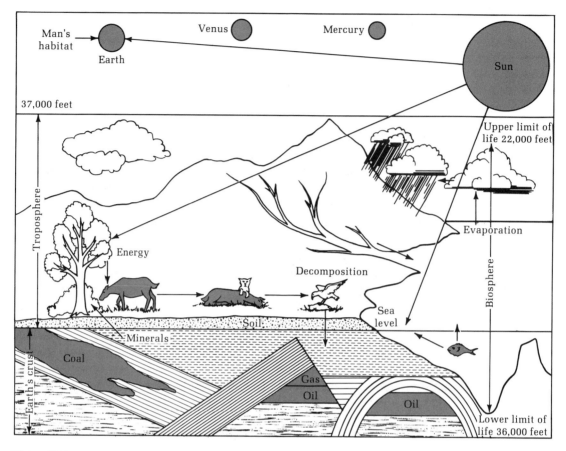

Figure 25.1
An ecosystem and its webs.

Figure by Robin Engle. Copyright © 1970 by the New York Times Company. Reprinted by permission.

the residents of the neighborhood and their use of natural resources. Thus, since ecosystems are inherently unstable, an input of energy is required in order to maintain equilibrium or *homeostasis*. This input of energy produces a closed and self-sustaining cycle whereby chains of interconnections arise. For example, life is nurtured from decomposition within the system, one species feeds off another, and so forth. All resources, by nature's rules, are recycled and continually reused in one form or another since energy is always constant.

In addition, ecosystems are in continuous interaction with one another and are joined by the actions of the various physical and biotic environments to form a total worldwide ecosystem called the *ecosphere* or *biosphere*. The ecosphere, although comprised of divergent, self-sustaining biological communities, is a single entity or system that relies on and shares a common well of natural resources (Odum, 1978).

The human species, unlike any other species, can extensively manipulate both the physical and biotic environments of ecosystems, indirectly affecting the ecosphere as a whole. While many of these alterations in and of themselves are not inherently damaging, the *cumulative* impact on the ecosphere has taken its toll and the natural recycling mechanisms have sometimes been overwhelmed. Ecologists have pleaded for all of us to develop a greater understanding of the scientific principles that govern ecosystems so that an increased awareness about our impact on the ecosphere will result. Then more of our decisions regarding the ways in which we choose to interact with the environment will be based on knowledge and logic rather than ignorance or greed. Ecologists have also warned of the grave danger facing our entire planet from depletion or pollution of its rich natural resources, which are finite and must be preserved for future generations.

POLLUTION OF THE ECOSPHERE

Pollution is the contamination of the environment that results from an overabundance of substances which render the physical surroundings unfit, unsafe, or unsanitary for use or habitation by the residents of the ecosystem. While pollutants may initially appear to directly affect only a limited or select population within the ecosystem, such as birds and marine life, these substances eventually have an impact on all members of the ecosystem because of the interdependence and interaction between organisms. Human activity is the major cause of environmental pollution, but humans often experience the results of contamination much less quickly than other members of the ecosphere. As a result, although pollution of the environment has been occurring for centuries, only relatively recently has an awareness developed that polluting constitutes self-destructive behavior. The most crucial areas of concern include problems caused by overpopulation, air pollution, water pollution, hazardous chemical pollution, solid waste pollution, radiation pollution, and noise pollution.

Overpopulation

Many environmental health problems arise not so much from misuse of technology but from the sheer numbers of people who exist. There are simply not enough natural resources to support an unlimited human population. Approximately 4.4 billion people live on earth now, and this figure is expected to reach 6 billion by the year 2000—less than 20 years away (Burton, Ramer, Thomas, & Thurber, 1978). This population explosion is a mid-twentieth century phenomenon since the most recent doubling of the world's population took only 50 years to occur. Historically, doubling of the world's population took much longer. It is estimated that the people who lived from the beginning of the world until the 1500s numbered a quarter billion. The half-billion mark was reached approximately 150 years after that, and the billion mark was reached 200 years later, around 1850. Between 1850 and 1925, a period of only 75 years, the figure doubled to two billion. Between 1925 and 1975, just another 50 years, the world population increased to 4 billion (Murdock, 1972). If this trend continues, the time interval taken to double the earth's population will continue to decrease, putting a greater and greater strain on available resources necessary to sustain the human population. In fact, world shortages of food have already been occurring since the population appears to be increasing twice as fast as the food supply. Even with advances in agricultural techniques and a more equitable balancing of food distribution and consumption, some ecologists believe that no relief is in sight. They feel the planet simply cannot support the disproportionate numbers of our species (La Place, 1978). The consequences of uncontrolled world population growth go beyond the issue of food. In addition to hunger, joblessness, environmental devastation, and uncontrolleld urban growth would result. It has been said that overpopulation would heighten global instability and promote authoritarianism (Russell, 1984).

In many countries in the last decade or two, attempts have been made to deal with the problem of overpopulation by means of governmental incentives to limit births. However, ethical and moral controversy surround the issue, which is understandably a very delicate and highly personal one to most individuals. Regardless of the ethical or moral considerations, however, overpopulation is a serious environmental problem that must be addressed—not only by governmental and private agencies but by the schools as well. Information about family planning and parenthood should be provided to junior high and high school students after a foundation about families and population has been provided at the elementary school level. Children need to understand that our planet will soon be unable to house the growing human population if reproduction rates continue at the present rate. While the solutions are not easy and decisions must ultimately be made by each individual, a world perspective should be provided as well. When one realizes that each minute approximately 132 births occur throughout the world and that the United States alone adds 3 million newborn babies each year, it becomes easier to conceptualize overpopulation as a legitimate environmental health problem (Carroll, Miller, & Nash, 1976).

Air Pollution

Human beings, all 4.4 billion of us, need air more desperately than any other material for survival. People can endure drought, famine, and drastic temperature changes, but oxygen deprivation will result in death after only a few minutes. Yet most of us think very little about the air we breathe, what it is composed of, or how as a finite supply it is replenished and kept clean. Almost no oxygen was present in the atmosphere at the earth's creation, but an abundance of carbon dioxide was available for sustaining plant life. Green plants, over an evolutionary period, were responsible for producing oxygen as a waste product of photosynthesis so that today the atmosphere is composed of approximately 80 percent nitrogen and 20 percent oxygen. While plants have been responsible for producing the oxygen humans and other animals need for life, humans have been largely responsible for polluting the atmosphere with a variety of harmful gases and other substances. The result is air pollution, an increasing environmental health problem in the United States and many other nations.

Exposure to high enough concentrations of air pollutants can cause a variety of health problems ranging from sneezing and coughing to labored breathing and death. Those individuals who are most sensitive to air pollution are usually older adults and people who have chronic respiratory or cardiovascular conditions. The chief air pollutants include carbon monoxide and nitrogen oxides, sulfur oxides, hydrocarbons, and particulate matter.

Carbon Monoxide and Nitrogen Oxides.   Carbon monoxide, which accounts for almost half of the total emission of air pollutants, is a colorless, odorless toxic gas whose chief source is the automobile. Because of hemoglobin's greater affinity for carbon monoxide than for oxygen, circulation is adversely affected upon exposure to the gas since the cardiovascular system is taxed more strenuously than normal in order to supply sufficient oxygen to tissue. An environment in which heavy traffic is present provides significant levels of carbon monoxide, and diminished physical and mental functioning can result from long-term exposure. Adverse effects include headaches, nausea and abdominal discomfort, visual impairment, and diminished judgment and motor coordination. According to Insel and Roth (1977, p. 25):

> In a person exposed to an atmosphere containing 80 ppm (parts per million) of carbon monoxide for eight hours, the capacity of the circulatory system to carry oxygen is lessened by about 15 percent. This condition is equal to the loss of more than a pint of blood. And in badly snarled traffic, the carbon monoxide content of the air may approach 400 ppm.

Nitrogen oxides, which account for about 6 percent of air pollutants, are chemically very similar to carbon monoxide, and poisonous nitrogen oxides, such a nitrogen dioxide and nitric acid, produce comparable physiological disturbances in the circulatory system. Nitrogen oxide combines with water vapor in the air to form nitric acid, a brown gas capable of corroding metal and destroying vegetation. As with carbon dioxide, the major emitter of nitric acid is the automobile.

Pollution from automobiles and other internal combustion engines is a major source of air pollution. This source produces most of the man-made carbon monoxide, about one-half the hydrocarbons and nitrogen oxides, and 90 percent of airborne lead in areas in which lead is not used or produced (Regenstein, 1982).

Sulfur Oxides.   Next to carbon monoxide, sulfur oxides are the most abundant air pollutant, accounting for 15 to 20 percent of all air emissions. When sulfur, released from industrial burning of materials like oil, rubber, paper, and especially coal, combines with oxygen in the atmosphere to form sulfur dioxide and sulfur trioxide, a very heavy gas is produced. In turn, sulfur dioxide and sulfur trioxide when combined with moisture form sulfuric acid, an extremely corrosive agent. Exposure to these sulfur compounds results in coughing, wheezing, and eye, nose, and throat irritation (Corman, 1971).

Hydrocarbons.   Although no specific ailments or irritations can be directly attributed to the release of hydrocarbons—compounds comprised of hydrogen and carbon—these substances constitute an important component of smog. They account for 10 percent to 15 percent of all air pollution emissions.

Particulate Matter.   Particulate matter refers to any nongaseous pollutant found in the air, whether liquid or solid. These pollutants include such substances as ash, soot, asbestos, and lead. It is estimated that particulate matter comprises approximately 8 percent of air emissions. Prolonged exposure to these pollutants can cause deterioration of the respiratory tract surfaces, particularly the cilia.

Lead.   Sources of airborne lead are primarily smelters and automobile exhausts. (Unleaded gasoline has eased the problem of automobile exhaust pollution somewhat.) Health hazards from high concentrations of lead include irritability, anemia, convulsions, severe intestinal cramps, loss of consciousness, and kidney and brain damage. Lead enters the body primarily through the respiratory tract and sometimes through the stomach walls. Signs of lead poisoning are behavior problems, anemia, decreased mental functioning, vomiting, and cramps.

Asbestos. In the past, asbestos was widely used in construction and manufacturing, and most exposures occur in occupational settings. Asbestos can cause serious respiratory problems, such as emphysema, and has been implicated in lung cancer.

Toxic substances, the final major source of air pollution, are generally the products of technology and have not been studied extensively. These substances include natural elements such as arsenic and mercury and man-made products such as polyvinyl chlorides, asbestos, and pesticides. Some are highly toxic, causing cancer and death.

Conditions Resulting from Air Pollution

Air pollution causes serious damage in terms of human well-being, property, and plant and animal life. In addition, two air pollution conditions can lead to serious environmental problems. They are acid rain and temperature inversions.

Pollution Damage. In terms of human welfare, air pollution negatively affects such respiratory illnesses as coughs, colds, asthma, pneumonia, and bronchitis, as well as cancer and even heart disease. Animals and plant life can also be severely harmed by air pollution. When pesticides are sprayed by crop dusters, only one-fourth lands on the crop, less than 1 percent may hit the target insects, and the rest drifts miles away. The insecticides kill birds, frogs, and predatory insects. Falcons and eagles have become extinct in some local areas, as a result of pesticide spraying. Herbicides sprayed on forest lands have caused miscarriages, cancer, and birth defects and often wipe out local wildlife as well as pets and livestock. Vegetation may change color or fail to pollinate. Animals grazing on affected land can be contaminated. Finally, our houses, apartments, and public buildings are damaged by air pollution. Buildings become darkened and discolored as a result of air pollution. Public works of art and monuments are damaged from contaminants. Unfortunately, today's high technology produces pollutants faster than the scientific community is able to study their results. These by-products may pose serious health problems that are currently unknown.

Acid Rain. The primary cause of acid rain is the burning of fossil fuels in electric generating plants. The sulfur in fuel is converted to sulfur oxides. If rain, snow, dew, or mist is present, sulfuric and nitric acids are formed. Most of the sulfur pollution originates east of the Mississippi River. Much of the pollution that originates in the United States is deposited in Canada. Throughout the eastern parts of Canada and the United States, acid rain changes soil acidic levels, ruins the eggs of amphibians and fish, and causes lakes and streams to become more acidic. As the water becomes more acidic, life begins to disappear from the water, thus disrupting the ecosystem and eventually affecting all of our lives.

Temperature Inversions. When a warm air mass moves over cooler air near the ground, a temperature inversion results. The cooler air cannot be dissipated. Temperature inversions decrease visibility and allow a buildup of pollutants, making the air unsafe for breathing. The pollutants are trapped and subjected to the acting of sunlight and produce other pollutants, such as ozone. The temperature inversion eventually disperses, but illness and even death have resulted from this condition.

Water Pollution

Like air, water is essential to life. Despite its importance, we dump everything from animal fertilizer and detergents to industrial wastes and sewage into our precious water supply. In addition, when pollutants are channeled into nonflowing bodies of water, such as lakes, *eutrophication,* or accelerated growth of algae, occurs. As algae growth skyrockets on a diet of inorganic pollutants, especially nitrogen and phosphorous, a blanket of slime covers the water. Eventual death of the algae results in bacterial decomposition that consumes the oxygen present. This oxygen deficit kills off fish and other lake inhabitants, many of which are valuable as food resources. Eventually, the body of water becomes contaminated beyond use. Even flowing bodies of water, such as streams and rivers, that undergo natural purification can be badly polluted if sufficient amounts of wastes are dumped.

There are numerous sources of water pollution. The main ones are industrial wastes, animal fertilizers, human sewage, and thermal pollution.

Industrial Wastes. Chemical byproducts from the manufacture of paper, steel, oil, pesticides, and the like account for more than half of the water pollution in this country. Despite water pollution laws, an abundance of diverse industrial wastes continues to be disposed of in lakes, streams, and rivers throughout the country. Many, like lead and mercury, are known to be toxic to humans. Of great concern regarding the danger of any industrial waste product is the length of time it takes to be broken down by the environment and the amount of concentration that is tolerable by given organisms, particularly humans.

Animal Fertilizers. Agriculture is one of the major sources of water pollution. Fertilizers, about 25 percent of which run off the soil and form silt beds in surrounding waterways, act as nutrients for bacteria, protozoa, and algae (Carroll, Miller, & Nash, 1976). Many animal fertilizers are particularly rich in nitrogen, thus adding to the problem of eutrophication and oxygen depletion of bodies of water.

Human Sewage. Although contamination of water from human waste is much less serious than it once was, it nevertheless can occur in varying degrees if a community's sewage treatment system is antiquated or not inspected regularly. It is recommended that sewage treatment consist of two stages: primary and secondary. The primary stage rids the water, which has been allowed to settle in a holding tank, of large objects through a filtration process of passing the liquid over a series of screens. During the secondary stage of treatment, smaller particles of organic material and microbes are removed through additional filtration techniques, dispersement over beds of stone, and chemical purification. The final step usually involves the addition of chlorine in order to disinfect the water of any remaining bacteria in order for it to be safe for recycling.

Thermal Pollution. Numerous industries, including those involved in generating nuclear power, use water as a coolant for their equipment. Water absorbs heat from the equipment and is channeled back to its source where it produces a rise in temperature of the source water itself. While this process seems harmless enough, the warmer water is, the less oxygen it will absorb, and the less oxygen absorbed, the less quickly the lake or river decomposes its organic material. Since power-generating plants in particular heat large volumnes of water, the parent waterway is certainly at risk. In addition, much of the aquatic life is drastically affected by extreme temperature variation from the norm.

The Effects of Water Pollution

Polluted water can be responsible for transmitting many pathogens. For example, typhoid fever, dysentery, cholera, and parasitic worms are just a few of the diseases that can be transmitted through polluted water. Viruses from human wastes carried in contaminated water can cause hepatitis. Bacteria found in polluted water can cause intestinal disorders. Other materials found in polluted water, such as asbestos fibers, can cause cancer.

Polluted water can be particularly harmful to fish, birds, and animals. For example, herbicides, phosphates, fertilizers, sewage, and industrial wastes kill numerous fish and birds. These products also promote the growth of algae, which changes the ecological balance. These same products produce odors and foul-tasting drinking water. In addition, fish may be affected by rising water temperature, which retards their reproduction, destroys their food supplies, or kills them.

The oil slicks of recent years have been widely publicized. The devastation to birds and fish has been apparent. The oil coats the gills of fish, thus killing them. Feathers of birds are coated so that they cannot fly. Oil-covered beaches are also expensive to clean, and the public loses recreational areas.

Hazardous Chemical Pollution

The hazardous chemicals that pollute our environment are numerous and varied. They include not only the toxins deposited in our air and waterways but also the pesticides sprayed on crops, the chemicals transported along our railways and highways for use in industry, and those contained in commonly used household products.

Pesticides. With the 1962 publication of Rachel Carson's *Silent Spring*, people began to become more conscious of the hazards of pesticides, toxic chemicals used to kill insects and other pests that destroy crops. In past decades, the harm caused by the widespread use of chlorinated hydrocarbons like aldrin, dieldrin, and DDT (dichlorodiphenyltrichloroethane) as pesticides was not fully recognized. These chemicals are particularly dangerous not only because they are toxic, but also because they accumulate in human tissue since they are fat-soluble. Traces of DDT are said to exist in all Americans. After these facts were discovered, DDT came under strict federal control in 1973 (Murdock, 1972). Chlorinated hydrocarbons decompose very slowly and remain toxic to a wide variety of animal life for long periods. Organophosphorous pesticides like diazinon, parathion, and malathion exhibit similar properties and are even more poisonous than the chlorinated hydrocarbons.

Although worldwide food production needs to be increased to meet the demands of a growing population, extensive use of pesticides can cause great harm to environmental health in the process. Questions still need to be answered concerning the implication of long-term exposure to moderate or even minimal levels of pesticides. There is evidence that these chemicals can damage the human reproductive and nervous systems, for example. It is obvious, therefore, that the use of pesticides must be limited and controlled in order to protect all inhabitants of our ecosphere.

Industrial Chemicals. One of the newer and most dangerous environmental threats is the transportation of industrial chemicals from state to state and from country to country. While transportation itself is not inherently deleterious, leakage or spills of chemical substances most certainly is. In fact, hardly a week goes by without news of such an accident that causes disability or death. Additionally, accidents involving the transportation of oil and other petroleum products have resulted in several major oil spills that have damaged some of our nation's most beautiful beaches and killed or endangered countless birds and marine life. Nearly 10 million tons of oil each year are accidently released into oceans all over the world (Huxley, 1974).

In response to this increasingly dangerous threat, many state governments as well as the federal government have formed special subcommittees to study the problem of transportation of industrial chemicals. Particularly in regard to the movement of radioactive material across states for industrial and burial purposes, many states have indicated an unwillingness to continue to allow such toxins to be brought in. More controls and safeguards need to be implemented in transporting hazardous chemicals of any kind, whether by trucks, ships, or trains.

Household Products.   Before the recent ban on spray cans containing propellant fluorocarbons and detergents containing phosphates, numerous household products served as contaminators of the environment by releasing these agents into the air and water, respectively. Fluorocarbons destroy the protective ozone layer of the atmosphere that shields us from damaging ultraviolet rays of the sun, while phosphates serve as excellent nutrients for bacteria, protozoa, and algae, promoting eutrophication of lakes, streams, and rivers. These examples serve as an excellent illustration of the dangers involved in releasing seemingly harmless compounds into our surroundings from heavily used household products like cleansers, polishes, waxes, and sprays of all kinds without first studying their environmental impact before marketing them.

Solid Waste Pollution

Today, we use more and more "convenience" products that are easily disposed of and replaced. Everything from disposable diapers, dishes, and food containers to plastic wraps, sanitary products, and paper napkins are available. The price of this convenience has been the growing problem of solid waste disposal. The unsightly junkyards, dumps, and scattered litter that dot our land are more than just an eyesore. They are a public health hazard as well.

Currently it is estimated that an excess of six pounds of solid waste is collected each day for each person living in the United States (Sittig, 1969). Many of these solid waste materials are not biodegradable and remain in the environment for long periods of time because they do not decay or cannot be burned easily. The piles of refuse serve as excellent breeding grounds for microorganisms, rats, insects, and other disease carriers. In addition, agricultural waste products from orchards, feedlots, and farms add significantly to the total solid waste that must be disposed of each year.

As our country becomes more heavily populated, more garbage is produced but less and less land is availabale for dump sites. In 1976, the Department of Health, Education and Welfare, reported that 94 percent of the disposal sites in this country were not acceptable (League of Women Voters, 1976). How then do we rid ourselves of all our refuse? Current methods primarily used include dumps, sanitary landfills, recycling, and incineration.

Dumps. Well over three-fourths of all the accumulated solid waste in this country is deposited in open, minimally managed dumping grounds where it is either left to decay, be transported by wind and weather, or eaten by scavenger animals (Carroll, Miller, & Nash, 1976). Some burning of garbage does take place in order to condense the material. Besides being extremely unsightly, open dumping grounds can pose a serious threat to a community's health if the insect or rodent population gets out of control. The widespread use of dumps results from the short-term cheapness of this method of solid waste disposal.

Sanitary Landfills. Unlike the procedures of open disposal in a dump, those in a sanitary landfill require that the solid waste be covered by dirt each day after it has been compacted. Once covered with dirt, the landfill is bulldozed in order to smooth out and compress the area. A properly operated sanitary landfill requires predetermined designing and engineering of the site as well as continued daily maintenance from a crew of workers within a city sanitation department. However, the benefits of a well-functioning landfill can be numerous. Because refuse is covered daily, risk of a contaminated water supply or of disease due to the breeding of flies, mosquitoes, rats, and the like is diminished considerably. Since burning is not necessary, the technique does not contribute to air pollution. In addition, after the location has been completely filled in, it can serve some other valuable purpose, such as a site for housing, recreation, or industry.

There are problems, nevertheless, associated with the use of sanitary landfills. Land itself is becoming more scarce and more expensive, not all types of terrain are suitable to serve as landfills, and the surrounding water table must be low enough. In addition, residents are often opposed to the establishment of a sanitary landfill nearby for fear that it will lower property values.

Recycling. Many products can be *recycled,* or reused in another mode. For example, paper, glass, and metal products can all be recycled. This method of solid waste control gained some popularity during the environmentally conscious era of the late 1960s and early 1970s. It is less in vogue today because waste materials must be sorted to recycle them. However, due to potential shortages as well as the need to decrease the volume of solid waste, recycling will likely gain a renewed foothold in the American lifestyle.

Incineration. Like dumping, incineration is a very old method of waste disposal that adds to environmental pollution because of the release of particular matter into the atmosphere during burning. Of particular danger is the release of hydrogen chloride from burning plastic materials, which are mainly composed of polyvinyl chloride. Upon contact with moisture in the air, hydrogen chloride forms hydrochloric acid, an especially corrosive agent that causes respiratory irritation.

However, the energy and heat produced as a byproduct of incineration can be used in homes and industry. Incineration of solid wastes has been employed successfully for this purpose in many locations throughout Europe and is now being used in the U.S. To accomplish this in the United States, many incinerators would have to be redesigned and rebuilt. As it stands, incineration is already one of the more costly waste disposal methods. Nevertheless, incineration as a generator of energy deserves more investigation.

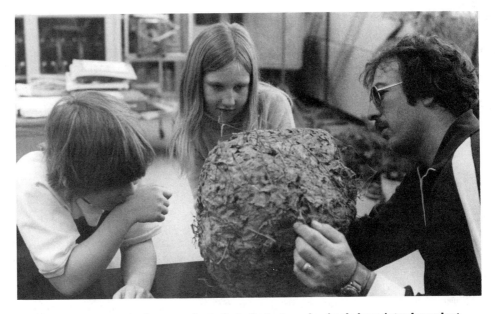

It is important to emphasize to students that all plants and animals have interdependent functions in our environment.

Radiation Pollution

Individuals are exposed to radiation daily both from natural sources, such as sunlight, and manmade sources. The manmade sources of radiation are of most concern. Radioactive materials release energy in the form of a stream of particles generally referred to as radiation. Alpha and beta radioactive particles do not easily penetrate the human body, but gamma radiation does. Gamma rays are much like X-rays. If an individual is exposed to a high enough dosage of gamma radiation, several adverse effects occur, ranging from nausea, hair loss, and diarrhea to cell mutation, anemia, and death.

In the United States, individuals come into contact with radiation mainly through medical testing and X-rays. Although X-rays are generally "safe," many instances of unnecessary exposure have been reported. Several month intervals should elapse before undergoing continued exposure to X-rays. Pregnant women, particularly during the first trimester, should avoid being X-rayed if at all possible because radiation can cause cell damage and mutation to the developing fetus.

Exposure to low-level radiation for a prolonged period is also of great concern for individuals whose work surroundings or home environment may be near a radioactive source. Research with military personnel exposed to radioactive fallout or people living near nuclear testing sites indicates that such individuals may be at greater risk in developing skeletal abnormalities, various types of cancer, and visual impairments. Research also suggests that the reproductive organs may be adversely affected by long-term exposure to low-level radiation (Odum, 1978). As a result, opponents to the use of nuclear power as an energy source are becoming more vocal. They fear both the potential for a nuclear accident like that which occurred at Three Mile Island in Pennsylvania in March 1979 and at the Chernobyl plant in the Soviet Union in April 1986, and the dangers of mishandling the disposal of nuclear wastes. On the other hand, supporters of nuclear power believe that through the implementation of the Nuclear Regulatory Commission's guidelines, nuclear power can be a safe, viable, and much needed energy source for the future.

Noise Pollution

With more and more of the American people living in metropolitan areas, the problem of noise as a pollutant is also growing. Noise pollution is a problem for almost every urban dweller, and a particular cause of concern among people living near airports, employees working in manufacturing or industry, and commuters who must endure hours of noise each week traveling in cars, trains, buses, and subways.

Noise levels are calculated in decibels (db), a logarithmic measurement for which 1 db represents the minimum level of hearing for humans. A sound that is 10 times as loud would be 10 db, another 100 times as loud would be 20 db, one 1000 times as loud would be 30 db, and so forth. Some typical noise levels include respiration (10 db) whispering (30 db), talking (60 db), automobile passing by (70 db) and airplane overhead (100 db). Temporary hearing impairment may result from even limited exposure to a loud noise source 80 db and above, while permanent hearing loss can result from lengthy or chronic exposure. High frequency hearing loss in particular seems to be affected. Sounds below 75 db appear relatively safe to the human ear, regardless of duration of exposure (Krier & Ursin, 1977).

Many detrimental effects apart from hearing impairment can occur due to noise because of its stressful nature. Headaches, difficulty in sleeping, increase in anxiety, and elevated blood pressure are just a few. As a result, increased efforts must be made toward minimizing noise pollution.

PRESERVATION OF THE ECOSPHERE

Conservation and protection of our natural resources must stem from both individual and public action. Both are needed to stabilize and eventually reverse the deleterious cycle of contamination that currently plagues the ecosphere. Legislation and implementation of healthier environmental practices have been instituted. The enactment of additional measures could serve to improve the quality of living for us and for future generations.

Population Control

The problems resulting from overpopulation are well recognized in such countries as China and India, where governmental incentives have been established to limit childbearing. Prior to the availability of the condom and the diaphragm in the nineteenth century, birth control methods were generally unsafe and did not enjoy widespread use. However, particularly with the introduction to the general public of the birth control pill and the intrauterine device (IUD) in the 1960s as well as improved female sterilization and male vasectomy techniques introduced in the 1970s, birth control has become more accepted throughout the world. In addition, dissemination of information about contraceptive methods has been increased to include preteens, teenagers, young adults, and older adults alike. Although some individuals and groups believe instruction about birth control is ill-advised in a school setting, many school systems nevertheless have incorporated such instruction into the curriculum. The establishment of various kinds of family planning services throughout the United States and in many other nations has also aided in increasing contraceptive education.

In the United States, population growth has stabilized. The average age for marriage has increased and many young couples delay parenthood in order to advance educationally or professionally. In Third World countries, where population control is more of a problem, efforts must be made to provide the same kind of education and services that are offered in the more technologically advanced nations. It must be recognized, however, that decisions about pregnancy are deeply personal, cultural, religious, and social in nature and should be based on free choice.

Air Pollution Control

On December 17, 1963, President Lyndon Johnson placed his signature on Public Law 88-206, the first federal Clean Air Act. He signed an additional piece of legislation on October 20, 1965 that as Public Law 89-272 gave the federal government even more influence in controlling air pollution. Then the Surgeon General of the United States, Dr. William Steward, as administrator of the Public Health Service, directed the first National Conference on Air Pollution in Washington, D.C. in December 1966. This landmark meeting sparked the 1970 passage of another amended Clean Air Act that mandated all states to submit a plan for achieving the act's air quality standards by January 31, 1972 to the Environmental Protection Agency (EPA), the federal environmental watchdog agency (Bernarde, 1973).

In addition, in 1976 the EPA set specific guidelines regarding reduction in the levels of carbon monoxide emitted from automobiles. One regulation required newly manufactured vehicles to be equipped with catalytic converters, which limit exhaust emissions although they also lower fuel mileage (Krier & Ursin, 1977). These measures have helped to control air pollution. However, the development of cleaner and more efficient source of fuel and energy would have a far greater impact.

Water Quality Control

Although federal controls regarding water pollution have not been as extensive as those for air pollution, the enactment of the Federal Water Pollution Control Act in 1973 was conceived as a means of developing a national system that would require any institution, industry, or company that discharges substances into waterways to meet EPA standards. Financial assistance from the federal government is available but enforcement of the law is a state responsibility (Krenkel & Novotny, 1980). In addition, recognition of the dangers of phosphates, nitrogen compounds, mercury, and lead and their subsequent removal from many industrial and household products have alleviated the water pollution problem somewhat. Further measures to improve water treatment techniques and to update, expand, and redesign city sewage treatment plants could also assist in preserving water quality.

Hazardous Chemical Control

With governmental regulation of DDT in 1973, national attention was focused on the dangers of pesticides in general. As a result, more sensible approaches to crop spraying have evolved. Nonetheless, the widespread use of pesticides still poses a danger to environmental health.

The control of transportation of hazardous chemicals has not yet been widely recognized as an issue of national concern, probably due to the fact that it is the newest environmental danger to surface. Even though uniform guidelines have not been established to control the type and amount of chemicals and the means by which they can be transported, the Disaster Relief Act of 1974 (Public Law 92-288) provides various types of assistance to victims of disaster, chemical spills included (Brownstone, 1977). This act could be strengthened by the inclusion of amendments that address the control and prevention issue rather than limiting concern to after-the-fact situations.

Solid Waste Control

Between 1966 and 1969, the Department of Health, Education, and Welfare was authorized to use more than $92 million at federal, state, and local levels for research in solid waste development, project and demonstration sites, and technique examination. This was made possible by the passage of the Solid Waste Disposal Act, Public Law 89-272, signed on October 20, 1965 by President Johnson (Hagerty, Pavoni, & Heer, 1973). As a result, advances have been made in ridding the environment of refuse in a healthier fashion. However, the majority of solid waste disposal measures still include either open dumps or inadequately designed or supervised sanitary landfills. Thus the United States, like many other nations, is still struggling with the problem. Until citizens recognize that many solid waste disposal programs are ineffective or unacceptabale the situation is unlikely to change. More public awareness and action are needed to draw attention to the problem of solid waste disposal. In addition, individual efforts toward decreasing the daily use of disposal products that are not easily biodegradable as well as efforts aimed at recycling can assist greatly.

Radiation Exposure Control

Guidelines exist that indicate allowable ranges of radiation exposure from medical testing, X-rays, and consumer products emitting small amounts of radiation, such as television sets. However, the long-term effects upon health of even low or "safe" levels of radiation are still poorly understood. Any radiation at all may in fact be deleterious to health. Certainly as individuals we must become more educated and aware of both the benefits and dangers of using radiation and nuclear power.

Noise Pollution Control

No uniform standards regarding acceptable noise levels for school, home, or work environments have been formulated. Therefore each individual must exercise personal judgment in deciding how much noise exposure is not only tolerable but safe. Employees in industry are, of course, issued protective ear devices, but the general public is not guaranteed the same protection on noisy highways or in neighborhoods near loud noise sources. Greater awareness of the harmful effects of noise, both physical and psychological, may lead to public action and legislation in the years ahead.

SUMMARY

All the individual efforts undertaken to maintain and promote personal health, no matter how responsibly and diligently they are enacted, cannot ensure high level wellness unless the environment in which one lives is free of dangerous levels of pollutants and therefore conducive to quality living—not just mere survival. In order to maintain the natural resources upon which all living things depend, it is essential that we understand how we interact with and influence our ecosystem, our immediate habitat.

Many manmade changes have caused havoc in the natural ecological chains or webs within ecosystems. Because ecosystems, like the residents within them, are interdependent and thus form one worldwide ecosphere, the deleterious impact of human growth and technology is felt through the entire planet. In sheer numbers alone, our species is stretching the capacity of land, water, and food supplies to accommodate us. In addition, particularly in the highly industrial nations, human lifestyles have resulted in an abundance of pollution problems that cannot be dealt with by the natural cycles within the ecosphere. With our automobiles, we release dangerous pollutants into the air. Industry adds still other toxins. Runoff from agriculture and industrial dumping contaminate our water. In addition, hardly a week goes by without some incident involving the accidental leakage or spilling of highly lethal substances being transported.

These environmental health problems, coupled with those of solid waste disposal, radiation exposure, and noise pollution, have resulted in ecological crises never before witnessed. Yet, through continued research and education, which will spark responsible action on the part of both governments and individuals, preservation of the ecosphere is possible. It is our job as educators to provide instructional and consciousness-raising experiences to the children we teach so that their children and grandchildren will enjoy continued health and well-being in a sound environment.

DISCUSSION QUESTIONS

1. Define and differentiate between the terms *environment* and *ecology.*
2. Identify three basic laws of ecology and tell how each affects the state of the environment.

3. What is the ecosphere and how do human beings interact with elements of the ecosphere?

4. What impact does overpopulation have upon the state of the environment and what problems directly or indirectly stem from overpopulation?

5. What are the major sources of air pollution? Describe the harmful effects of specific air pollutants upon human health.

6. Why are pesticides a particularly dangerous form of pollution?

7. What steps can be taken to more effectively manage and control solid waste?

8. What threats to environmental health does the transportation of hazardous substances pose?

9. What is noise pollution? How does it affect environmental health?

10. How can each individual help to preserve the ecosphere? Give specific suggestions.

REFERENCES

Bernarde, M. *Our precarious habitat.* New York: W. W. Norton, 1973.

Brownstone, J. et al. Disaster relief training and mental health. *Hospital and Community Psychiatry, 28:* 1, 1977.

Burton, R., Ramer, B., Thomas, M., & Thurber, S. *Key issues in health.* New York: Harcourt Brace Jovanovich, 1978.

Canby, T. "Our most precious resource," *National Geographic 158,* August 1980.

Carroll, C., Miller, D., & Nash, J. *Health: The science of human adaptation.* Dubuque, Iowa: Wm. C. Brown, 1976.

Corman, R. *Air pollution primer.* New York: National Tuberculosis and Respiratory Disease Association, 1971.

Dasman, R. *Planet in peril.* New York: World Publishing, 1972.

Hagerty, D., Pavoni, J., & Heer, J. *Solid waste management.* New York: Van Nostrand Reinhold, 1973.

Huxley, J. *Man, nature, and ecology.* Garden City, N.Y.: Doubleday, 1974.

Insel, P. & Roth, W. *Core concepts: Health in a changing society.* Palo Alto, Calif.: Mayfield, 1977.

Krenkel, P. & Novotny, V. *Water quality management.* New York: Academic Press, 1980.

Krier, J. & Ursin, E. *Pollution and policy.* Berkeley: University of California Press, 1977.

La Place, J. *Health.* Englewood Cliffs, N.J.: Prentice-Hall, 1978.

League of Women Voters of the United States. *Solid waste—It won't go away.* Publication 675, Washington, D.C., 1976.

Murdock, W. (Ed.) *Environment: Resources, pollution, and society.* Stamford, Conn.: Sinauer Associates, 1972.

Odum, E. *Fundamentals of ecology.* Philadelphia: W. B. Saunders, 1978.

Regenstein, L. *America the poisoned.* Washington, D.C.: Acropolis Books, 1982.

Russell, G. "People, people, people." *Time, 124,* August 6, 1984.

Sittig, M. *Water pollution control and solid waste disposal.* Park Ridge, N.J.: Noyes Development, 1969.

Stoler, P. "Pulling the nuclear plug." *Time 123,* February 13, 1984.

26. Techniques for Teaching Environmental Health

Although the works of nature are innumerable and all different, the result or expression of them is similar and single. Nature is a sea of forms radically alike and even unique. A leaf, a sunbeam, a landscape, the ocean, make an analogous impression on the mind. What is common to them all . . . is beauty.—Ralph Waldo Emerson, *Nature*

FOSTERING ENVIRONMENTAL APPRECIATION

Every species of plant and animal has had to adapt to its environment or face extinction. This adaptation has resulted in an amazing variety of life forms on the planet. Thick-skinned cacti have adapted to the harsh environment of our deserts. Self-luminescent fish live successfully in the perpetual darkness of the ocean depths. Polar bears carry on their life cycles in the frozen landscape beyond the Arctic Circle.

Human beings have also had to adapt to the physical environment. But unlike any other form of life on the planet, human beings can also extensively adapt the environment to suit their needs. We build cities, dam rivers, mine the earth, and farm the land. To a large extent, we can manipulate and control our environment. This unique ability has sometimes resulted in the misconception that we are the masters of our environment. This has led to abuse of natural resources and consequent pollution, waste, and lowering of environmental quality.

In the last few decades, we have become more aware that human beings are not free to alter the environment without paying a price. We have recognized that we are part of a worldwide ecosystem, interacting and interrelating with every other part.

This increased environmental awareness has not come too soon. We now know all too well that nature's resources are finite and must be conserved and used wisely. We have begun to see that change to any part of the environment can have wide-ranging impact on many other parts. Failure to understand the consequences could mean disaster not only for ourselves but for the entire planet.

Children need to learn about the importance of healthy environment. They must recognize that it is up to each of us to maintain the environment. By doing so, high level wellness will be more easily fostered. Instruction about environmental health should build a sense of appreciation for all life and natural resources and encourage personal practices that will help to ensure the continued preservation of the ecosphere. The suggested activities in this chapter will help you attain this goal for your students.

Concepts to be Taught

- High levels of personal wellness can only be sustained if the environment is conducive to well-being.

- All the animals, plants, and natural resources in any particular habitat form a self-sustaining ecosystem.

- All parts of an ecosystem are interdependent.

- Each ecosystem is linked to all other ecosystems to form a global network called an ecosphere. Thus change in one ecosystem has the potential to affect any other ecosystem and the ecosphere as a whole.

- Because human beings have the ability to alter and manipulate the environment, human activities have the greatest impact on ecosystems.

- Human activities have caused extensive harm to the environment, which has affected environmental health.

- The major sources of pollution are air impurities, water contaminants, hazardous chemicals, solid waste, radiation, and noise.

- Overpopulation has also resulted in environmental problems.

- Conservation of natural resources, preservation of ecosystems, and protection of the environment from pollution are essential for preserving the ecosphere.

- Preservation of the ecosphere must stem both from individual and public action.

Cycle Plan for Teaching Topics

Topic	Grade Level						
	K	1	2	3	4	5	6
Ecosystems and the Ecosphere	*	*	**	**	*	***	***
Air Pollution	*	*	**	**	***	**	*
Water Pollution	*	*	**	**	**	***	**
Hazardous Chemical Pollution	*	*	*	**	*	**	***
Solid Waste Pollution	*	**	*	**	**	**	*
Radiation Pollution	*	*	*	**	*	***	**
Noise Pollution	*	**	*	*	**	**	***
Overpopulation Problems	*	*	*	**	**	***	*
Preservation of the Ecosphere	*	**	**	**	**	**	***

Key: *** = major emphasis, ** = emphasis, * = review.

VALUE-BASED ACTIVITIES

Nature Watch

Group students into threes and place each group in a spot on or near the school premises in as "natural" an environment as possible. Have each group *silently* observe the happenings in the environment for 10 to 15 minutes, particularly those associated with plants and animals. Then have each group discuss their observations. Later, ask the members of the class as a whole to focus on their feelings and attitudes about nature based on this observation experience.

Activities and Their Environmental Effects

Ask each student to list ten hobbies or activities he or she enjoys doing. After listing the activities, students should examine each activity in terms of its effects, if any, on the environment. As a result of this exercise, students will observe the relationship between their behavior and the environment in which they live.

Me and My Surroundings

Ask each student to keep a daily log for a week about his or her perceptions of environmental influences by writing a short paragraph that describes each day in terms of environmental awareness. Students should emphasize not only facts but also feelings about these influences. For example, "Heavy rain against my window last night sounded nice. The noisy and crowded school bus made me feel irritable." At the end of the week, divide the class into small discussion groups, each one representing one day of the week. Have groups compare their logs for that day and summarize major perceptions about surroundings. One group member should then present a five-minute report to the class outlining summary findings.

Environmental Stories

Select a colorful, eye-catching, and appropriate picture depicting an aspect of the environment. Have each student write a story about the picture. Allow about 20 minutes and encourage both creativity and the exploration of values. Several volunteers may want to read their stories to the class.

Resource Reduction

Divide the class into small groups and assign each group a common environmental product or resource, such as paper, plastic, water, electricity, or natural gas. For a few days, ask each group member to keep a daily list of his or her specific uses of the resource. Then have group members compare lists and prepare a master list on wall-size sheets of paper outlining the most typically used products, frequency or most common uses, amount students think has been used by the total group, and ways to reduce the use. Tack the master lists to the wall. Lists might look something like this:

Product	Frequency	Amount	Ways to reduce
Paper napkins	Every day—at every meal	120	Use cloth napkins
Facial tissues	Rarely—used only by members who had colds	1½ boxes	Use handkerchief
Toilet paper	Every day	6 rolls	None
Notebook paper	Every school day	200 sheets	Write on both sides Don't doodle Use scratch paper completely

Environmental Newswatch and Commentary

Divide students into small groups. Provide each student with three sheets of colored construction paper and ask students to paste a newspaper or magazine article on each sheet that deals with an environmental topic. Use of newsletters, supplementary magazines, and books that are written for the students' grade level should be encouraged. Underneath each article, have the students write a caption that describes the "moral" or "lesson" of the article. Have each group then compile their articles into a booklet. Similar articles should be grouped within the booklets.

Global Goals

Have students draw a large circle on a sheet of paper. The circle represents the earth and ecosphere. Eight divisions should be made and numbered as shown in figure 26.1.

Ask each student to draw or illustrate his or her ideas in the appropriate section about the following:

1. Most important environmental resource
2. Most abundant environmental resource
3. Most depleted environmental resource
4. Most dangerous environmental threat to the world
5. Most environmentally helpful family measure practiced

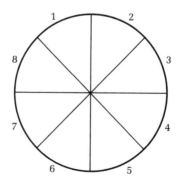

**Figure 26.1
Environmental worksheet.**

6. Least environmentally helpful family measure practiced
7. Most environmentally helpful personal measure practiced
8. Least environmentally helpful personal measure practiced

Let students share their global pictures with each other to compare ideas.

Decision Stories

Present decision stories such as these, using the procedures outlined in chapter 5.

The Fishing Trip

Johnny is going fishing with his grandfather. He is very excited. They have fixed a picnic lunch because they plan to stay all day. Johnny and his grandfather drive to the river. As they walk along the riverside, Johnny notices some dead fish floating in the water. "Grandfather, what killed those fish?" Johnny asks. "They were killed because people put garbage into the river," Grandfather replies. Then they sit down and start to fish. Johnny and his grandfather catch several fish apiece.

Focus Questions: Should they take the fish home and cook them? Why or why not? What can Johnny and his grandfather do to make the river cleaner?

A Bird's Nest

Jim and Richard are good friends who live next door to one another. They are now old enough to walk home from school, and today is their first time to do so. On the way home they cut through a small park. Richard discovers a bird's nest with three eggs in it. He wants to take it home. Jim has been taught to respect living things. He knows it is important not to disturb the natural surroundings, but Richard is such a good friend.

Focus Question: What should Jim do?

Is Recycling Worth the Work?

Kathy has heard about a recycling center in her town. People can bring bottles and aluminum cans there. The material is crushed and then sold to industry to be used again. Kathy tells her mother about the recycling center and asks if the family can bring in their bottles and cans. "It sounds like a good idea," Kathy's mother says. "But it's too much work. We would have to clean and sort all our old bottles and cans. Anyway, the recycling center has enough bottles and cans without us."

Focus Questions: Should Kathy try to convince her mother that recycling is worth the effort? How could she do this?

Bad Air

One day, Sarah's mother comes home from work coughing and wheezing. "What's wrong, Mom?" Sarah asks. "It's all that dirty air I have to breathe riding the bus to and from work," her mother replies. "Maybe you could find a job closer to home," Sarah says. "It's not that easy to find jobs these days," her mother says. "I guess I'll just have to put up with the bad air on the bus."

Focus Questions: Is there anything Sarah can do to help her mother? Who can Sarah contact to find out about lowering air pollution?

DRAMATIZATION

Plants and Animals Need Protection, Too

Divide students into groups and use a story like "Smokey the Bear," "Bambi" or any other suitable example for the specific grade level to trigger students to role play a community of plants and animals who are in danger from an environmental threat. Tell students not only to voice their concerns as the animals and plants, but to also try to decide whether they as plants and animals can do anything to either prevent or diminish the environmental threat.

Home Hunting

Divide the class into small groups. Each group is responsible for describing a home in a neighborhood that is for sale. One or two people in the group act as the sellers, while one or two people act as the buyers. The buyers come to look at the house and ask all sorts of questions, many of which focus on environmental concerns, such as: What is the average monthly heating bill? Cooling bill? How many miles from downtown is the neighborhood? How far away are the schools and shopping centers? Where is the nearest industrial site? Is there much noise in the neighborhood? Give only minimal guidance, such as a few examples of environmentally related questions. Allow each group five minutes for the presentation and keep track of the commonly asked questions. Then summarize by emphasizing the importance of living in a safe, wholesome environment.

Future Lifestyles

Divide students into small groups. Assign each group a different social role. For example, one group could be factory workers, another group business professionals, and a third group small farmers. Ask groups to portray what they think life will be like for their members 50 years in the future, paying particular attention to possible environmental changes and their influences on the surroundings.

City Crisis

Provide the class with a hypothetical dilemma involving a voting question about a proposed city ordinance concerning an environmental issue. Give enough detailed information about the city and its problems so that the viewpoints of various special interest groups can be developed. This may best be accomplished with a descriptive ditto outlining pertinent information about the city. Then divide the class into three groups. Assign two groups the task of presenting a scenario and possible solution to the problem at a town meeting. Let students within each group volunteer to role play identical characters, such as meeting moderator, mayor, union representatives, conservation spokespersons, and so forth. Allow both groups a few days to prepare a 15-minute dramatization. Dramatizations are presented as the third group acts as observers. Following the presentations, the third group then objectively critiques the ideas by highlighting strong points of each presentation and suggesting additional alternatives.

Disaster Preparation Practice

Divide the class into moderate size groups and assign each group to research an environmental disaster that could affect communities, such as an air pollution crisis, train derailment of hazardous chemicals, or a highly toxic pollutant entering municipal water system. Ask each group to dramatize a preparation plan that demonstrates the actions that should be taken or contributions that could be made by various community organizations in dealing with the environmental danger, should it ever occur.

Alien Impressions

Divide the class into groups of about five students. Tell each group that they are aliens from outer space who have suddenly landed in the heart of the city. Ask the groups to act out their reactions to our earthly surroundings, placing special emphasis on impressions about noise levels, traffic, air pollution, crowding, and use of natural resources.

DISCUSSION AND REPORT TECHNIQUES

Environmental Definitions

Depending upon age level, have students either describe or write their own definitions for terms such as the following:

environment	smog
ecosystem	chemical dumping
food chains	noise
ecology	decibel
pollution	conservation
overpopulation	preservation

Ecosystem Explanation

Using the dairy cow as an example of the relationships that exist in an ecosystem, explain with pictures, posters, and diagrams how milk results from grass eaten by cows to produce what we drink. Then ask each student to think of another animal that is part of a food chain and have the students describe the workings of that food chain.

Population Problems

To stimulate discussion about the concerns of overpopulation for very young students, have them recite the nursery rhyme, "There was an old woman who lived in a shoe. She had so many children she knew not what to do." Have students tell you what this rhyme means to them. Older students can be asked to make a graph of the world's population increases since the beginning of recorded time. Note especially the curve for the last 20 years. Then provide further information about the problem of overpopulation and have students discuss suggestions to curb overpopulation.

Hunger Hurts

As a class, have students research information about the impact of hunger on children throughout the world. This may be done by asking the librarian to suggest a few sources that each class member can read. Also have students determine the three leading causes of death among infants and children in America as compared to those of several other countries you select. Be sure to include both European and third world countries. Allow students to discuss their ideas concerning the reason for these differences.

General Pollution Problems

Divide the class into several small groups and assign each group a different major pollution problem. After researching the general aspects of the problem, each group should give a short oral panel presentation. Within the groups, each member is then assigned a specific aspect of the given pollution problem, such as oil spills, effects of sulfides in the air, or the banning of DDT. Have the students prepare individual written reports.

Energy Savings

Have a general class discussion concerning ways Americans can save energy. Discuss how rising costs of fuel have made Americans more energy conscious in recent years. Individual students may wish to volunteer how their families are doing more to save energy.

Individual Research Papers

Suggested topics for individual reports include the following:

Endangered Species	Environmental Protection Agency
The Green Revolution	Misuse of Land by American Pioneers
Zero Population Growth	Results of Atomic Bombs in World War II
Food Chains	Alternative Energy Sources
Dinosaurs	Neighborhoods

EXPERIMENTS AND DEMONSTRATIONS

Animal Adaptations

Collect pictures of various animals and bring them to class. Ask students to identify each animal and describe where it lives (its habitat) and what features the animal has to help it live in its surroundings (color, fur, feeding adaptations, body size). Be sure to incorporate ideas like migration of birds in winter and hibernation of cold-blooded animals. Then ask how humans adapt.

Seasonal Adjustments

Divide students into small groups and ask each group to select a favorite tree or shrub in the school yard to observe once a month for the school year. Let groups record their observations in relation to environmental influences on the changes of the tree or shrub.

Plant Properties

Let students plant several pots of geraniums (or any other flower) and place each pot in a different environment based on temperature. Have students observe changes and make comments after a few weeks. Suggest other controlled experiments along these lines. For example, instead of temperature, the variable can be amount of water, type of soil, or amount of light.

Terrariums and Aquariums as Ecosystems

As a class project, help students make a terrarium and an aquarium. Refer to science texts as resources to help you do this. Use the terrarium and aquarium to demonstrate the interrelationships that exist between residents in each particular ecosystem.

The Water Cycle in Nature

Place water that is almost boiling in a drinking glass and rotate the glass so that the sides are moistened. At an angle on top of the glass, place a Florence flask filled with cold water. Water will evaporate, condense on the cool surface of the flask, and fall in droplets back into the glass. This illustrates evaporation, condensation, and precipitation. Discuss this cycle and relate it to other cycles within the ecosphere.

Air Pollution Around Us

Let each student paste a white sheet of construction paper to posterboard or sturdy cardboard. Ask the students to take the paper home overnight, put petroleum jelly on it, and leave it outside. Particles will collect on the surface. Also put out sheets at several school sites and busy streets as well as more remote areas to compare differences.

How Air Pollutants Travel

Clap two dusty chalkboard erasers together so that students can see the particles of chalk dust traveling through the air and have them note the various places the dust reaches. Relate this to major air pollutants that eventually get carried by air currents to most parts of the world.

Water Impurities

Have each student bring in a small jar of water from a tap at home. Even though the water may all come from the same municipal supply, there will be differences in the samples because of rust or chemical residues in the water pipes in each home. Discuss implications of impurities in drinking water.

Chemicals and Their Effect on Water

Fill several jars with water and place various substances in them such as dirt, polishes, bleach, and cleansers. Let children observe the appearance of each jar and compare it with a jar filled with clean water. Discuss their reactions. As an additional demonstration, obtain several types of laundry detergents and place some of each in a different jar of water. Shake the jars and let students decide which ones are the most polluting (the ones that have the most suds).

Effects of Oil Spills

Pour some grease or oil on a piece of cloth and let students try to remove it with water. Also pour the oil into a jar of water and let them observe what happens. Discuss the results.

Water Purification Demonstration

Use a bottomless bell jar and plug it with a one-hole stopper with a glass tube that fits into the opening. As shown in figure 26.2, layer the jar from the top to the bottom in an inverted position with the following: cotton, clean pebbles, coarse sand (washed), fine sand (washed), charcoal paste, and muddy water. Allow the muddy water to filter through the layers, collect the residue, and observe the results.

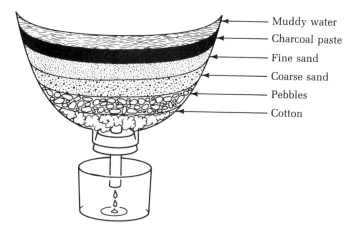

Figure 26.2
Water purification apparatus.

Wasted Water

Help students locate one or several leaky faucets in school. During a one-hour interval, ask them to measure the amount of water leaking out. Let them calculate the amount wasted in one day, one week, one month, and one year. Discuss the importance of conservation.

Crowding Problems

Divide students in groups and give each group two milk cartons with a few holes punched in the bottom for drainage. Ask students to fill each carton about two-thirds full of potting soil and in one carton plant two or three bean seeds about one inch apart and just under the surface of the soil. In the other carton, students should plant 15 seeds about one-half inch apart. Let them water the cartons every four days and record their observations. Discuss the problems of overcrowding as it relates to the use of natural resources. As an extension of this activity, crowd students into a confined space for a few minutes and then ask them to describe how it felt.

Throwaway Blues

As a class project, ask students to collect litter from the school grounds for a few days. Have them dump all litter into large cardboard boxes so that the class can see the amount of solid waste being dumped. Older students may choose to sort litter into two piles: recyclable and non-recyclable.

Noise Levels

Use a decibel meter to check noise levels in varous locations throughout the school. Noise levels will vary during different times of day. Which locations are noisiest? Are there any sources of particularly loud sounds, such as school bus engines? Ask students to suggest ways to diminish noise pollution in their school environment.

Soil Conservation

Take students to an undisturbed, wooded area and let them collect some topsoil in pails. Then have them dig further until they reach the subsoil and can take samples of it as well. Upon returning to class, ask students to observe the differences in the two soil samples. After doing so, plant some seeds or flowers in each sample and check the results in a few weeks.

Explain that topsoil is best for growing plants and demonstrate the concept in the following way. Ask small groups to each collect a sample of grass sod clumps growing in topsoil and a sample of bare topsoil to represent land devoid of trees and plants. Groups should make each sample into a mound and sprinkle water on it to represent rainfall. Ask the students to observe the differences in the two mounds of soil. A similar demonstration can be done to illustrate the effect of wind erosion.

Recyclable Resources

Display the following objects:

notebook paper	rubber stopper
a dime	ladies' nylons
plastic wrap	piece of jewelry
a leaf	cotton ball

Ask each student to identify the natural resource from which each of these objects originated and decide which of the resources are recyclable.

PUZZLES AND GAMES

If I Were, I Could

List names of various plants, animals, and natural resources on separate slips of paper. Go around the room and let each student draw a name and answer "environmentally" within a few seconds. Example: "If I were a *giraffe*, I could *reach the tree-tops for food.*" Students who answer quickly enough get to go through additional rounds.

Food Web

Divide students into two groups and line them up facing each other. Pin the name of a plant or animal on each student. Starting at the head of one line, ask the student to go to a person in the other line who represents a food source for his or her organism. Connect the two with a string. Then go to the next student at the head of the other line and repeat the procedure. Keep going until a great many combinations have been connected.

Food Chain Puzzle

Divide students into small groups. In a sealed packet, provide each group with pictures of plants and animals that can be linked together to form a food chain. At your signal, each group opens the packet, and the first group to arrange their pictures in the correct sequence wins.

Recycling Relay

On opposite ends of the chalkboard, place posterboard labeled "Recyclable" and "Nonrecyclable" respectively. Divide students into two lines and between the lines place a table with pictures of objects. At your signal, the first two challengers reach for a picture, quickly place it accordingly, and then run back to line to tag their next team member, who repeats the procedure. You act as referee. Students who mislabel objects must try again until they are correct. First team to finish wins.

Pollution Word Find

Have students find the following hidden words listed horizontally, vertically, or diagonally.

AIR
ECOSPHERE
ENVIRONMENT
NOISE
POLLUTION
SOLID WASTE

FOOD CHAIN
OVERPOPULATION
RECYCLING
WATER
ECOLOGY
ECOSYSTEM

```
X A S K Q M O E O A N T J H R U D Z V Y R L Y F Z P J G Z U X A
K D L G S U X H B Q H M Z A D M L V S Y Y T S Y W C V Q W A N T
T X J Z Q O F R M H K U J A B H O D V N Z A J Y Z Z F O A I A R
E V E W D Q A T I T K L O H C V V G V V V L W B R R U S C E H F
M N X X S O U Z A P Y L U O P O E T B S H R A J P K M F S D L H
W J G S H Y U V Z B H J E N V I R O N M E N T I O P B R N Y T T
K V Z D B N F T X T C M B A D V P A Z Q R P E X V H L X G I M N
Q O M M N K I X Q O W N P V F D O I V R R I R G Z P Y F G A X B
W K L Y R Y T B M E C L K V P F P H I E X L Z M E K R B C B Q F
F O O D   C H A I N B U C D Z L U A Q D Q O F S Z X E P Q M K B
N A E D Z P E I A G A X T R B M L H J D J E C O S Y S T E M F D
Z A J P M S T R V F E T P P Y N A A A A D G U L D X U Y Z D O F
I W T G X O F G C I V G N N E O T N F Z A N R I C E M B A T K T
G I L N T U R V O U R C H K W L I F U O K G L D H K A N S V H N
K K I R Y Y D Q A U O G Q R S X O D H M F C Q   M W R Y A   L U
A Z B R T Z H C J U Z R P E C T N W Z O L L Z W V I D Y G W K G
X E E J H S D H H V Q W R C J I Q N C W F J J A A G Z N W P E J
L I V E Q N C O B D Z E H N N E J F G V L O I S N Z I Y T Q W D
I F Q Q L S Y N I A H V Q T T X T N L U A J S T Q L Q T G F Y A
D M T P Y G X C U P I S A L B T N S N T W T I E C U N N W E T M
E I M W V J T N S Y K B L A D J P S L E W R Q Y E S I J S K P O
P Z L M Z J B O I U R N A M O S G Y E J O K C G T M A T H G M N
O R B A O D C F V F O F P L K W V I D S J E P D K E G P D R S E
L X C R A E Y F W C M G T S C O J G U Y R I L O T E C O B Y U T
D V C P S U P V H A Y D D O I V E W U R V L B F L V I U S Y U W
R Z V C G J C R I P Z P A A R G C L T V Q T Q Y P L M P T Y G T
A S Z Z S J U G M S C P Y B P H Q V V W L Q G Q S N U P K D K R
H V D E D L O G M U N C N N K X J F V Y A O Z W A D T T D U L Q
T C F Z Q X C B H V Q P R Z B C T Q M Z L S H U O W B M I L P Q
D N O I S E B S D J T W Z N W V B T N O I C P L V D N P S O O X
O K N R O W Q P H J I N R G T E L F C U F U V C C H I H Y S N W
A Z L Z W K G R T L S M M I W L Q E O E Q N Y H G S X V O N O Q
```

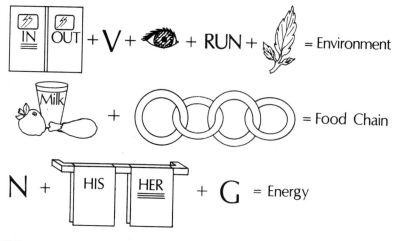

Figure 26.3
Picturegrams.

Pollution Identification

On separate slips of paper write the names of various pollutants or words associated with pollution, such as hydrogen sulfide and DDT. Each student draws a slip of paper and indicates the correct category of pollution, whether it be air, water, noise, or other classification. Make a master list on the chalkboard as words are grouped. For each correct answer, a student gets three points. For each incorrect answer, subtract two points. Play several rounds in order to determine the top scorers.

Master Sentence

Using the sentence here as the master sentence, ask each student to form as many one-word combinations as he or she can in five minutes that refer to environmental health.

> PROTECTION OF THE SURROUNDINGS IS EVERYONE'S RESPONSIBILITY.
> Examples: noise, decibel, ecology, sound, energy, conservation, radiation

Picturegrams

Provide picturegrams such as those shown in figure 26.3 for students to solve. Then have them make similar picturegrams as challenges for their classmates.

BULLETIN BOARDS

Litter Lovelies

Using the litter obtained from the Throwaway Blues activity described earlier, ask the class to make a creative bulletin board display.

Environments

Divide the bulletin board into four or six sections. Group students and ask each group to illustrate a different environment, such as ocean, woodland, desert, prairie, and mountain.

Conservation Is the Key

Have students design a bulletin board display so that "conservation" is written vertically using large letters. The beginning of each letter should serve as the first word for an ecological principle or statement, as in this example.

> Conserve gasoline by combining errands.
> Oxygen is a vital resource made by plants.
> Nature is a delicate balance.
> Save electricity by turning off lights.
> Ecosystems are interdependent.
> Recycle paper, aluminum cans, and glass bottles.
> Vigilant action is necessary to protect our environment.
> All ecosystems are parts of the ecosphere.
> Turn down the thermostat to 68 degrees F.
> Insulate your house for winter weather.
> Overpopulation causes environmental problems.
> Natural resources are finite and expendable.

Other Topics for Bulletin Boards

Have students prepare bulletin board displays with these themes:

> Endangered Animals
> Natural Resources
> Pollution Solutions
> Laws of Ecology

OTHER IDEAS

Commercial Writing

Divide students in small groups of three or four. Ask each group to write an ecological commercial that could be used as a one-minute television or radio commercial. Encourage the use of familiar tunes or jingles. Have the students present their commercials in front of the class.

Poster Contest

Ask each student to make a poster entitled "Energy." Give minimal details about what might be included. Let the students use their creativity. Number each poster anonymously and tack them around the room. Have another class view the posters and select the five best.

Field Trips

Arrange a field trip to a recycling center, the city dump, a power generating plant, or a water treatment plant. Prepare the class for what they will see and have each student develop a list of questions he or she would like to have answered on the field trip.

Preservation Pictures

Provide the students with posterboard and ask each to illustrate one way in which individuals can help preserve the environment.

Survival Lists

Divide students into small groups. Ask each group to prepare two lists. One should include necessary supplies for a family of four to survive on the earth for the next year in the event of a disaster. The other list should include the 20 most important items to take on a trip to outer space. Let groups compare lists and discuss ideas. Try to make a class master list if enough agreement can be reached.

Group Surveys

Divide students into small groups. Ask each group to construct a short survey that they in turn give to their parents, peers, and others. The survey should contain opinion questions about environmental issues. Help in the construction of the survey so that scaled or forced choice responses appear rather than open-ended questions. Allow groups to administer their surveys, collect the opinions, and report the results.

27. Death and Dying

To everything there is a season, and a time to every purpose under the heaven:
A time to be born, and a time to die;
A time to kill, and a time to heal;
A time to break down, and a time to build up;
A time to weep, and a time to laugh;
A time to mourn, and a time to dance.
   —Ecclesiastes 3:1-4

CONSIDERING DEATH

Death is as much a part of human existence, of human growth and development, as birth. Death sets a limit on our time in this world and life culminates in death. Recognizing that death is a natural end to life can have a profound influence on our lives. Our lifestyles can depend on our attitudes toward death. Elizabeth Kubler-Ross (1975) says, "Dying and the time of death is our final chance to grow in this life, to become more truly who you really are, and to become more fully human."

This natural end comes suddenly for some, lingers for others, early in life for some, and very late in life for others, cruelly for some, and peacefully for others. Further, each person responds to her own dying uniquely. It is a natural end to our existence—one that cannot be denied or avoided.

Still, most people fear dying and death. They fear the unknown as well as a fear the process of dying. These feelings are complicated by fears of the possibility of humiliation and pain, and the prospects of separation from loved ones. Dying in our society now is not like it used to be. Rather than dying at home, as was often the case at the turn of the century, many people now die in hospitals surrounded by strangers and machines, with relatives often kept away by restricted visiting hours. As a result, Americans do not share the intimacy of death as they once did. In some ways, they have lost contact with the reality of death.

Much information on death and dying is now available. Many misconceptions and problems concerning issues of death and dying still exist. For example, many physicians and clergy members have had little training in caring for the emotional needs of dying persons and their families. Physicians are trained to cure, but they are lacking in ability to be caring and comforting. Often, they avoid the crucial issues, thereby complicating the dying process. Even today, such courses are conspicuously absent at many of the seminaries and medical schools in our country (Leviton, 1985).

Another problem with death and dying concerns children of elementary school age. Parents often "protect" their children from the trauma of death-related events, thinking they are doing the best thing for the child. However, this treatment tends to propagate fears and misconceptions. For example, children of elementary age tend to regard death as happening only to the old. This is a product of parents telling them not to worry about death until they are older.

In this chapter, we shall examine these and other death-related issues. We shall also look at attitudes toward death, the needs of dying persons and their families, the grief experience, funerals and related rituals, and death education for children.

COMMON ATTITUDES TOWARD DEATH AND DYING

Otherwise mature individuals often find themselves unable to cope with the thought of death. These individuals generally choose to try to ignore death, to pretend on a subconscious level that they are immortal. This attitude is assumed primarily out of a fear of death.

Further, other peoples' deaths remind us of our own vulnerability, causing us to feel totally helpless, as if nothing we can say or do can change a thing.

Many people try to avoid even mentioning death. When it is brought up in conversation, it is usually in the form of a joke. When the subject of personal death, or the death of someone close comes up, there are often looks of dismay and discomfort, until someone changes the subject, much to everyone's relief. When people refer to death, they often use euphemisms that do not imply the finality, totality, and complete separation from life that death is. These euphemisms include "expired," "passed away," "departed," "gone to his rest," and "gone to her great reward." Such phrases make it easier to talk about and think about death, since they soothe the harshness of its reality. The use of euphemisms is an extension of the denial attitude that many Americans take toward death. This denial is carried over to other aspects of death as well. For example, the embalming of a body is requested by many families so the body in the casket will "look alive" and "seem real."

These attitudes toward death can have a profound influence on people's lives. If death is nothing but fear, and if fear prevents people from thinking and acting, they then become less than human. Also, if the fear of death does limit an individual's view of the future, this negative attitude can hinder the person's ability to plan ahead, to anticipate both hazards and opportunities in life.

PERSONAL BELIEFS

Personal beliefs are helpful in coping with the reality of death and dying, whether these beliefs are called ethics, thoughts, meditations, or religion. People rely on personal beliefs to find comfort in the face of death. Some use religious beliefs as an escape, as if to gain personal exemption from the reality of death. However, belonging to any religious group does not guarantee that death will be faced any more positively. Research does appear to show that maintaining a *strong* religious belief system does diminish the fear of death (Kalish, 1985).

In searching for personal answers to questions about death, it is helpful to look at the way in which others respond to it. Even though the problem of death is universal, different cultures and religions respond very differently to the issue. Some people believe we return to dust as we started, that this life is the end of existence, while others believe we continue to exist in some form whether it be reincarnation in a body or in a spirit form. The perception that a personal belief is true, regardless of what that belief is, helps many people cope with the reality of death by demystifying it to some degree.

NEEDS OF A DYING PERSON

Most Americans, when asked how they would want to die, will say they wish to die in a sudden, unexpected way, or in their sleep. In other words, they want to die without knowing what is happening; however, the majority of Americans will die of chronic illnesses.

Those in this situation tend to feel powerless over their own destiny. They begin to realize their own mortality and sense a loss of independence.

Fear is the most typical psychological response that a dying person experiences. Dying persons often fear humiliation—that others will have to care for them when they lose control of their bodily functions. For this reason, self-worth usually suffers. The dying person might also have a sense of failure accompanied by much anxiety. This is partially explained by a loss direction. Having spent a lifetime looking to the future, to something better, the dying person sees that now nothing is out there but death, and that is mysterious and uncertain. Other common fears of the dying are the fear of the unknown (i.e., not knowing what will happen after death), fear of being disfigured, fear of pain, fear of suffocation, a fear of insanity, and a fear of abandonment by friends and relatives (Hamrick, 1986).

In a sense, dying people have no model to follow. They feel like strangers to the healthy living because no one understands either what they are going through or what they are going to face in the near future. Modern medicine has done little to meet the emotional needs of the dying person. As mentioned, many physicians and other helping professionals avoid the issue of death with their dying patients. Yet when studies were made of what terminally ill patients desired to know, a large majority said that they would like to be told of such a diagnosis (Bok, 1980). Dying persons usually know they are dying even though they have not been told. They can interpret the truth from the secrecy, body language, conversation, and avoidance of issues by their visitors and medical staff. Most dying people want to talk about death and their own illness, but unfortunately, sometimes they cannot find anyone willing to discuss these matters.

Adjusting to Dying

Elizabeth Kubler-Ross (1975) has devised a five-stage model describing the process many dying persons go through in coming to terms with their own death. According to Kubler-Ross, the five stages are denial and isolation, anger, bargaining, depression, and acceptance, or resolution. Understanding these stages of adjustment to impending death is critical in understanding the needs of the dying person. It should be noted that the relatives of the dying person also go through these stages of adjustment, as will be discussed later in the chapter.

It should also be noted that there have been some changes in the interpretation of these stages of adjustment since originally presented. Each person is unique in death as in life, and everyone responds differently. Some may progress naturally through these stages while others might reach a latter stage of adjustment, then regress. Further, all dying persons will not reach a stage of acceptance or resolution before they die.

In the first stage, denial and isolation (sometimes referred to as shock), the patient, upon learning of the diagnosis of a terminal condition, reacts with disbelief. This is not surprising, since most people go through their whole lives pretending that they are not going to die. However, the diagnosis or statement brings the reality of one's death to a conscious level, and does so with a tremendous impact. The person reacts by stating that surely the diagnosis is wrong and that recovery is bound to occur. Some individuals, sadly, remain stuck in this stage until they draw their dying breath.

If the first stage of adjustment can be characterized by the statement, "No, not me, I couldn't be dying," then the second stage, anger, can be characterized by "Why me?" During this stage, the reality of impending death is beginning to seep into consciousness. The individual gets angry at the doctors for not having a cure, at the nurses for not providing enough attention, at relatives for isolating, abandoning, or otherwise not meeting the person's needs, and at God for the injustice of impending death.

The third stage, bargaining, can be characterized by "Yes, me, but. . . ." The patient is accepting the fact of death but tries to bargain for more time before actually having to face death. If a holiday or a special occasion, like a wedding, is coming up soon, the person asks God for more time. The person makes a promise, but then rarely keeps that promise, because when the first occasion comes and goes, the person often strikes another bargain with God.

The next stage of adjustment is depression: "Yes, me." The patient is saddened by the fact that death is approaching, and then starts the preparatory grief process for the losses death will bring. This time of adjustment is sometimes very confusing and frustrating for relatives or helping staff because the dying person wants nothing to do with anyone. The individual is taking care of unfinished emotional business and is preparing for the arrival of death.

The stage of depression can lead to the final stage of adjustment, acceptance, or resolution. The person has come to terms, or has resolved, the meaning of death for his own life. If this stage of emotional adjustment is achieved, the person can usually die peacefully.

THE FAMILY OF A DYING PERSON

Impending death affects family members of the dying person in various ways. Sometimes there is a strong prohibition in the family against talk of death because they

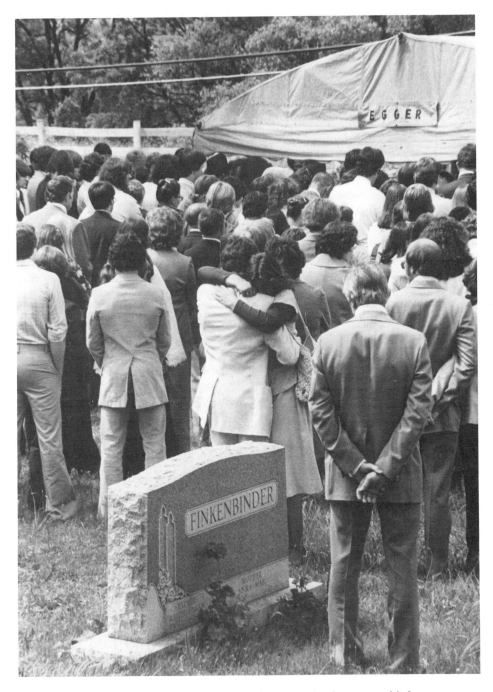

Death is as much a part of human existence, growth, and development as birth.

feel this may bring about death more quickly. Some family members think that a discussion of death would make the others more uncomfortable, and any discussion may seem to be related to an undue interest in the estate of the dying person. The loss of an important family member, like the head of a household, can threaten certain social and psychological arrangements. This can lead to enormous stresses and cause tension among all remaining members.

Besides grief, emotional reactions to the death of a family member may range from guilt and anger to fear, anxiety, and money worries. Sometimes the anger is directed toward the person that died: "He died and left me with these all debts" or "She deserted us during a crucial time of our lives." Further, death is a reminder of the survivors' own vulnerability, which evokes fear in itself. If the dying person lives in the home before death, tension and resentment can develop. When family members have to sacrifice their own friends and activities to provide care, feelings of hostility and anger toward the dying person develop. Then, the anger turns to guilt, which has been described as anger turned inward. Some family members tend to feel inadequate when confronted with this overwhelming situation. They tend to want to protect themselves and the dying relative by not speaking to the person. This is wrong because it leads to emotional abandonment, making the situation all the more difficult for the dying person. Compassion, not isolation, should be given.

The family can help the most by, when circumstances permit, maintaining an emotional and social environment consistent with the person's past life. This means keeping the person at home rather than in a hospital or nursing home. The family should include the dying relative as a participant in every discussion, especially those that involve decisions about that person's care and welfare. The family should do all they can to show their love and concern without doing it in ways that make the person feel guilty for being a burden to them. Family members should not allow their inability to face death to hinder the dying person's adjustment. When the person is ready to accept the reality of dying, the family should share that acceptance. An absence of support at this crucial time will mean that the person will die without dignity.

THE GRIEF EXPERIENCE

Grief is usually described as sorrow, mental distress, emotional agitation, sadness, suffering, and related feelings caused by a death. *Bereavement* refers to a state of experiencing grief. *Mourning* is comprised of culturally defined acts that are usually performed when death occurs.

Research has shown that the closer the relationship of the bereaved to the deceased, the stronger the emotional response (Eddy & Alles, 1983). Among these emotions and patterns of behavior are sadness, anger, fear, anxiety, guilt, loneliness, tension, loss of appetite, weight loss, loss of interest in things once interesting, a decrease in socialization, and disrupted sleep. These responses are usually greater when the death is unexpected.

Grief, bereavement, and mourning are generally much less formal in the United States than in some other cultures, or than it was in early America. Because of the lack of formal social codes of conduct, conflict sometimes arises among the survivors in defining appropriate mourning behavior (DeSpelder and Strickland, 1983).

Studies of mourning show that it is therapeutic for survivors to talk about the deceased, and work through their death-related problems in counseling sessions (Leviton, 1985). Another therapy involves going to work, going to school, or participating in organizational activities.

Americans seem in need of much more elaboration of death ceremonies than many other cultures. This helps explain why many in our society place a strong emphasis on the rituals of funerals and burials.

Funerals and Related Rituals

The funeral is an organized, group-centered response to death. It involves a ritual and ceremonies during which the body of the deceased is present. The traditional funeral includes speaking to the needs of the mourners. Some religions include a eulogy of the deceased, and some include an open casket that survivors view as part of the ceremony.

An alternative to the traditional funeral is a memorial service. Memorial services are sometimes held in conjunction with a cremation (with the urn present or absent) or when the body is not present for some reason (such as being donated to a medical school immediately upon death). This service is held in a church, chapel, home, or whatever place considered appropriate by the family. The service is not a eulogy but a chance to show thankfulness for having known the person. It also gives an opportunity for the expression of grief and sharing with family members. Generally, individuals who hold a memorial service are using this time to celebrate the life of the deceased while on earth as opposed to a mourning. Memorial services are most common among families who have strong religious convictions and the belief in life after death.

A primary purpose of the funeral is to dispose of the body. It also meets many emotional needs, like grief and mourning, of the survivors. The visitation part of the funeral ceremony is important for friends to show their respect for the deceased and support for the survivors. Also, viewing the casket, which is part of some funeral home visits, is important to some for realization (seeing is believing) and recall (providing an acceptable image for recalling the deceased). For these reasons, the funeral home visitation can be therapeutic for friends as well as family.

Cemeteries, with markers for each grave, formerly were thought of as very sacred places where relatives could go in quiet and peace to show their respects to the dead. Now, though, many cemeteries are crowded, congested, and impersonal. The relatives of the deceased might also live many miles from the burial site. For these reasons, cemetery visits are less common than they once were. This ritual is not used as often in working out grief and mourning among the survivors.

ISSUES SURROUNDING DEATH

Some topics related to death have become the focal point of controversy in recent years. These issues include the definition of death, the right to die, organ transplants and donations, wills, and suicide.

Definitions of Death

For thousands of years, the concept of the time of death was clearly defined as the cessation of the functions of life. Now, however, with advanced medical technology, life can be sustained beyond when death formerly would have occurred. The problem of defining it is much more complex. For example, at what point is the brain completely, irreversibly dead? The problem is not just knowing when a person is dead, but being able to determine the exact moment of death. This is important in the case of potential organ transplants, when every second is critical.

Death is a process, not a clearcut action; the brain dies in stages, not all at the same time. Part of the brain might be dead while another part still controls heartbeat and breathing. Some say that a person is "brain dead" when the entire brain is dead, even if respiration and circulation could be maintained artificially. Others argue that a person is dead when the outer surface of the cerebrum of the brain has ceased to function. (This individual may still breathe spontaneously via control of the brain stem, but thinking and reasoning ability would have ceased.)

Definitions of death center around "brain," "heart" or "physiological" death—when various organs cease to function—and "clinical" death—when there is a total lack of response to any external or internal stimuli, lack of spontaneous respiration, fixed and dilated pupils, lack of brainstem reflexes, and a flat EKG (no heartbeat). The significance of the definition of death is not just for the purpose of organ transplants. It also indicates which human lives can be saved, possibly with life-support systems such as heart-lung machines.

Organ Donation and Transplants

Some people wish to donate their organs or entire body for scientific and medical uses. This sometimes involves an urgent decision at the time of the donor's death. Biological, medical, and legal ethics are all involved in this issue. For those who wish to donate an organ, the Uniform Anatomical Gift Act of 1978 sets guidelines underlying the donor laws of each state. Some individuals donate their entire bodies to medical schools for dissection. This is valuable in the training of doctors, as a single donated body may give two or more students the information needed to save thousands of lives during their careers. Other parts of the body that can be donated include eyes, for corneal transplants; ear bones, to temporal bone banks for use in research into ear diseases; kidneys, for kidney transplants; pituitary glands, for use in producing growth hormone for those who lack this vital substance; and hearts, for heart transplants.

Virtually no religion in our country places any restrictions on organ donations to help another patient regain health. Further, the donation of an organ does not have to interrupt or modify the planned funeral service for the donor in any way. A donor needs to have a signed and witnessed donor card, usually carried at all times. These donor cards are available from many agencies in the community, such as the local dialysis or kidney clinic.

The Right to Die and Euthanasia

The term euthanasia has come to imply a contract for the termination of life in order to avoid unnecessary suffering at the end of a fatal illness. Direct euthanasia is defined as a deliberate action to shorten life. It involves a procedure like injecting air into the bloodstream. This is termed mercy killing and is still considered murder in our country, though some feel it should be permissible. In indirect, or passive, euthanasia, death is not induced; it is permitted death accomplished through the omission of an act or acts rather than commission of a life-taking act. For example, doctors might halt treatments that would prolong the life of a patient, or they might withhold treatment altogether. According to a Harris poll (Hemlock Society, 1985), 61 percent of Americans support passive euthanasia.

Rapid advances in medical technology have given the medical profession the ability to sustain or prolong life through extraordinary methods, so that those who might have died quickly now have a chance of survival with life-sustaining artificial support mechanisms. An adult in this country is considered to have the right to determine whether this type of medical technology should be employed. The person has the right to expressly prohibit life-saving surgery or other medical treatments. In other words, the right to die is inherent for every individual, as much so as the right to live. Some individuals fear the indignity and humiliation of existing merely as a vegetable, with others making decisions for them and caring for their every need. These people would rather die a "good death" than exist in this manner. For this reason, courts in many states are deciding on euthanasia cases. The proponents of euthanasia, or the right to die, state that saving a life is not always the same as saving people, as some do not wish to go on living or be revived. They argue that further extension of life should not be forced on the person just so life itself is preserved. This places an emphasis on the quality of life rather than just the literal existence of life.

Some states have passed laws to ensure their citizens of the right to die. This type of legislation provides death with dignity to those who sign a legal document known as a living will, as shown in figure 27.1. Signers of a living will anticipate a time when they cannot make or communicate decisions about their condition and treatment, but wish to reject artificial means of prolonging life and ask, in most cases, for such treatment to be withheld. California became the first state to enact such legislation on September 30, 1976 (Russell & Purdy, 1980). Many other states have since passed similar legislation or are currently considering such a bill.

Wills

It is not surprising most Americans, even many with sizeable estates, do not have a will since writing a will reminds people of their own mortality. The last will and testament is a legal instrument declaring a person's intentions concerning the disposition of property, the guardianship of children, or the administration of the estate after the person's death.

A will is needed to ensure that personal property gets distributed as the testator desires, to avoid the consequences of estate and inheritance taxes, and to have some control over one's estate after death. For individuals who die without wills, property passes according to state law. In other words, the state will decide which relatives get which part of the estate, even if the deceased person may have wished otherwise.

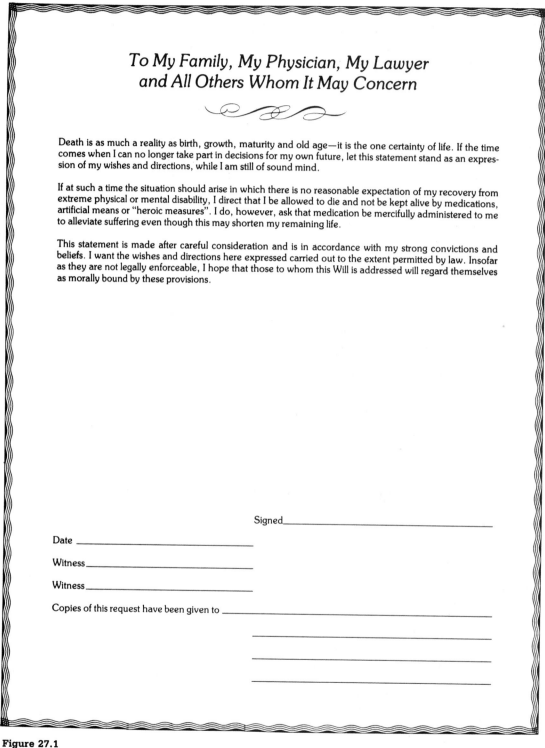

*To My Family, My Physician, My Lawyer
and All Others Whom It May Concern*

Death is as much a reality as birth, growth, maturity and old age—it is the one certainty of life. If the time comes when I can no longer take part in decisions for my own future, let this statement stand as an expression of my wishes and directions, while I am still of sound mind.

If at such a time the situation should arise in which there is no reasonable expectation of my recovery from extreme physical or mental disability, I direct that I be allowed to die and not be kept alive by medications, artificial means or "heroic measures". I do, however, ask that medication be mercifully administered to me to alleviate suffering even though this may shorten my remaining life.

This statement is made after careful consideration and is in accordance with my strong convictions and beliefs. I want the wishes and directions here expressed carried out to the extent permitted by law. Insofar as they are not legally enforceable, I hope that those to whom this Will is addressed will regard themselves as morally bound by these provisions.

Signed_____

Date _____

Witness_____

Witness_____

Copies of this request have been given to _____

_____

_____

_____

**Figure 27.1
A living will.**

Hospice

A hospice is a program, type of care, or facility that cares for the terminally ill and their families. Sometimes hospice care is given in the patient's home and, at other times, in a separate wing of a hospital. Generally, the goal of hospice care is to enhance the quality of a dying person's life during the last days and to allow the person to live as comfortably and inexpensively as possible.

Hospice care employs the concept of holistic care, in which the patient is treated with dignity. The patient is encouraged to take an active role in the decisions regarding treatment. Families of the patient are allowed to visit as often and as long as possible.

Suicide

Suicide at any age is always an enormously tragic event for the survivors, but when the self-inflicted death occurs in a young person, the grief is accentuated. Children of school age are most likely to attempt suicide (Hals, 1985). There is more guilt associated with suicide than with any other type of death. The parents or relatives feel they

Table 27.1
Common Myths about Suicide

American society harbors many misconceptions concerning suicide. To help clear up some of the myths, the following list has been developed:

Myth: People who talk about suicide won't commit suicide.
Fact: Statistics indicate that eight out of ten individuals who commit suicide give definite warnings of their intentions.

Myth: Suicidal people are fully intent on dying.
Fact: Most suicidal people are ambivalent about living or dying. They are often willing to gamble with death in order to get the attention or help they desire.

Myth: Once an individual attempts suicide, he is suicidal forever.
Fact: People are usually suicidal for only a short period of time.

Myth: Improvement following a suicide attempt means that the crisis is over.
Fact: Most suicides that follow attempts occur within three months from the beginning of "improvement," or the initial lessening of the threat of suicide. The appearance of improvement may mean that the individual now has the energy to put his suicidal thoughts into action.

Myth: Suicide occurs most often among the poor.
Fact: Suicide is neither the rich man's curse nor the poor man's disease. It is represented proportionately throughout all strata of society.

Myth: Suicide is inherited and runs in families.
Fact: Suicide is an individual pattern and does not run in families.

Myth: Suicidal people are mentally ill, and the act is a psychotic one.
Fact: Although suicidal persons are extremely unhappy and depressed, they are not necessarily mentally ill.

Myth: Asking whether a person is considering suicide will lead him to make an attempt.
Fact: Asking a person directly will often minimize the suicidal feeling and act as a deterrent to the act.

Source: *Health*, Hamrick, Anspaugh, & Ezell (Columbus: Merrill, 1986, p. 191)

are somehow to blame for needless death. Some feel that a suicide reflects badly upon the parents and family, but this is not always the case. Some hold a religious view that suicide is morally wrong or that one who commits suicide cannot enter heaven.

There is no single answer as to why a person wishes to put an end to life. The reasons are many and complex, but usually center around loss, revenge, hopelessness, failure, loneliness, aggression, and depression. Family problems, identity problems, and drugs can also contribute to feelings of anonymity and isolation leading to suicide (Hals, 1985).

Any suicidal threat, however subtle, must be taken seriously. Most individuals who commit suicide provide significant clues to their contemplated action. These include obvious changes in mood or behavior, excessive use of drugs, changes in any set of habits, preoccupation with personal health, decreased academic performance, and insomnia.

There are four commonly recommended steps for helping someone who seems in danger of suicide. First, talk to the person who threatens suicide and determine how deeply troubled the individual really is. Second, do not challenge the individual to act on the threat. Such a challenge may force the person to act to prove the validity of the threat. Third, help the person postpone the decision. Offer other options to consider. Fourth, be knowledgeable about resources that can provide aid. The person might have exhausted all personally known avenues of assistance and might need professional help.

Suicide prevention is a community responsibility, and everyone can play an important part in its resolution. However, many people hold various misconceptions regarding suicide. Some of these misconceptions (and the truths) are shown in table 27.1.

CHILDREN AND DEATH

Children in our society no longer experience many aspects of the life cycle. Most do not live with grandparents or on farms, so they do not observe aging and death in their immediate environment. Death education is necessary for the proper development of elementary school children. Death education should be viewed as a natural topic for inclusion in the child's education because children are not immune to experiencing the death of a loved one, a pet, or classmate. Future elementary teachers should be extremely well prepared to teach death education since considerable mental harm to children could occur if the teacher were incompetent to teach the topic (Molnar-Stickels, 1985).

Children have a temporary concept of death until a certain age. They might be able to grasp some of the concepts of finality, but they remain confused. For example, the cartoon characters children watch get smashed in one scene and are up and around in the next. The leading character who was killed in the movie last night is doing a commercial tonight. A child's conception of death is entirely dependent upon age, intelligence level, and cultural background.

There are definite stages in a child's understanding of death (Eddy & Alles, 1983), as seen in table 27.2.

Table 27.2
Children's Understanding of Death

Stage	Age	Concepts of Death
1	3 to 5 years	Temporary and sleeplike Unable to comprehend finality of death Deceased can return to life
2	5 to 9 years	Comprehends finality of death Caused by external force which can be avoided Death perceived as a personality Death not seen as inevitable
3	9 and above	Seen as part of life cycle Can occur at any time Can occur to anyone Death is inescapable Understands psychological significance of death

Children respond to their own imminent deaths within the framework of the stages just described. A dying child needs to be assured that death is not punishment for something the child did or said.

Death Education for Children

Death is a universal part of living even though it is a taboo topic in our society. Children are interested in knowing more about the subject of death, but they are generally shielded from such exposure. Many parents are reluctant to talk with their children about death because they wish to protect their children (and themselves) from the pain of loss. Children are often prohibited from some hospital wards, health care institutions, and other places where people are dying. As a result, they tend to learn about death through the media, which can be confusing and misleading.

Sooner or later, children must confront death—to understand the needs of the dying, to have some preparation for the experience, and to deal with their own feelings.

Health Highlight: Children and Grief

A child's grief response depends on three factors.

1. The family situation. If children receive adequate affection and security from the family, their reaction is much healthier.
2. The way in which the person died. Sudden, unexpected death of a parent may cause a more severe grief response than an anticipated death in which the child has the time and opportunity to gradually adapt to the situation.
3. The developmental age and past experiences of children. The more mature and more experienced with death the child is, the better the child is able to cope with a death.

Some common reactions of children toward death are:

- denial
- isolation and withdrawal
- physiological distress
- guilt
- hostility
- fear and panic

Source: Eddy, J. M. and Alles, W. F. *Death Education.* St. Louis: The C. V. Mosby Company, 1983, p. 33).

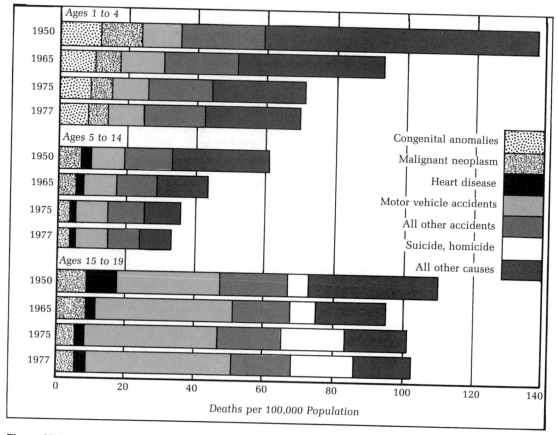

Figure 27.2
Death rates for children and teenagers.
Source: U.S. Department of Commerce, Bureau of the Census, *Social Indicators III*, p. 74.

Education about death *is* a legitimate subject for children. It is an important topic worthy of open, informed, and sensitive discussion. Death education can guide students toward greater understanding about death and dying, and, even though it might be painful for them and for the teacher, gaining such understanding can be essential for sound mental health.

In death education, you should come to terms with your own feelings about death and not just learn the material. You need to be aware of your students' willingness to express their feelings on this sensitive topic and be ready to let them discuss the subject openly and frankly. Never tell children they should wait until they are older to talk about death. Many times, adults use this ploy as an excuse to avoid their own insecurities about death. Answer any question at their level of understanding. Feelings and emotions related to death (yours and the students) should also be allowed to be expressed in the classroom, even encouraged. Use experiences in the classroom, such as the death of a flower, a pet, or a classmate to teach students about death feelings and rituals.

SUMMARY

Death is the natural end to life, yet many in our society try to deny its existence. Death is mysterious because we do not know what is beyond death. Many people fear death and refuse to discuss the topic openly and frankly. Everyone, however, has personal beliefs about death. Some of these beliefs are helpful in facing death because they help demystify it but facing death is still a traumatic experience for the dying person and survivors alike. The dying person has many emotional needs that often go unmet by relatives and the medical profession. This may leave the dying person very lonely and feeling abandoned. The individual goes through various stages of adjustment to impending death. If we understand these stages, we can better help the dying person.

Many controversies and issues surround death, including the definition of death, the person's right to die, organ donation and transplants, wills, and suicide. Most children in our society do not experience death close to home anymore. These children go through definite stages in their understanding of death. Children are interested in knowing more about the subject of death. Thus, death education is a legitimate, worthy topic in elementary schools.

DISCUSSION QUESTIONS

1. Discuss the fears of a dying person.
2. How is our society a "death-denying" society?
3. How are personal beliefs important in facing dying and death?
4. Discuss the stages of adjusting to dying.
5. How can family members help a dying person adjust to dying?
6. Differentiate between grief, bereavement and mourning.
7. Discuss the purposes of the funeral.
8. Discuss the goals of hospice care.
9. Differentiate between direct and indirect euthanasia.
10. How should death and dying be discussed in the classroom?

REFERENCES

Bok, S. "Lies to the sick and dying." In Schneidman, E. (ed.). *Death: Current perspectives,* second edition. Palo Alto, Calif.: Mayfield, 1980.

DeSpelder, L. & Strickland, A. *The last dance: Encountering death and dying.* Palo Alto, California: Mayfield Publishing Company, 1983.

Eddy, J. & Alles, W. *Death education.* St. Louis: The C. V. Mosby Company, 1983.

Hals, E. "Suicide prevention." *Health Education. 16, 4,* August/September, 1985.

Hamrick, M., Anspaugh, D., & Ezell, G. *Health.* Columbus: Merrill, 1986.

Hemlock Society. "61% Say Doctors Should Help Dying." *Euthanasia Review,* Issue 18, April, 1985.

Kalish, R. *Death, grief, and caring relationships,* second edition. Monterey, California: Brooks/ Cole Publishing Company, 1985.

Kubler-Ross, E. *Death: The final stage of growth.* Englewood Cliffs, N.J.: Prentice-Hall, 1975.

Leviton, D. "Counseling the bereaved or dying: An aspect of health education." *Health Education. 16,* 4, August/ September, 1985.

Molnar-Stickles, L. "Effect of a brief instructional unit in death education on the death attitudes of prospective elementary school teachers." *Journal of School Health, 55,* 6, August, 1985.

Russell, R. & Purdy, C. *Coping with death and dying.* Glenview, Illinois: Scott, Foresman and Company, 1980.

28. Techniques for Teaching about Death and Dying

There are so many new books about dying that there are now special shelves set aside for them in bookshops, along with the health-diet and home-repair paperbacks and the sex manuals. Some of them are so packed with detailed information and step-by-step instructions for performing the function that you'd think this was a new sort of skill which all of us are now required to learn. The strongest impression the casual reader gets, leafing through, is that proper dying has become an extraordinary, even an exotic experience, something only the specially trained get to do.—Lewis Thomas, The Medusa and the Snail

OBJECTIVES OF DEATH EDUCATION

The death of a relative, or even a pet, *can* be traumatic to people of all ages, including children. For this reason, some parents approach the problem by trying to shield their children from experiences related to dying and death. Rather than solving the problem, this avoidance leaves the child unprepared to face a natural part of the life cycle.

The current treatment of dying patients in hospitals and nursing homes also tends to remove us from dying and death experiences. This further limits our contact with the reality of dying and lessens our chances of coming to grips with our feelings about death.

Because of our society's negative attitude toward death and the atmosphere of avoidance, children need education about death. Many children, though they may not have an accurate concept of death, want to know about the many aspects of life related to dying and death, such as funerals and cemeteries. Death education in the elementary schools can help meet this need. Its objectives are to allow children to clarify their values about death and dying, to provide factual information about the subject, and to encourage children to discuss openly the vital issues concerning the natural end of the life cycle.

Concepts to be Taught

- Death is a natural end to the life cycle.
- There are many different ways to determine the exact moment a person dies.
- Our society generally avoids the topics of death and dying in discussion and conscious thought.
- Personal beliefs about death and dying can affect mental health and lifestyle.
- There are vastly contrasting views on what happens to us after we die.
- There are many misconceptions about how to treat a dying person.
- Dying people have special needs.
- The family of a dying person also has special needs.
- Grief and bereavement naturally follow the death of a close friend or relative.
- Funeral and burial rituals have significant meaning in our society.
- People are choosing alternative methods of burials and funerals in order to save money.
- Wills and testaments are beneficial legal documents.
- The right to die is a basic human right.
- Suicide attempts among young people are increasing.
- There are ways each of us can help a friend who is contemplating suicide to reconsider the action.
- Organ donation can be considered an "ultimate gift of life."

Cycle Plan for Teaching Topics

Topic	Grade Level						
	K	1	2	3	4	5	6
Society's Attitude toward Death	*	**	**	**	**	*	*
Death as a Natural End to Life	***	***	**	**	*	*	*
Coping with Death and Dying	**	**	***	***	***	***	**
Causes of Death Among the Young	*	**	**	**	*	*	*
Funeral and Burial Rituals	*	*	**	**	**	*	*
Grief and Bereavement	**	**	**	**	*	*	*
Needs of the Dying Person	*	*	*	*	**	**	**
Medical and Legal Ethics	*	*	*	*	**	**	***

Key: *** = major emphasis, ** = emphasis, * = review.

VALUE-BASED ACTIVITIES

Values Statements

Have the students complete each of the following statements with their first reactions. Afterwards, discuss how different individuals react and feel about each issue raised in the statements.

1. When I think about death, I _____ .
2. To me, death means _____ .
3. If I could choose how I will die, I would _____ .
4. My greatest fear about dying is _____ .
5. When I think about relatives who have died, I _____ .
6. Every living thing dies, so _____ .
7. The human life cycle means _____ .
8. Grief is _____ .
9. People who are dying need _____ .
10. Living and dying _____ .

Personal Views on Suicide

Have students answer and discuss these questions.

1. Do you feel that an individual has the right to make the ultimate decision as to whether he or she should live or die?
2. What would you do if a friend said to you, "I think I might commit suicide—would you help me?" Would you:
   a. Call the police.
   b. Do nothing.
   c. Ask why.
   d. Call a doctor.
   e. Send your friend away with the statement. "Sorry, but I am unable to help you!"
   f. Try to help by talking.
   g. Other.
   Could you explain your answer just a little more here?
3. What do you feel might be one possible answer to suicide prevention?

On Living and Dying

Have students look over the various statements below. They relate to death, dying and living. Have the students ask themselves, "Would this idea be acceptable or unacceptable to me?" They can use a rating scale as follows:

1 = Very acceptable
2 = Acceptable
3 = Unsure
4 = Unacceptable
5 = Not acceptable at all

1. Being killed in an auto accident.
2. Living forever.
3. Dying slowly.
4. Dying of cancer.
5. Being saved through medical help but unable to walk again.
6. Being able to choose when you will die.
7. Dying before your spouse.
8. Living to age 110.
9. Dying after your spouse.

10. Choosing how you will die.
11. Living but unable to function.
12. Dying at home.
13. Dying quickly.
14. Dying before you are 50 years old.
15. Giving up your life for another person.
16. Giving up your life to save someone else.
17. Dying in your sleep.
18. Being very sick and close to death but not being told.
19. Dying with the hope that there is a life after.
20. Trying a new "miracle" drug that may save you or kill you instantly.

Write Your Own Epitaph

Give children the chance to write their own epitaphs. Prepare a handout with a drawing of a tombstone.

Euthanasia Questionnaire

Have students answer the following questions. Discuss their answers afterwards.

1. You just read that a 19-year-old boy was in a car accident that left him completely paralyzed with some degree of brain damage. Would you: (mark one)
   a. Refrain from giving him medication that may save his life?
   b. Keep him alive as long as vital signs are normal and/or stable.
   c. Ask him if he would like to live or die?
   d. Tell him of the consequences and then ask him what the doctors should do?
   e. Let him die?
2. You and your spouse just had your first child. The doctor has informed you that your baby has Down syndrome and also has a small hole in her heart. With several expensive operations and much treatment, she may eventually be saved but will need constant care. What would you do?
   a. Allow her to die?
   b. Refuse to allow the operation and medication and take what comes?
   c. Use any means possible to keep her alive but if she lives, place her in an institution?
   d. Use any means to keep her alive, and if she lives, keep her?
   e. Tell the doctors it is up to them?
3. You have just been told that you have an illness that will get progressively worse. In a few weeks or so, you will go into a coma and remain that way until you die. The doctors tell you that there is a machine that could keep you alive for about three to seven months but you will have to remain in bed and there is no guarantee that you will ever come out of the coma. Would you want
   a. To be given a medication that would induce death?
   b. The doctors to refrain from giving you a medication that would prolong your life?
   c. To be allowed to die slowly?
   d. To use any means possible to keep you alive as long as possible?

Value Voting

Present a series of statements such as the following to your class. First, explain that each statement represents the way some people feel about death-related issues. Then ask students to raise their hands if they *basically* agree with the stance or to keep hands down if they disagree. After each show of hands, allow students who wish to comment on the statement to do so. Follow the activity with a general discussion of issues that came up.

1. I do not fear death.
2. I refuse to go to funerals.
3. I would like to donate my body to science when I die.
4. Sometimes suicide is the only answer to overwhelming problems.
5. I think funerals help people handle their grief better.
6. I can discuss death and dying openly with my family.
7. I am more afraid of death than anything else.
8. I would be afraid to be around a dying person.
9. I accept death as a natural end to life.
10. Dying can be done with dignity.

Rank Ordering*

By assigning a rank order to each of the following three-item sets, your students may become more aware of their priorities and attitudes on particular issues.

1. A favorite pet of yours has a very bad (and very painful) disease. You would:
   a. let it die naturally, despite its pain
   b. have it put to sleep
   c. ask to have its body frozen, in hopes of some future medical breakthrough
2. Of the following positions, you would choose to be:
   a. a hangman
   b. a member of a firing squad
   c. an electrocutioner in a prison
3. You would most willingly accept:
   a. the death of a parent
   b. the death of a good friend
   c. your own death
4. You would prefer:
   a. short but exciting life
   b. a long but dull life, with a peaceful death
   c. a long, exciting life, with a painful death

The Fallout Shelter†

Imagine that our country is under threat of immediate nuclear attack and that you are in a position of command. There is a fallout shelter nearby that can hold 6 people, but there are 12 people trying to get in. It is up to you to decide which 6 to allow to enter the shelter. As you can see from the list below, very little is known about the 12 individuals. The persons include:

1. a 25-year-old female lawyer
2. the lawyer's 29-year-old husband, who has a serious disease and is expected to live no more than a year (he and his wife have agreed to go in together or stay out together)

---

*Source: Simon, Sidney and Goodman, Joel, "Study of Death," in *Learning,* March, 1976, p. 72.
†Source: Simon, Sidney and Goodman, Joel, "Study of Death," in *Learning,* March, 1976, p. 74.

3. a 40-year-old female violinist who is a suspected drug pusher
4. a 34-year-old male architect who is very skilled but has a reputation for building houses that leak when it rains
5. a 38-year-old female doctor who cannot stand being closed in
6. a 65-year-old priest
7. a 22-year-old female black militant
8. a 48-year-old male scientist who has just been released from a mental institution
9. a 19-year-old female student who is a known shoplifter
10. a 27-year-old male professional athlete who seems to have been blessed with very little common sense
11. a 39-year-old female movie star who is a bigot
12. a 30-year-old ex-policeman who was thrown off the force for committing acts of brutality and who refuses to enter the shelter without his gun

For each person you admit to the fallout shelter, try to make a values statement about your life. Your statements might start with such phrases as: "Judging from this choice, I seem to value. . . ." or "I strongly believe in this case that. . ." Next, identify the criteria you used in deciding which people to leave out. These statements will probably reflect some values you were protecting.

Decision Stories

Follow the procedures outlined in chapter 5 for presenting decision stories such as these.

Grandmother's Grief

Linda's grandfather died last night and everyone in Linda's house was very sad. Her grandmother came over to stay the night. Linda's parents are trying to console her grandmother and Linda thinks that she should say something, too. But she doesn't know what she could say or do.

Focus Question: What could Linda say or do?

Staying Away from Sam

When Sam didn't show up at school for two days, Larry wondered what was wrong. Then Sam returned. Larry found out that Sam's younger brother had been found to have cancer and was dying. Sam was very sad. But Larry noticed that some of the other kids started avoiding Sam after that. It seemed that they didn't want to be around him because they knew Sam's brother was dying. Maybe they were right, Larry thought. Maybe everybody should just leave Sam alone. But Larry wasn't sure.

Focus Question: What should Larry do?

What Would You Do?

A teenage boy attended a party where he took several drugs. As a result of the drug overdose, the boy lapsed into a coma and had to be placed on a respirator to help his heart beat and lungs breathe. Medical tests showed that there was no activity in his brain—he was essentially "brain-dead." The boy has stayed in a coma for several months with no sign of improving.

Focus Questions: If you were the boy's parents, what would you do? If you were the doctor, what would you do?

A Gift of Life

Loretta is dying of kidney disease. She knows it and has accepted the fact of her coming death. Now, her doctors would like to use her heart in a transplant operation. They tell her that her heart could be used to help another person to live. Loretta isn't sure about the matter.

Focus Question: What should Loretta do?

Herb's Brother

Herb's brother is dying of leukemia. The doctors say there is nothing more they can do. Herb's brother is at home. He is still strong enough to take part in some family doings. One day Herb asks his friend Bill to come over to the house to play Monopoly. "My brother wants to play, too," Herb says. Bill knows that leukemia is not contagious. But he is uneasy about being in the same room with Herb's brother. He doesn't know how to act. Should he pretend that Herb's brother is okay? Should he ask about how it feels to be dying? Or should he make an excuse to Herb and go home?

Focus Question: What should Bill do?

DRAMATIZATION

Talk Can Help

Have one student play the part of a dying patient in a hospital. Have another play the role of a close friend who comes to visit. Role play the situation for five minutes per pair of students. Ask each student to play the part in the way that seems most comfortable and natural. Discuss the different approaches used in acting out this situation.

Only One Week To Live

Have volunteers role play an interviewee who has just been asked what he or she would do if he or she only had one week to live. This activity could be spontaneous or you could allow the volunteers some time to think about the activities and list them.

A Memorial Service

If a well known personality whom the students are familiar with has died recently, have them hold a brief memorial service in that person's honor. Participants in the service should discuss what the deceased person meant to them and why this person is being mourned. Explain to your students that the activity is not a religious ceremony but rather a commemoration of the deceased person's life.

Consoling Others

Let one student play the part of someone who has just lost a close friend or relative. Have two or three other students role play how they would console the person and help the grief process. Afterwards, have a general discussion of how people can aid one another in handling the death of someone close to them.

DISCUSSION AND REPORT TECHNIQUES

My Pet Died

Most students have had pets that died, either dogs, cats, hamsters, or other small animals. Ask students who have had the experience of having a pet die to write a short report about the event. The reports should emphasize the things about the pet that the child liked most. Explain that we can remember those qualities and talk about the pleasure or companionship of a past pet even though the pet will never return to us. Note the comfort that such fond memories can bring.

Different Mourning and Funeral Customs

Have students research mourning customs in different cultures and present oral reports about their findings. This is a good library project. Children may wish to find out about funeral and mourning customs in Arab nations, in the Orient, and in Latin America. After the presentations, discuss different customs in class. For example, black is the usual mourning color in Western nations, but white is the mourning color in China, Korea, and Japan. In Arab countries, there is no visitation and the body must be buried by sunset of the day the person died. In Tibet, dead bodies are cut up and fed to vultures. This is called celestial burial. The belief is that only when the entire body is disposed of can the spirit of the deceased be released to go to heaven.

Death is a Part of Life

Have students keep a three-day diary of events and occurrences that happen to them that are related to death. The diary can contain any mention in conversation about death, stories on television, or cartoons that mention death or in which someone dies, or any pictures on billboards they see of death. After three days, either collect the diaries and discuss them with the class, or have the students relate their own experiences.

Death Notices*

Provide groups of students with copies of death notices and obituaries from newspapers. Ask them to respond to the following questions:

> What are some reasons for including death notices in the paper?
> What are some things we think people should be remembered for?
> What was the most unusual death notice?
> Which death notice contained the most information?

Follow up this activity by asking the students to write their own obituary. Hang the obituaries around the room as examples.

---

*Source: Eddy, James M., and Alles, Wesley F. *Death Education*. St. Louis: The C. V. Mosby Company, 1983, p. 267.

Euphemisms*

On a chalkboard or a large poster, list the following euphemisms for and other expressions about dying and death:

Kicked the bucket	Scared to death
Went to their reward	Never say die
Passed on	Dead center
Dead tired	Kill the ump
I wish I could die	Deadbeat
Dead wrong	Deadly sin
Killing time	

Brainstorm reasons why these euphemisms are used, and consider how they reflect our attitudes toward death. Conduct a discussion on the meaning of these euphemisms.

Life After Death†

Have the students draw two pictures—one symbolizing death, and the other symbolizing what might happen after death. These drawings will demonstrate the students' conceptions of death. Then, have volunteers discuss their drawings with the class.

Causes of Death In Young People

Assign students to research the causes of death in young people and then present a panel discussion on the subject. Different students should look into various causes of death, such as accidents, degenerative diseases, and contagious diseases. Allow time for a question and answer session after the panel presentation.

Organ Donation

Ask students to prepare individual reports on some aspect of organ donation. Some students may wish to investigate heart or kidney transplants. Others can look into cornea transplants or other donations. Still others should find out about the procedures used to make organ transplants. Select representative reports from each area and have the students read them to the class. Follow with a general discussion.

---

*Source: Eddy, James M. and Alles, Wesley F. *Death Education.* St. Louis: The C. V. Mosby Company, 1983, p. 266.

†Source: Dahlgren, Toni and Prager-Decker, Iris, "A Unit on Death for Primary Grades," In Osness, Donna and Thompson, Karen (editors). *Health Education Teaching Ideas: Elementary.* Reston, Virginia: American Alliance for Health, Physical Education, Recreation and Dance, 1983, p. 72.

How Funerals Make Me Feel

Ask students who have attended funerals to prepare reports on how they felt. Point out that although a funeral is a sad occasion, it also has therapeutic benefits for the survivors. Therefore students should include any positive feelings they experienced as well, such as a feeling of emotional release by openly expressing grief or comfort in hearing the eulogy about the deceased person.

Suicide Prevention

Ask a representative of the local suicide prevention agency to address the class on the topic of suicide among young people. Before the guest arrives, prepare the class by explaining how such resources as suicide prevention agencies can help prevent needless deaths. Be sure that your guest emphasizes the different resources in the community that a young person considering suicide can turn to for help and counseling.

EXPERIMENTS AND DEMONSTRATIONS

Plant Comparisons

Have the children plant some bean seeds in a large container filled with potting soil. Let them observe the life cycle of the plants. Typically, although most the seeds will sprout, some will die before others. Observe dying plants closely and compare them with others that continue to thrive. Explain the possible causes of early death among some of the plants and note that plants, like animals, live for varying lengths of time.

Observing a Life Cycle

Raise a short-lived animal in class, such as a mouse. Let the children observe the life cycle of the animal from youth to old age. If the animal dies, plan and carry out an appropriate funeral for it.

Across
1. Lives 70 or more years.
2. Can live 10 to 15 years.
3. Some live more than 150 years.
4. Lives only a few days.

Down
5. Lives as long as 2000 years.
6. Lifespan of about one year.
7. Lives for several months.

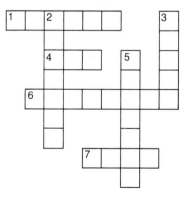

**Figure 28.1
Crossword puzzle.**

PUZZLES AND GAMES

Lifespan Crossword

Discuss the varying lifespans of different species of plants and animals. Then have the children complete a crossword puzzle similar to the one shown in figure 28.1. Afterwards, discuss the different lengths of time different species typically live. Note that although some live quite a long time, eventually every organism dies.

BULLETIN BOARDS

Death is a Natural Part of the Life Cycle

Have students collect news stories, magazine articles, and pictures that relate to dying and death. Assemble them on a bulletin board with captions to demonstrate that dying and death are natural parts of the life cycle.

Cemeteries

With the assistance of the students, prepare a bulletin board display of different kinds of cemeteries. Use pictures cut from old magazines. Include pictures of cemeteries from different cultures and nations.

Suicide Prevention Week

Have the class declare a specific week as Suicide Prevention Week. Let them research suicide prevention agencies in the community and then make a bulletin board display illustrating their findings. These should include the names and telephone numbers of specific resources, such as suicide prevention centers, the police department, community hotline services, and counseling services. A separate display can be made listing symptoms of possibly suicidal behavior or intentions. Use the displays as the basis for a discussion of how we can all help prevent needless death by suicide.

OTHER IDEAS

Wills

To emphasize the importance of a will, ask students to list their most important possessions and decide to whom they would leave these possessions if they were to die. Relate this activity to a discussion of the legal aspects of actual wills.

Cemetery Visit

If feasible, take the class on a field trip to a nearby cemetery. If the cemetary is an old one, this activity can be done as part of a unit on local history as well as part of your death education teaching. Ask students to look for the oldest graves in the cemetery. When did the first burials take place? What do the grave markers tell about the individuals buried there? Note the dates of birth and death. Did people live longer or shorter many years ago? Do any grave markers indicate the cause of death? How have styles changed in grave markers over the years? Afterwards, have students write reports on what they learned from the cemetery visit about death customs.

Poetry

Some of the greatest works of poetry in literature concern death and dying. Find short poems appropriate to the level of your class and read them aloud. Discuss the meaning of each poem. Then ask the children to write poems of their own on aspects of death and dying. Post the completed poems around the room for all to see and appreciate.

What Does a Funeral Director Do?

Invite a funeral director to speak to the class about how funeral arrangements are made. Ask your guest to explain what is done, how costs are determined, and how family members are involved. The funeral director should explain any special considerations that must be taken into account for religious, cultural, or family reasons. Allow time for a question and answer session after the presentation.

Distorted Images of Death

"Death" occurs nightly on popular television programs. Every police and detective drama usually includes one or more violent deaths. Ask the class to note such instances in recent programs they have seen. Then discuss the distorted images of death that are usually presented in such programs. For example, grief is often absent or minimized. As a result, the audience also considers the death as a casual matter simply included to advance the plot. Contrast the images of death as presented on television with the actuality of real death.

A. Appendix: Sources of Free and Inexpensive Health Education Materials

When writing for health education materials be specific in your request, tell the age level for whom the material is intended, and write your request on school letterhead paper. Typing the request makes for a more professional appearance. The authors caution that the addresses listed may have changed.

Code:
A/D = Alcohol and Drugs
COM = Communicable Diseases
PERS = Personal Health
F/LF = Family Life
H/C = Health Courses
F/A = First Aid

CR = Chronic Disorders
CON = Consumer Issues
ENV = Environmental Health
NUTR = Nutrition
M/H = Mental Health

1. Abbott Laboratories
   Dept. 383
   Abbott Park
   North Chicago, Ill. 60064
   A/D, CR, COM

2. Aetna Life and Casualty Co.
   151 Farmington Avenue
   Hartford, Conn. 06115
   A/D, F/A

3. A. H. Robins Co., Inc.
   Public Affairs Dept.
   1407 Cummings Drive
   Richmond, Va. 23220
   NUTR, M/H

4. Allergy Foundation of America
   801 Second Avenue
   New York, N.Y. 10017
   CR

5. American Academy of Family
   Physicians
   1740 West 92nd Street
   Kansas City, Mo. 64114
   CON, H/C

6. American Automobile Association
   Traffic Engineering & Safety Dept.
   Falls Church, Va. 22042
   A/D, ENV, F/A

7. American Cancer Society
   (contact local office)
   CR, H/C, A/D

8. American Dental Association
   Bureau of Dental Health Education
   211 East Chicago Avenue
   Chicago, Ill. 60611
   PERS, CON, NUTR, H/C, A/D

535

9. American Diabetes Association
   600 Fifth Avenue
   New York, N.Y. 10020
   CR

10. American Foundation for the Blind
    115 West 16th Street
    New York, N.Y. 10011
    PERS

11. American Heart Association
    (consult local office)
    CR, NUTR

12. American Hospital Association
    840 North Lake Shore Drive
    Chicago, Ill. 60611
    CON

13. American Institute of Baking
    P.O. Box 1448
    Manhattan, Ks. 66502
    NUTR

14. American Institute of Family Relations
    5287 Sunset Boulevard
    Los Angeles, Cal. 90027
    F/LF, M/H

15. American Insurance Association
    Engineering and Safety Services
    85 John Street
    New York, N.Y. 10038
    F/A

16. American Lung Association
    (consult local office)
    CR, ENV, A/P

17. American Medical Association
    Bureau of Health Education
    535 North Dearborn Street
    Chicago, Ill. 60610
    A/D, CR, COM, CON, F/LC, PERS, H/C,
    F/A

18. American Mutual Insurance
    Institute for Safer Living
    Wakefield, Mass. 01880
    F/A

19. American National Red Cross
    National Headquarters Library
    17th and D Streets, N.W.
    Washington, D.C. 20006
    F/A

20. American Optometric Association
    7000 Chippewa Street
    St. Louis, Mo. 63119
    PERS

21. American Podiatry Association
    Department of Public Affairs
    20 Chevy Chase Circle, N.W.
    Washington, D.C.
    PERS

22. Arthritis Foundation
    3400 Peachtree Road, N.E.
    Atlanta, Ga. 30326
    CR, CON

23. Ayerst Laboratories
    685 Third Avenue
    New York, N.Y. 10017
    CR

24. Better Vision Institute, Inc.
    239 Park Avenue
    New York, N.Y. 10017
    PERS

25. Bicycle Manufacturers Association of
    America, Inc.
    1101 15th Street, N.W.
    Washington, D.C. 20005
    F/A

26. Center for Disease Control
    1600 Clifton Road, N.E.
    Atlanta, Ga. 30353

27. Connecticut General Life
    Insurance Co.
    Advertising and Public Relations
    Hartford, Conn. 06115
    F/A, PERS, A/D, COM

28. Department of Citrus
    State of Florida

Florida Citrus Commission
Lakeland, Fl. 33802
NUTR

29. Eli Lilly and Co.
P.O. Box 100B
Indianapolis, Ind. 46206

30. Epilepsy Foundation of America
1828 L. Street, N.W., Suite 406
Washington, D.C. 20036
CR

31. General Mills, Inc.
Nutrition Department
P.O. Box 1113
Minneapolis, Minn. 55440
NUTR, CON

32. Institute of Makers of Explosives
420 Lexington Avenue
New York, N.Y. 10017
F/A

33. Johnson and Johnson
Consumer Services
New Brunswick, N.Y. 08903
FAM, PERS, F/A

34. Juvenile Diabetes Foundation
3701 Conshohocken Avenue
Philadelphia, Penn. 19131
CR

35. Kimberly-Clark Corp.
The Life Cycle Center
2001 Marathon Avenue
Neenah, Wis. 54956
F/LF, PERS

36. Lederle Laboratories
Public Affairs Department
Pearl River, N.Y. 10695
COM, NUTR, M/H

37. Licensed Beverage Industries, Inc.
155 East 44th Street
New York, N.Y. 10017
A/D

38. Mental Health Materials Center
Information Resources Center
419 Park Avenue, South
New York, N.Y. 10016
F/LF, M/H

39. Metropolitan Life Insurance Co.
Health and Safety Education Division
One Madison Avenue
New York, N.Y. 10010
A/D, COM, PERS, F/A

40. Muscular Dystrophy Association, Inc.
810 Seventh Avenue
New York, N.Y. 10019
CR

41. National Association for Mental Health
1800 North Kent Street
Rosslyn, Va. 22209
A/D, M/H, F/LS

42. National Clearinghouse for Drug
Abuse Information
P.O. Box 1635
Rockville, Md. 20850
A/D

43. National Congress of Parents and
Teachers
700 North Rush Street
Chicago, Ill. 60611
A/D, F/LS

44. National Council on Family Relations
1219 University Avenue S.E.
Minneapolis, Minn. 55414
F/LS, M/H

45. National Cystic Fibrosis Foundation
60 East 44th Street
New York, N.Y. 10017
CR

46 National Fire Protection Association
470 Atlantic Avenue
Boston, Mass. 02210
F/A

47. National Health Council
    1740 Broadway
    New York, N.Y. 10019
    H/C

48. National Institute of Health
    National Institute on Aging
    Public Inquiries
    Bethesda, Md. 20014
    PERS, F/LS

49. National Institute of Health
    National Institute of Arthritis,
        Metabolism, and Digestive Diseases
    Building 31, Room 9A04
    Bethesda, Md. 20014
    CR

50. National Institute of Health
    National Institute of Child Health and
        Human Development
    Public Inquiries
    Bethesda, Md. 20014
    CR, PERS, F/LS

51. National Institute of Health
    National Institute of Dental Research
    Public Inquiries
    Bethesda, Md. 20014

52. National Institute of Health
    National Institute of Environmental
        Health Science
    Public Inquiries
    Bethesda, Md. 20014
    ENV

53. National Institute of Health
    National Institute of Neurological and
        Communicative Disorders
        and Stroke
    Public Inquiries
    Bethesda, Md. 20014
    CR

54. National Multiple Sclerosis Society
    205 East 42nd Street
    New York, N.Y. 10017
    CR

55. National Safety Council
    444 North Michigan Avenue
    Chicago, Ill. 60611
    A/D, F/A, PERS

56. National Society for the Prevention of
        Blindness
    79 Madison Avenue
    New York, N.Y. 10016
    PERS, CR

57. National Tay-Sachs and Allied
        Diseases Association
    122 East 42nd Street
    New York, N.Y. 10017
    CR

58. Personal Products Co.
    Miltown, N.J. 08850
    PERS, F/LS

59. Pfizer, Inc.
    235 East 42nd Street
    New York, N.Y. 10017
    CD, M

60. Pharmaceutical Manufacturers
        Association
    Consumer Affairs
    1155 Fifteenth Street, N.W.
    Washington, D.C. 20005
    A/D, CON

61. Prudential Insurance Company of
        America
    Public Relations Department
    Prudential Plaza
    Newark, N.J. 07101

62. Procter and Gamble Company
    P.O. Box 14009
    Cincinnati, Ohio 45214
    FAM, PERS

63. Public Affairs Committee, Inc.
    381 Park Avenue, South
    New York, N.Y. 10016
    F/LS, A/D, COM, CR, CON, PERS,
    NUTR, M/H

64. S.I.E.C.U.S.
    137–155 North Franklin
    Hempstead, N.Y. 11550

65. Smith, Kline and French Laboratories
    Drug Abuse Literature-E60
    1500 Spring Garden Street
    Philadelphia, Penn. 19101
    A/D

66. Tampax, Inc.
    Lake Success, N.Y. 11040
    F/LS, PERS

67. United Cerebral Palsy Association
    66 East 34th Street
    New York, N.Y. 10016
    CR

68. U.S. Consumer Product Safety
    Commission
    Washington, D.C. 20207
    CON, F/A

69. U.S. Department of Agriculture
    Cooperative Extension Service
    (consult local office)
    NUTR

70. U.S. Department of Energy
    Office of Marketing and Education
    Washington, D.C. 20545
    CON

71. U.S. Department of Health and Human
    Services
    Food and Drug Administration
    5600 Fishers Lane
    Rockville, Md. 20852
    A/D, CON, NUTR, F/A

72. Upjohn Company
    Public Relations Department
    7000 Portage Road
    Kalamazoo, Mich. 49001
    A/D

73. Wheat Flour Institute
    710 North Rush Street
    Chicago, Ill. 60611
    NUTR

B. Appendix: Some Federal Consumer-Oriented Agencies

1. U.S. Consumer Product Safety
   Commission (CPSC)
   Washington, D.C. 20207
   (Toll free hotline in the continental
   United States 808-638-8326.)
   CPSC's primary goals are to protect the
   public against unreasonable risks of injury
   associated with consumer products in or
   around the home, schools, and recreational
   areas; to assist consumers in evaluating the
   comparative safety of consumer products.

2. Food and Drug Administration (FDA)
   Department of Health and Human
   Services
   5600 Fishers Lane
   Rockville, Maryland 20857
   (301-443-3170)
   FDA enforces the Federal Food, Drug and
   Cosmetics Act and related laws to insure
   the purity and safety of foods, drugs, and
   cosmetics, the safety of therapeutic
   devices, and the truthful, informative
   labeling of such products.

3. National Highway Traffic Safety
   Administration (NHTSA)
   Department of Transportation
   400 7th St., S.W.
   Washington, D.C. 20590
   (202-426-0670, toll free hotline 800-424-
   9393)
   NHTSA writes and enforces safety
   standards which set minimum performance
   levels for certain parts of motor vehicles and
   for the vehicle as a unit. Its jurisdiction
   includes automobiles, trucks, buses,
   recreational vehicles, motor cycles,
   bicycles, mopeds and all related accessory
   equipment.

4. Federal Aviation Administration (FAA)
   800 Independence Ave., S.W.
   Washington, D.C. 20591
   (202-426-1960)
   FAA sets mandatory safety standards for
   aircraft construction, flammability of
   aircraft interior finishes, and aircraft safety
   in general. FAA is part of the Department of
   Transportation.

5. Federal Trade Commission (FTC)
   6th and Pennsylvania Ave., N.W.
   Washington, D.C. 20580
   (202-523-3598)
   FTC enforces antitrust and warranty laws
   and consumer protection statutes including
   those prohibiting false advertising and
   fraud in credit (lending). The agency also
   requires labeling on various products, such
   as care labeling for fabrics.

6. Public Health Services (PHS)
   Department of Health and Human
   Services
   200 Independence Ave., S.W.
   Washington, D.C. 20201
   (202-245-6867)
   The Public Health Service is concerned
   with: health research, through the National
   Institutes of Health; regulation of health-
   related products through FDA; prevention
   of disease through the Center for Disease
   Control; delivery of health care through the
   Health Service Administration.

7. Agriculture Department
   Food Safety and Quality Service
   (Meat and poultry inspection 202-447-3473)
   (Meat and poultry, egg, dairy, fruit, and vegetable grading 202-447-5231)
   Food and Nutrition Service (food stamps, nutrition information 202-447-8138)
   Extension Service (202-447-2750)
   Independence Ave., between 12th and 14th Street, N.W.
   Washington, D.C. 20250

   The Agriculture Department, through its subdivisions, inspects and grades meats, poultry, fruits, and vegetables; provides some nutrition information to consumers through labels required on meat, poultry, fruits, and vegetables; provides food to poor families through programs such as food stamps; carries out studies on human nutrition, home economics, and farm-oriented science; and works with adult and youth education programs in the 50 states.

8. U.S. Postal Service
   475 L'Enfant Plaza, S.W.
   Washington, D.C. 20260
   (202-245-4144)

   The U.S. Postal Service is an independent Federal establishment responsible for mail delivery and related activities. Most special requests and complaints are handled locally. Mail fraud allegations may be presented to local postmasters. Complaints which cannot be handled locally should be referred to the Consumers Advocate of the U.S. Postal Services.

9. Environmental Protection Agency (EPA)
   401 M. St., S.W.
   Washington, D.C. 20460
   (202-755-0707, toll free number to explain the regulation under the Toxic Substances Control Act: 800-424-9065; this number cannot help with general information.)

   EPA has the power to set standards for air, water, and noise pollution, and for toxic substances. The agency guides Federal and state environmental policies affecting manufacturing plants, automobiles, hazardous wastes, and solid waste disposal. EPA also regulates the manufacture and use of pesticides in the U.S. to insure environmentally safer and more effective pest control.

10. Federal Communications Commission (FCC)
    1919 M St., N.W.
    Washington, D.C. 20554
    (202-632-7000)

    The FCC monitors the programming of radio and TV, regulates the licensing of radio and TV stations, and sets standards for the use and availability of cable TV, and licenses communications satellites.

11. Interstate Commerce Commission (ICC)
    Constitution Ave. and 12th St., N.W.
    Washington, D.C. 20423
    (202-275-0860, toll free hotline 800-424-9312)

    The ICC regulates surface transportation by truck, bus, rail, oil pipeline, express company, and freight forwarded when goods are transported across state lines. The ICC sets standards for quality and cost of interstate transportation.

12. Occupational Safety and Health Administration (OSHA)
    Department of Labor
    200 Constitution Ave., N.W.
    Washington, D.C. 20210
    (202-523-8151)

    OSHA has responsibility for safety and health in the workplace. There are some exceptions—in the case of state and municipal employees, and for work covered by other laws such as mine safety, atomic energy and railroads. OSHA is part of the Department of Labor.

13. U.S. Office of Consumer Affairs
    621 Reporters Bldg.
    300 7th St. S.W.
    Washington, D.C. 20201
    (202-755-8810—for information
    202-755-8820—for complaints)

    The U.S. Office of Consumer Affairs coordinates and advises other Federal agencies on issues of interest to consumers. Its primary function is to represent the interests of consumers in proceedings of Federal agencies and to provide support to the Special Assistant to the President for Consumer Affairs.

Index

WE VALUE YOUR OPINION—PLEASE SHARE IT WITH US

Merrill Publishing and our authors are most interested in your reactions to this textbook. Did it serve you well in the course? If it did, what aspects of the text were most helpful? If not, what didn't you like about it? Your comments will help us to write and develop better textbooks. We value your opinions and thank you for your help.

Text Title _____ Edition _____

Author(s) _____

Your Name (optional) _____

Address _____

City _____ State _____ Zip _____

School _____

Course Title _____

Instructor's Name _____

Your Major _____

Your Class Rank _____ Freshman _____ Sophomore _____ Junior _____ Senior

_____ Graduate Student

Were you required to take this course? _____ Required _____ Elective

Length of Course? _____ Quarter _____ Semester

1. Overall, how does this text compare to other texts you've used?

_____ Superior _____ Better Than Most _____ Average _____ Poor

2. Please rate the text in the following areas:

	Superior	Better Than Most	Average	Poor
Author's Writing Style	_____	_____	_____	_____
Readability	_____	_____	_____	_____
Organization	_____	_____	_____	_____
Accuracy	_____	_____	_____	_____
Layout and Design	_____	_____	_____	_____
Illustrations/Photos/Tables	_____	_____	_____	_____
Examples	_____	_____	_____	_____
Problems/Exercises	_____	_____	_____	_____
Topic Selection	_____	_____	_____	_____
Currentness of Coverage	_____	_____	_____	_____
Explanation of Difficult Concepts	_____	_____	_____	_____
Match-up with Course Coverage	_____	_____	_____	_____
Applications to Real Life	_____	_____	_____	_____

3. Circle those chapters you especially liked:

1   2   3   4   5   6   7   8   9   10   11   12   13   14   15   16   17   18   19   20

What was your favorite chapter? _____

Comments:

4. Circle those chapters you liked least:

1   2   3   4   5   6   7   8   9   10   11   12   13   14   15   16   17   18   19   20

What was your least favorite chapter? _____

Comments:

5. List any chapters your instructor did not assign. _____

6. What topics did your instructor discuss that were not covered in the text?_____

_____

7. Were you required to buy this book? _____ Yes _____ No

Did you buy this book new or used? _____ New _____ Used

If used, how much did you pay? _____

Do you plan to keep or sell this book? _____ Keep _____ Sell

If you plan to sell the book, how much do you expect to receive? _____

Should the instructor continue to assign this book? _____ Yes _____ No

8. Please list any other learning materials you purchased to help you in this course (e.g., study guide, lab manual).

_____

9. What did you like most about this text? _____

_____

10. What did you like least about this text? _____

_____

11. General comments:

May we quote you in our advertising? _____ Yes _____ No

Please mail to: Boyd Lane
                College Division, Research Department
                Box 508
                1300 Alum Creek Drive
                Columbus, Ohio 43216

Thank you!